THE SURGICAL CLINICS OF NORTH AMERICA

Minimal Access Surgery, Part II

CAROL E. H. SCOTT–CONNER, MD, PhD, and
KEMP HOWARD KERNSTINE, MD, PhD
GUEST EDITORS

VOLUME 80 • NUMBER 5 • OCTOBER 2000

W.B. SAUNDERS COMPANY
A Harcourt Health Sciences Company
PHILADELPHIA   LONDON   TORONTO   MONTREAL   SYDNEY   TOKYO

W.B. SAUNDERS COMPANY
A Harcourt Health Sciences Company

The Curtis Center • Independence Square West • Philadelphia, Pennsylvania 19106
http://www.wbsaunders.com

THE SURGICAL CLINICS OF NORTH AMERICA   Volume 80, Number 5
October 2000   ISSN 0039–6109
Editor: Joe Rusko   Production Editor: Michael Pittard

The ideas and opinions expressed in *The Surgical Clinics of North America* do not necessarily reflect those of the Publisher. The Publisher does not assume any responsibility for any injury and/or damage to persons or property arising out of or related to any use of the material contained in this periodical. The reader is advised to check the appropriate medical literature and the product information currently provided by the manufacturer of each drug to be administered to verify the dosage, the method and duration of administration, or contraindications. It is the responsibility of the treating physician or other health care professional, relying on independent experience and knowledge of the patient, to determine drug dosages and the best treatment for the patient. Mention of any product in this issue should not be construed as endorsement by the contributors, editors, or the Publisher of the product or manufacturers' claims.

The Surgical Clinics of North America (ISSN 0039–6109) is published bimonthly by W.B. Saunders Company. Corporate and Editorial Offices: The Curtis Center, Independence Square West, Philadelphia, PA 19106–3399. Accounting and Circulation Offices: 6277 Sea Harbor Drive, Orlando, FL 32887–4800. Periodicals postage paid at Orlando, FL 32862, and additional mailing offices. Subscription price is $96.00 per year (US students and residents), $146.00 per year (US individuals), $171.00 per year (Canadian individuals), $195.00 per year (US institutions), $199.00 per year (foreign individuals), $237.00 per year (foreign institutions), and $237.00 per year (Canadian institutions). To receive student/resident rate, orders must be accompanied by name of affiliated institution, date of term, and the *signature* of program/residency coordinator on institution letterhead. Orders will be billed at individual rate until proof of status is received. Foreign air speed delivery is included in all *Clinics* subscription prices. All prices are subject to change without notice. POSTMASTER: Send address changes to *The Surgical Clinics of North America*, W.B. Saunders Company, Periodicals Fulfillment, Orlando, FL 32887–4800. **Customer Service: 1-800-654-2452 (US). From outside of the US, call 1-407-345-4000.**

The Surgical Clinics of North America is also published in Spanish by McGraw-Hill Interamericana Editores S.A., P.O. Box 5-237, 06500 Mexico D.F., Mexico; and in Portuguese by Interlivros Edicoes Ltda., Rua Comandante Coelho 1085, CEP 21250, Rio de Janeiro, Brazil; and in Greek by Paschalidis Medical Publications, Athens, Greece.

The Surgical Clinics of North America is covered in *Index Medicus, EMBASE/Excerpta Medica, Current Contents/Clinical Medicine, Current Contents/Life Sciences, Science Citation Index,* and *ISI/BIOMED.*

Printed in the United States of America.

GUEST EDITORS

CAROL E. H. SCOTT-CONNER, MD, PhD, Professor and Head, Department of Surgery, University of Iowa Health Care, Iowa City, Iowa

KEMP HOWARD KERNSTINE, MD, PhD, Associate Professor, Division of Cardiothoracic Surgery, Department of Surgery, University of Iowa Health Care, Iowa City, Iowa

CONTRIBUTORS

AL ALY, MD, Assistant Professor, Division of Plastic and Reconstructive Surgery, Department of Surgery, University of Iowa Health Care, Iowa City, Iowa

G. JAMES AVERY II, MD, Vice Chairman, Department of Cardiac Surgery, California Pacific Medical Center, San Francisco, California

EDUARDO AVILA, BS, Medical Student, University of Iowa Health Care, Iowa City, Iowa

REDMOND P. BURKE, MD, Chief, Division of Cardiovascular Surgery, Miami Children's Hospital, Miami, Florida

ALBERT E. CRAM, MD, Professor, Division of Plastic and Reconstructive Surgery, Department of Surgery, University of Iowa Health Care, Iowa City, Iowa

NICK H. GABRIEL, DO, Postdoctoral Fellow, and Clinical Instructor, the Endo-Laparoscopic Center, Department of Surgery, Yale University School of Medicine, New Haven, Connecticut

JEFFREY J. GOATES, MD, Department of Pathology, Rose Medical Center, Denver, Colorado

ROBERT L. HANNAN, MD, Attending Surgeon, Division of Cardiovascular Surgery, Miami Children's Hospital, Miami, Florida

STEPHEN R. HAZELRIGG, MD, Division of Cardiothoracic Surgery, Southern Illinois University School of Medicine, Springfield, Illinois

SEAN P. HEDICAN, MD, Assistant Professor and Director, Laparoscopy, Department of Urology, University of Iowa Health Care, Iowa City, Iowa

B. TODD HENIFORD, MD, Chief, Minimal Access Surgery, Carolinas Laparoscopic Advanced Surgery Program, Department of Surgery, Carolinas Medical Center Charlotte, North Carolina

JAMES R. HOWE, MD, Department of Surgery, University of Iowa Health Care, Iowa City, Iowa

WILLIAM E. KELLEY, MD, Director, Minimal Access Surgery Fellowship, Richmond Surgery Group, Richmond, Virginia

RODNEY J. LANDRENEAU, MD, Director, Division of General Thoracic Surgery, Allegheny General Hospital, Pittsburgh, Pennsylvania

ISADOR H. LIEBERMAN, BSc, MD, FRCS(C), Department of Orthopaedic Surgery, The Cleveland Clinic Foundation, Cleveland, Ohio

JEFFREY C. LIN, MD, Division of General Thoracic Surgery, Allegheny General Hospital, Pittsburgh, Pennsylvania

DEMETRIUS E. M. LITWIN, MD, FRCSC, Associate Professor and Director, Minimally Invasive Surgery Services, and Endosurgery Center, University of Massachusetts Medical Center, Worcester, Massachusetts

†GREGORY A. LOWDERMILK, MD, formerly Assistant Professor, Division of Cardiothoracic Surgery, St. Louis University Health Sciences Center, St. Louis, Missouri

MICHAEL J. MACK, MD, Chairman, Cardiopulmonary Research Science Technology Institute, Dallas, Texas

JAMES W. MAHER, MD, Professor and Director, Gastrointestinal Surgery, Department of Surgery, University of Iowa Health Care, Iowa City, Iowa

BRENT D. MATTHEWS, MD, Fellow, Carolinas Laparoscopic Advanced Surgery Program, Department of Surgery, Carolinas Medical Center, Charlotte, North Carolina

ROBERT C. McINTYRE, Jr, MD, Associate Professor, Department of Surgery, University of Colorado Health Sciences Center; and the Department of Surgery, Veterans Affairs Hospital, Denver, Colorado

ROBERT J. McKENNA, Jr, MD, Head, Section of Thoracic Surgery, Cedars Sinai Medical Center, Los Angeles, California

G. RODNEY MEEKS, MD, Professor, and Winfred L. Wiser Chair in Gynecologic Surgery, Department of Obstetrics and Gynecology, University of Mississippi Medical Center, Jackson, Mississippi

MICHINORI MURAYAMA, MD, PhD, Postdoctoral Fellow, the Endo-Laparoscopic Center, Department of Surgery, Yale University School of Medicine, New Haven, Connecticut

---

†Deceased.

KEITH S. NAUNHEIM, MD, Professor, Division of Cardiothoracic Surgery, St. Louis University Health Sciences Center, St. Louis, Missouri

CHRISTOPHER D. RAEBURN, MD, Resident, Department of Surgery, University of Colorado Health Sciences Center, Denver, Colorado

JAMES C. ROSSER, Jr, MD, Associate Professor, and Director of Laparoscopy, the Endo-Laparoscopic Center, Department of Surgery, Yale University School of Medicine, New Haven, Connecticut

ANDRAS SANDOR, MD, Resident, Department of Surgery, University of Massachusetts Medical School, Worcester, Massachusetts

BARBARA S. SCHWARTZBERG, MD, Associate Clinical Professor, Department of Surgery, Rose Medical Center, Denver, Colorado

ZOLTAN SZABO, PhD, Director, Microsurgery and Operative Endoscopy Training Institute, San Francisco, California

FORTHCOMING ISSUES

RECENT ISSUES

VISIT THESE RELATED WEB SITES

MD Consult—A comprehensive online clinical resource:
http://www.mdconsult.com

For more information about Clinics:
http://www.wbsaunders.com/periodicals/clinics/index.htm

CONTENTS

The technological advances of endoscopy have benefited many
surgical specialties. Endoscopy is particularly suited for cosmetic
and reconstructive procedures because of its emphasis on aesthetics. This article describes three plastic surgery procedures in
which endoscopic techniques have been applied: the brow lift,
transaxillary breast augmentation, and abdominoplasty. Endoscopic techniques are compared to more traditional techniques,
which they may replace.

Today, many patients with abnormal breast lumps or suspicious
mammograms are evaluated with minimal access breast biopsy
procedures, including fine needle aspiration, needle core biopsy,
vacuum-assisted biopsy, and large core cannula biopsy. Breast
cancer therapy also offers several minimal access procedures, of
which the sentinel lymph node biopsy has gained the greatest
publicity and acceptance.

More surgeons are performing unilateral exploration for primary
hyperparathyroidism (HPT) than ever before. This article reviews

the factors that have led to the trend toward less invasive surgery. Discussion includes the history of unilateral exploration for HPT, the advent of magnetic resonance sestamibi imaging, and the development of intraoperative assays for parathyroid hormone. Results of minimally invasive techniques, including radio-guided parathyroidectomy, endoscopic parathyroidectomy, and outpatient parathyroidectomy, also are presented

The adrenal gland lends itself to laparoscopic removal because it is small, and adrenal tumors are most often benign. Similarly, most endocrine tumors of the pancreas are small and benign, or are slow-growing malignancies that permit removal by enucleation or distal pancreatectomy by laparoscopy. Laparoscopic adrenalectomy, though requiring advanced laparoscopic surgical skills, has become the procedure of choice for benign adrenal lesions because it results in less pain, a shorter hospital stay, comparable safety, and more patient satisfaction. The laparoscopic approach to pancreatic endocrine tumors, however, does not as yet have clearly established benefits over the open approach, and should be considered primarily investigational at this point.

Minimally invasive gynecologic surgery began with tubal sterilization, which was performed laparoscopically. Advances in laparoscopic technology have allowed increasingly complex procedures to be performed. Laparoscopically assisted hysterectomy is now a common procedure, and procedures for correcting urinary incontinence and pelvic organ prolapse have been developed and are currently under evaluation.

Advances in laparoscopic equipment and instrumentation have led to new applications in nearly all fields of surgery. This article describes the major laparoscopic procedures being performed in urology in the year 2000. Laparoscopic applications range from simple staging and diagnostic procedures, such as pelvic lymphadenectomy and assessment of the nonpalpable testis, to major extirpations for malignancy, including radical nephrectomy and nephrourectomy. Laparoscopic operations for benign renal disease, such as cyst decortication, pyeloplasty, and simple donor nephrectomy, also are presented. As the volume of cases and the length of follow up increase, these procedures will continue to challenge the "gold standard" therapies of urologic disease in the new millennium.

Laparoscopic Lumbar Interbody Spinal Fusion

B. Todd Heniford, Brent D. Matthews, and
Isador H. Lieberman

In the surgical management of spinal disorders, the role of the general surgeon increased dramatically in response to the need for collaboration with skilled laparoscopists to perform laparoscopic anterior lumbar spinal fusion. Initial enthusiasm for this technique was fostered by the development of interbody fusion devices and laparoscopy's ability to improve exposure and visualization while minimizing collateral tissue damage and injury to healthy tissue. Preliminary studies have demonstrated the feasibility of laparoscopic anterior lumbar spinal fusion, offering minor technical advantages versus open techniques when using current implants and bone grafting techniques for single-level disc disease. General acceptance of laparoscopic anterior lumbar spinal fusion awaits further investigation.

Thoracoscopic Esophagomyotomy for Achalasia

James W. Maher

Achalasia is characterized by the absence of peristalsis in the distal two thirds of the esophagus, failure of receptive relaxation of the lower esophageal sphincter, and dysphagia to both solids and liquids. Diagnosis is confirmed by barium swallow, esophageal manometry, and flexible endoscopy. Treatment is based primarily on disruption of the lower esophageal sphincter, which can be achieved by forceful dilation of surgical esophagomyotomy. Esophagomyotomy produces relief of symptoms in more than 90% of patients.

Video-Assisted Thoracic Surgery for Diseases within the Mediastinum

Jeffrey C. Lin, Stephen R. Hazelrigg, and
Rodney J. Landreneau

A minimally invasive thoracic surgical approach to mediastinal pathology often is an appropriate alternative to open invasive techniques. This article describes the indications and technical aspects of these video-assisted procedures.

Thoracoscopic Evaluation and Treatment of Thoracic Trauma

Gregory A. Lowdermilk and Keith S. Naunheim

Video-assisted thoracoscopy has become a reality since the evolution of endoscopic instrumentation began in the early 1990s.

These technologies provide more thorough and precise visualization of the thoracic cavity and its contents. In 1993, video-assisted thoracoscopic surgery (VATS) was introduced into trauma care in a series that evaluated diaphragmatic injury. Today, VATS is being used in a variety of pulmonary, chest wall, mediastinal, neurologic, and cardiac surgical procedures. VATS has been added to the trauma armamentarium for treating hemothorax, diaphragmatic injuries, posttraumatic empyema, and persistent air leaks.

Thoracoscopic Evaluation and Treatment of Pulmonary Disease
Robert J. McKenna, Jr

The expectations for minimally invasive thoracic procedures have been that they would reduce morbidity, mortality, and hospital stay, and result in patients' returning rapidly to regular activities after undergoing procedures that formerly required major incisions. These expectations have yet to be proven conclusively, although some of the early results are encouraging, and video-assisted thoracoscopic surgery (VATS) is a common part of the practice of thoracic surgery. The techniques for lung resection (wedge resection, lobectomy, and pneumonectomy) with VATS are evolving, and this article presents details about current approaches.

Suturing and Knotting Techniques for Thoracoscopic Cardiac Surgery
Zoltan Szabo, G. James Avery II, Andras Sandor, and Demetrius E. M. Litwin

Microvascular anastomosis for endoscopic coronary artery bypass grafting has become the latest technique in the evolution of advanced endoscopic surgery. Although the construction of the anastomosis is a particularly challenging technique, adhering to certain principles enables the surgeon to accomplish this task safely. Topics of critical focus include endoscopic suturing principles and approach, methods for improving efficiency, needle control, and suturing instrumentation. The intracorporeal knot tying technique, using the classic convertible square knot, is described and illustrated.

Coronary Surgery: Off-Pump and Port Access
Michael J. Mack

Attempts to minimize the invasiveness of cardiac surgery have focused on decreasing access trauma and eliminating cardiopulmonary bypass. The initial procedures, minimally invasive direct coronary artery bypass (MIDCAB, limited access beating heart) and port access (limited access arrested heart), have become niche procedures. Off-pump coronary artery bypass (OPCAB, median sternotomy beating heart) presently accounts for approximately 15% of all coronary bypass operations performed in the United States. Morbidity and cost appear to be decreased with these procedures. Feasibility trials of endoscopic coronary bypass surgery using robotic devices are underway in many centers. It is anticipated that over the next 5 years the alternative approaches to conventional coronary artery bypass surgery will continue to grow as methods of coronary revascularization.

Harnessing new technology, surgeons are steadily modifying approaches, in an effort to reduce surgical trauma to the repair of congenital heart defects. Operating through small incisions and using an array of enabling instrumentation, it is possible to repair many congenital heart lesions without thoracotomy or sternotomy, and without sacrificing operative precision or surgical outcomes.

Despite its tremendous impact, minimally invasive surgery faces challenges for which guidelines have been developed that must be implemented. New educational strategies and techniques that are assisted by the integration of cost-effective technology are needed.

In Memoriam

As this issue was going to press, the editors learned of the sudden and tragic death of one of the contributors. Dr. Gregory A. Lowdermilk, Assistant Professor of Surgery in the Division of Cardiothoracic Surgery at the St. Louis University School of Medicine, co-authored *Thoracoscopic Evaluation and Treatment of Thoracic Trauma*. We know his article will be enjoyed by our readers. It is our hope that this issue, containing his contribution, will serve to honor his memory and a promising career untimely ended.

Gregory A. Lowdermilk, MD
June 19, 1963–July 26, 2000

An excellent surgeon, compassionate physician, and a loving husband, father, son, and friend, he will be sadly missed by all who knew him.

PREFACE

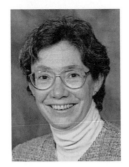 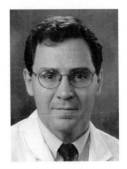

CAROL E. H. SCOTT–CONNER,   KEMP HOWARD KERNSTINE,
MD, PhD   MD, PhD

Guest Editors

Much has changed since Carl Langenbuch performed the first open chole-cystectomy in 1882, and Kelling performed the first celioscopy in 1901. Although gynecologic surgeons embraced operative laparoscopy, general surgeons did not take the next step until 1987 when Mouret performed the first laparoscopic cholecystectomy (LC).

Indeed, laparoscopy was still a new tool for many surgeons in 1992 when *The Surgical Clinics of North America* devoted an entire issue to the subject. Four years later, a concise update stressed new developments. But now in the year 2000, even two volumes barely suffice—our editor at W.B. Saunders is still dismayed at the number of pages, as each volume exceeds initial projections.

The first volume revisited familiar procedures, such as laparoscopic chole-cystectomy, from new viewpoints and also discussed many new operations. Laparoscopic surgeons continue to push the envelope of the possible. The issue appropriately began with those situations that render laparoscopy difficult— massive obesity, pregnancy, and previous abdominal surgery—conditions listed as contraindications to laparoscopic surgery not so long ago.

Because LC (the operation that started it all) is now routine, the adjuncts of laparoscopic ultrasonography and ERCP were given coverage to complement this workhorse procedure, and a clinical pathway was offered next.

Subsequent articles discussed benign liver disease, esophageal surgery, para-esophageal hernia, gastric and colon resections, and other advanced procedures. The two concluding works looked to the future, discussing cost containment and advanced technology.

This volume contains additional minimal access procedures of interest (such as breast, adrenal, parathyroid) to the general surgeon and a variety of thoraco-scopic procedures.

It has been a pleasure bringing this two-volume issue together. We and the many contributors hope you find it interesting and valuable.

CAROL E. H. SCOTT–CONNER, MD, PhD, and
KEMP HOWARD KERNSTINE, MD, PhD
Guest Editors

Department of Surgery
University of Iowa Health Care
200 Hawkins Drive, #1516 JCP
Iowa City, IA 52242–1086

0039–6109/00 $15.00 + .00

ENDOSCOPIC PLASTIC SURGERY

Al Aly, MD, Eduardo Avila, BS, Albert E. Cram, MD

Although plastic surgery was not one of the earliest specialties to incorporate endoscopic surgical techniques, it is probably the specialty with the greatest demand on reducing the size of access incisions because of the emphasis on aesthetics. Initially, certain anatomic obstacles and technologic limitations prevented plastic surgeons from using minimal incision endoscopic surgical techniques.[11] An optical cavity is essential for the use of endoscopes, and other specialties have benefited from the presence of natural potential cavities, such as joint spaces and the peritoneal cavity. In the most commonly performed endoscopically assisted plastic surgery procedures, spaces are created surgically between tissue planes because no natural cavities are present. The optical cavity then is maintained by retracting the soft tissues using balloons or umbrella-like retractors or externally with the use of sutures, adhesives, or skin hooks. Various instruments are needed to accomplish endoscopic plastic surgical procedures and many have been adapted from other specialties; however, as the demands of particular procedures are realized, instrument development has progressed, leading to highly specialized tools for the specialty.

In three procedures, endoscopes are more commonly used in plastic surgery: (1) forehead or brow lifts, (2) transaxillary breast augmentation, and (3) abdominoplasty. Each of these procedures is discussed with reference to surgical indications and desired results, traditional technique, endoscopic technique, and a comparison of the two techniques.

FOREHEAD AND BROW ENDOSCOPIC LIFT

Surgical Indications and Desired Results

Candidates for forehead and brow endoscopic lift include men and women who have descent of the eyebrows relative to the supraorbital ridges, patients

From the Division of Plastic and Reconstructive Surgery, Department of Surgery, University of Iowa Health Care, Iowa City, Iowa with troublesome glabellar frown lines, and those who have mild to moderate skin laxity of the upper eyelids caused by brow descent.[3] The procedure is performed to elevate the brows to a higher position and reduce wrinkling in the forehead and glabellar regions.

Traditional Method

Conventional brow lift surgery, or coronoplasty, is accomplished through a lengthy bicoronal incision extending from ear to ear across the frontal scalp (Fig. 1A).[6] The scalp is elevated down to the supraorbital rims (Fig. 1B). The underlying muscles contributing to frowning, the corrugators and procerus muscles, usually are excised or scored in an attempt to limit their activity. The elevated scalp tissues then are re-draped and pulled in a cephalad direction, the excess is excised, and the incision is closed, elevating the brows (Fig. 1C).

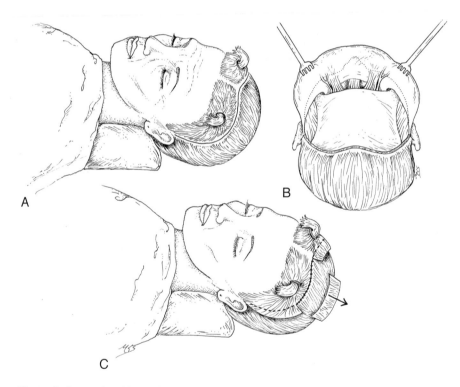

Figure 1. Conventional brow lift surgery. *A,* Conventional brow lift surgery is accomplished through a lengthy incision extending from ear to ear across the frontal scalp. *B,* The forehead skin and underlying soft tissues are elevated down to the supraorbital rims. *C,* The elevated scalp tissues are then re-draped and pulled in a cephalad direction; the excess is excised (*arrow*), and the incision is closed, elevating the brows.

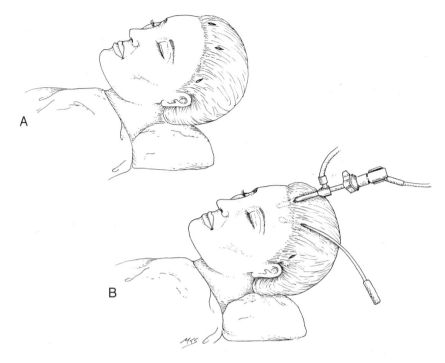

Figure 2. Endoscopic forehead lift. *A,* Usually five incisions are made behind the hairline: one in the midline, two at the horizontal level of the highest point of the eyebrows, and two temporal incisions. *B,* Most of the dissection is done without the aid of the endoscope, but once the supraorbital area is approached anteroinferiorly, the endoscope is used for direct visualization.

Endoscopic Technique

The endoscopic forehead lift was the first clinical application introduced and the most widely performed plastic surgery endoscopic procedure.[9] Usually five incisions are made behind the hairline: one in the midline, two at the horizontal level of the highest point of the eyebrows, and two temporal incisions (Fig. 2*A*). Through these incisions, the scalp, at a subperiosteal level centrally and just superficial to the temporalis fascia laterally, is elevated off of the underlying structures. The dissection is carried to the vertex of the scalp posteriorly. Most of the dissection is done without the aid of the endoscopes, but when the supraorbital area has been approached anteroinferiorly, the endoscope is used for direct visualization (Fig. 2*B*). The dissection then proceeds to identify and protect the supraorbital neurovascular bundles. The procerus and corrugator muscles are scored or transected after incising the periosteum that overlies them. Periosteal release is performed lateral to the neurovascular bundles to allow for elevation of the brows. To maintain elevation of the scalp, and thus the brows, the whole scalp is rotated posterosuperiorly and may or may not be fixated to the outer cortex of the cranium.

Discussion

The traditional brow lift produces excellent elevation of the brows but at the expense of numbness of the scalp posterior to the incision, a lengthy scalp incision, and the possibility of significant hair loss adjacent to the suture line. Endoscopic brow lift achieves elevation of the brows through small scalp incisions, with minimal hair loss and without significant scalp numbness, and, like the open approach, addresses the muscles responsible for frowning.[7] It is gaining popularity, and many surgeons prefer it to the traditional open brow lift technique.[2]

ENDOSCOPIC-ASSISTED BREAST AUGMENTATION

Indications and Desired Results

The primary indication for breast augmentation is inadequate volume of the breast. Many women, particularly young women who have hypomastia or women who have had several children and found that their breast volume has decreased, seek the procedure. Physically the desired result varies depending on the age and anatomy of the patient; however, most patients would like an increase in volume that appears natural for their body type and an inconspicuous scar. The most popular placement of the implant is in the subpectoral plane to increase soft-tissue cover and maintain a higher position of the implant on the chest wall.

Traditional Method

Typically breast augmentation is performed through one of three approaches: (1) inframammary, (2) periareolar, or (3) transaxillary (Fig. 3). A subpectoral pocket then is dissected. The medial and inferomedial attachments are released to prevent lateralization of the implant when the pectoralis muscle contracts, which can be difficult through the transaxillary approach. The implant then is inserted into the pocket, and the incision is closed.

Endoscopic Technique

The inframammary and perioareolar approaches do not require endoscopic assistance because the pocket dissection is close to the incision sites. Thus the endoscope mainly is used to achieve control of pocket dissection and bleeding with the transaxillary approach.[4] A small axillary incision is made, and dissection is carried deep to the pectoralis muscle. When the subpectoral plane is entered, a pocket is dissected with a blunt dissector, such as a urethral sound (Fig. 4). The endoscope-retractor unit is inserted through the incision into the subpectoral space (Fig. 5A), and the medial and inferomedial borders of the pectoralis muscle are visualized and incised with cautery to allow for the appropriate release of the muscle (Fig. 5B). Bleeding points are cauterized under direct vision. After the appropriate space is created, the implants are inserted and checked for symmetry, and the wounds are closed.

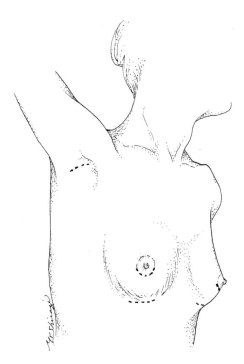

Figure 3. Breast augmentation approaches. Typically breast augmentation is performed through one of three approaches: inframammary, periareolar, or transaxillary.

Discussion

Some surgeons prefer the transaxillary approach, but there had been some degree of dissatisfaction with this procedure because of difficulties in achieving symmetry and accurate implant placement.[8] Using the endoscope, more control is possible through the transaxillary approach, so more surgeons are willing to use it. The major disadvantage of this approach is that if subsequent revision surgery is required, reoperation through the axilla is difficult.

ENDOSCOPIC-ASSISTED ABDOMINOPLASTY

Indications and Desired Results

Patients present for abdominoplasty for various reasons. Most patients present with excess abdominal skin and fat and with abdominal wall muscle laxity. A small subset of patients present with no skin laxity or excess fat but with a fairly lax abdominal wall (Fig. 6A). These patients typically are fairly thin women who have had multiple pregnancies and develop a significant rectus diastasis (Fig. 6B). Only this group of patients benefits from endoscopically assisted abdominoplasty.[1] The goal of the surgery is to tighten the abdominal wall to attain a flat belly contour with minimal scarring.

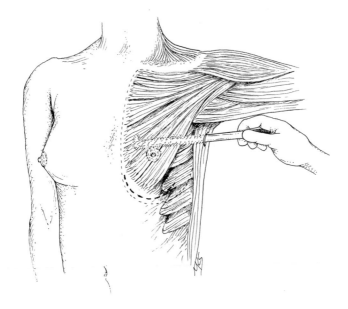

Figure 4. Endoscopic transaxillary breast augmentation. Once the subpectoral plane is entered, a pocket is dissected with a blunt dissector such as a urethral sound.

Traditional Method

An incision usually is made from one anterosuperior iliac spine to the other through the suprapubic crease (Fig. 7A). An abdominal flap of skin and fat is elevated superiorly to the level of the xiphoid and costal margins, detaching the umbilicus from its base or incising around it. The anterior rectus sheath then is plicated in a vertical direction to tighten the abdominal wall (Fig. 7B). The umbilicus is reattached to its base or sewn back in its original position, depending on how it was handled initially.

Endoscopic Technique

A transverse incision approximately 4 cm in length is made in the suprapubic crease, and another is made around the umbilicus. With the assistance of the endoscope, fat is dissected off of the anterior rectus sheath from the pubic area to the umbilicus and from the umbilicus to the xiphoid. Anterior rectus sheath plication then is performed superior and inferior to the umbilicus with the assistance of the endoscope (Fig. 8).[12] The plication may be performed with surgical staples or specialized needle holders. The incisions then are closed.

Discussion

Although this technique is applicable in only a few patients who present for abdominoplasty, it has the advantage of limited scarring. Considerably less dissection is associated with this technique, and because of an overall decrease

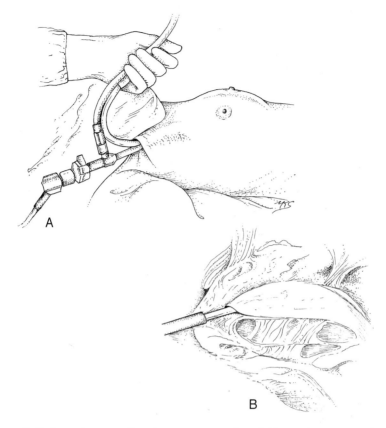

Figure 5. Endoscopic transaxillary breast augmentation. *A*, The endoscope-retractor unit is inserted through the incision into the subpectoral space. *B*, The medial and inferomedial borders of the pectoralis muscle are visualized and incised with cautery to allow appropriate release of the muscle.

in tissue injury, patients usually experience a quicker recovery.[1] As with any other endoscopically assisted procedure, the learning curve is steep, and an initial investment in the endoscopes and related instruments is necessary.

SUMMARY

This article discusses three of the most popular endoscopic procedures in plastic surgery. Brow lift, transaxillary breast augmentation, and abdominoplasty are all cosmetic procedures with a high demand on inconspicuous scars; however, many investigators are working on reconstructive endoscopically assisted procedures. The treatment of many facial fractures involving the upper third of the facial skeleton usually requires long bicoronal incisions similar to the incisions used in the traditional brow lift. Attempts are under way to use endoscopically assisted minimal-access techniques to reduce and fixate these fractures.

Many flaps used in plastic surgery require long scars for harvest, as in the

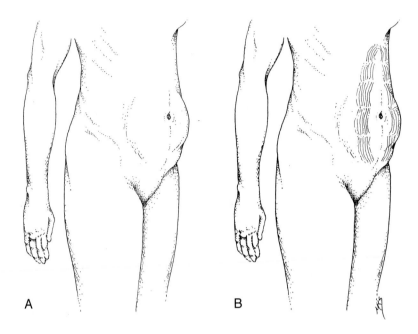

Figure 6. Endoscopic-assisted abdominoplasty. *A,* There is a small subset of patients who will present with no skin laxity or excess fat but have a fairly lax abdominal wall. *B,* This usually occurs in fairly thin women who have had multiple pregnancies and develop a significant rectus diastasis.

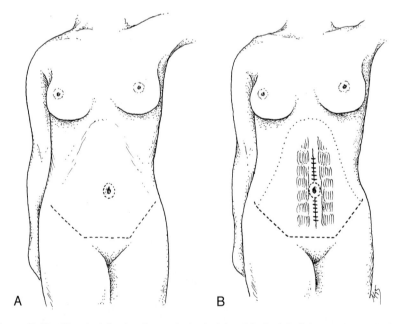

Figure 7. Traditional abdominoplasty. *A,* An incision (*dashed line*) is usually made from one anterosuperior iliac spine to the other through the suprapubic crease. *B,* The anterior rectus sheath is then plicated in a vertical direction to tighten the abdominal wall.

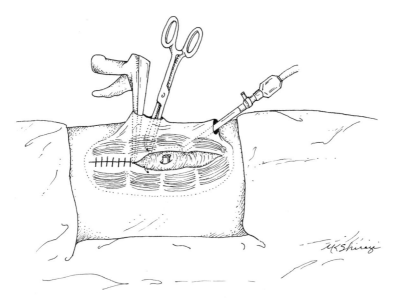

Figure 8. Endoscopically assisted abdominoplasty. A transverse incision approximately 4 cm in length is made in the suprapubic crease, and another is made around the umbilicus. Anterior rectus sheath plication is then performed above and below the umbilicus with the assistance of the endoscope. In this example, plication is performed with surgical staples.

case of the latissimus dorsi muscle flap. A relatively long incision on the back is needed to gain access to the muscle so that it can be elevated from structures superficial and deep to it. Although it is unpopular, investigators have reported harvesting latissimus dorsi muscle flaps through fairly small incisions with the assistance of balloon dissectors and endoscopes.

In the field of hand surgery, carpal tunnel release surgery has had more than one method proposed to transect the carpal ligament using endoscopes and special instrumentation.[10] Although some reported series[10] claim excellent results, many hand surgeons are reluctant to use endoscopes because of associated complications and a high recurrence rate of carpal tunnel syndrome.

Plastic surgery has special demands that emphasize aesthetics in cosmetic and reconstructive procedures. Although the lack of natural optical cavities has slowed the incorporation of endoscopic surgery in the specialty, surgically created cavities are used to allow for minimal access incisions. The future of plastic surgery will include an ever-increasing number of endoscopically assisted procedures. Cosmetic and reconstructive procedures will benefit from this new technology.

References

1. Core GB, Mizgala CL, Bowen JC III, et al: Endoscopic abdominoplasty with repair of diastasis recti and abdominal wall hernia. Clin Plast Surg 22:707–722, 1995
2. Core GB, Vasconez LO, Graham HD III: Endoscopic browlift. Clin Plast Surg 22:619–631, 1995

3. Daniel RK, Tirkanits B: Endoscopic forehead lift: Aesthetics and analysis. Clin Plast Surg 22:605–618, 1995
4. Eaves FF III, Bostwick J III, Nahai F, et al: Endoscopic techniques in aesthetic breast surgery: Augmentation, mastectomy, biopsy, capsulotomy, capsulorrhaphy, reduction, mastopexy, and reconstructive techniques. Clin Plast Surg 22:683–695, 1995
5. Faria-Correa MA: Endoscopic abdominoplasty, mastopexy, and breast reduction. Clin Plast Surg 22:723–745, 1995
6. Fisher JC, Guerrerosantos J, Gleason M: Manual of Aesthetic Surgery. New York, Springer-Verlag, 1985, p 89
7. Guyuron B, Michelow BJ: Refinements in endoscopic forehead rejuvenation. Plast Reconstr Surg 100:154–160, 1997
8. McCain LA, Jones G: Application of endoscopic techniques in aesthetic plastic surgery. Plastic Surgical Nursing 15:149–157, 1995
9. Poindexter BD, Vasconez LO: The present status of endoscopy. Ann Plast Surg 41:779–783, 1998
10. Sellers DS: Endoscopic carpal tunnel release. Clin Plast Surg 22:775–780, 1995
11. Vasconez LO, Core GB, Oslin B: Endoscopy in plastic surgery: An overview. Clin Plast Surg 22:585–589, 1995
12. Zukowaski ML, Ash K, Spencer D, et al: Endoscopic intracorporal abdominoplasty: A review of 85 cases. Plast Reconstr Surg 102:516–527, 1998

Address reprint requests to

Al Aly, MD
Plastic Surgery
UIHC
200 Hawkins Drive
Iowa City, IA 52242

e-mail: al-aly@uiowa.edu

MINIMAL ACCESS BREAST SURGERY

Barbara S. Schwartzberg, MD, Jeffrey J. Goates, MD,
and William E. Kelley, MD

The increasing prevalence of breast cancer in our society has produced an ever-greater demand for new diagnostic and therapeutic technologies. Today, patients ask not only that these new technologies offer improved diagnostic and treatment capabilities but also that the procedures are convenient, cost-effective, and less invasive than conventional techniques. Understandably, patients want procedures that minimize pain and trauma and have the least potential for side effects. In response, the medical community has come forward with various new technologies designed to improve the diagnosis and treatment of breast cancer while being more acceptable to patients.

Routine mammography is the best screening procedure for the early diagnosis of breast cancer. Additional diagnostic tools, such as sonography, magnetic resonance imaging, and scintimammography, are now available. The additional information afforded by these technologies is intended to limit the number of patients who need further evaluation with breast biopsy.

Patients requiring breast biopsies for palpable lumps now are offered minimal access procedures, such as fine-needle aspiration (FNA) or needle core biopsies, as alternatives to excisional breast biopsies. Patients with nonpalpable abnormalities are offered image-guided FNA, core needle biopsies (CNBs), vacuum-assisted procedures, or large CNBs.

Breast cancer treatment has gone through two major evolutions: (1) a shift from mastectomy to lumpectomy and (2) the development of the sentinel lymph node biopsy. Both surgical procedures are minimal access, providing patients with equal, if not superior, treatment while allowing for more rapid recovery and less pain, trauma, and side effects.

From the Departments of Surgery (BSS), and Pathology (JJG), Rose Medical Center, Denver,
    Colorado; and the Minimal Access Surgery Fellowship Program, Richmond Surgery
    Group, Richmond, Virginia (WEK)

MINIMAL ACCESS BREAST BIOPSIES OF PALPABLE BREAST LUMPS

Excisional breast biopsies long have been the gold standard for management of palpable breast masses. Many patients still opt for this approach. Palpable masses also may be sampled by FNA, CNB, or incisional biopsy. These techniques are safe and reliable when performed by trained, experienced surgeons.

FNA can be performed on an outpatient basis using local anesthesia, a 10-mL or 20-mL syringe, and a 22-gauge needle.[105] The diagnostic accuracy of FNA with palpable breast masses has been reported at approximately 80%.[75] Others report a sensitivity of 96.0% to 97.7% and a specificity of 99% to 100%.[4, 6] False-positive results are rare, 0% to 0.4%.[4, 60] The false-negative rate of FNA ranges from 0.7% to 22.0%.[4, 134] Most of these cases result from a lack of diagnostic tumor cells in the needle aspirate. The risk for false-negative results is reduced by increasing the number of aspirates. The tumor type also may be a factor, with lobular cancer having a higher false-negative rate than other tumor types. Any suspicious breast mass not yielding the diagnosis of cancer by FNA should be retested with a CNB or incisional or excisional biopsy.

Palpable breast masses may be sampled using Tru-Cut (Travenol, Deerfield, IL) or similar-style needles. The procedures are performed on an outpatient basis with local anesthesia, with five fragments of tissue being removed from the mass. A 14-gauge needle is the most common size used, removing fragments measuring approximately 2 mm by 10 mm. Specificities of 90% to 100% and sensitivities of 90.0% to 96.6% have been reported.[6, 27] CNBs essentially have replaced incisional biopsies in the evaluation of breast masses. Incisional biopsies still are used to make the diagnosis of inflammatory cancer and Paget's disease.

IMAGE-GUIDED BREAST BIOPSY

Since the introduction of the radical mastectomy by Halsted in 1894,[55] the advent of screening mammography has been the most important factor in reducing the mortality rate of patients with breast cancer. Randomized studies have documented a 30% reduction in the breast cancer mortality rate for women involved in mammography screening programs.[123, 128, 129] Traditional mammographic needle or wire localization with surgical biopsy has been the standard procedure for the diagnosis of nonpalpable breast abnormalities. Large series of wire-localized breast biopsies have reported a positive biopsy rate or positive predictive value (PPV) of 10% to 40%.* Centers with expertise in mammography and breast surgery have reported results in the range of 35% to 40%.[53, 103, 111, 127] Programs achieving a PPV of 35% miss approximately 1% to 2% of early breast cancers, relegating them to short-term follow-up mammography. Most missed cancers are ductal carcinoma in situ (DCIS) or early infiltrating cancers for which a 6-month delay in treatment is unlikely to alter prognosis. Also, a miss rate of 1% to 2% parallels the surgical miss rate of wire-localized breast biopsy[4, 53, 54, 97]; however, the pressures of patient and referring physician expectation, strong malpractice risk factors, and the desire to maximize sensitivity have made radiologists and surgeons willing to accept a PPV of 20%. One study[20] of 50 community-based practices found an average PPV of 21% for wire-localization biopsy. The induced costs of follow-up studies and diagnostic procedures com-

---

*References 12, 20, 53, 54, 56, 103, and 135.

prise the major expense of mammography screening programs.[32] These induced costs may jeopardize the economic feasibility of screening programs. Women have suffered the anxiety and cosmetic sequelae of surgical biopsy for a 20% likelihood of diagnosing malignancy.

In 1977, two reports from the Karolinska Institute in Sweden[15, 106] described FNA biopsy and a drill-like needle biopsy technique for small-specimen histologic diagnosis directed by mammographic stereotactic radiography guidance. Stereotactic FNA biopsy requires no incision, is cost-effective, and is accurate in experienced hands; however, FNA is operator dependent, and the best results require a highly skilled cytopathologist to prepare the slides on site and to interpret the cytology. Results in large series have been highly variable, with sensitivities of 77.2% to 95.0% and specificities of 72.0% to 99.8%, while false-negative rates have ranged from 0.6% to 32%, and specimens inadequate for interpretation, 2% to 40%.* Cote et al[29] reported 243 cases of FNA, all with histologic confirmation. Excluding 26.4% of specimens inadequate for diagnosis, they found 8.8% false-negative cytologies. Initial reports of 20-gauge and 18-gauge CNBs produced results similar to those of FNA biopsy.[12, 39]

In 1991, Parker et al[114] reported on a series of 102 stereotactic large CNBs with 14-gauge automated cutting needles. All cases were confirmed by open wire localization biopsy. Parker et al[114] found a sensitivity of 96%, a specificity of 100%, and a false-negative rate of 1.2%. Five subsequent studies[8, 18, 33, 40, 49] of large CNBs with histologic wire localization biopsy confirmation have shown sensitivities of 85% to 96%, specificities of 96% to 100%, and false-negative rates of 2.1% to 3.1%. Most studies of stereotactic CNBs have provided only partial histologic confirmation or have suffered from inadequate mammographic follow-up but have shown comparable results.†

Stereotactic CNB studies document results that are competitive with the literature for open wire localization biopsy. The literature on open wire localization published from 1976 to 1997 reveals an average lesion miss rate of 2.6%, with a range of 0% to 6% (exclusive of one study, which reported 17.9% missed lesions).[4, 65, 69, 97] The false-negative rate averaged 0.67%, with a median of 0.4%, and calculating benign wire localization biopsies that missed cancers.

Cosmetic advantages of a 4-mm needle biopsy scar versus a surgical incision are self-evident. The cost savings for stereotactic CNB over wire localization biopsy have been documented in the range of $1000 to $1600 per procedure.[31, 37, 87, 93, 119, 135] Taking into account repeat biopsies, the overall cost savings for making a tissue diagnosis by stereotactic CNB is estimated to be 50%.[87, 119]

All physicians who manage patients with stereotactic CNBs must recognize the limitations of core needle histology and the indications for repeat biopsy. The weaknesses of CNB arise from sampling errors and from the hazard of misinterpretation or underinterpretation of results. Jackman et al[63] emphasized the importance of following all needle biopsies of atypical ductal hyperplasia (ADH) with a large-tissue biopsy. Fifty-eight percent of patients with stereotactic CNBs yielding ADH were found to have cancer after subsequent excisional biopsy. A review of 14 series of stereotactic CNBs reveals an average 50% prevalence of malignancy when large-specimen biopsy is performed after CNBs showing ADH (range, 17.0–87.5%).‡ Dershaw et al[38] were among the first groups to emphasize a comprehensive critical evaluation of the pathology results and the importance of reconciling each pathologic diagnosis with its corresponding

---

*References 35, 39, 66, 67, 101, 110, and 131.
†References 3, 7, 12, 41, 46, 61, 80, 97, and 112.
‡References 2, 3, 8, 21, 33, 46, 47, 63, 82, 92, 99, 102, 116, and 130.

mammographic abnormality. Dershaw et al[38] reported an 18% rebiopsy rate in 314 consecutive stereotactic CNBs. Among 50 patients whose stereotactic CNBs revealed apparently benign diagnoses, including ADH, benign entities that were nonconcordant with radiographic findings, or inadequate specimens, 44% of repeat biopsies documented malignant lesions. Using the same critical evaluation of stereotactic CNB pathology and correlation with mammographic findings, five subsequent studies[11, 79, 99, 102, 116] have reported 14% to 19% rebiopsy rates. The prevalence of malignancy approaches 50% in CNBs revealing ADH, radial scar, and nonconcordance with radiographic findings. Highly cellular fibroadenomas found by CNB may represent phylloides tumors. All of these pathologic diagnoses obtained by CNB require mandatory repeat biopsy, usually by large-tissue biopsy. Finally, a CNB diagnosis of DCIS underdiagnoses infiltrating duct cancer in approximately 26% of cases (range, 19–47%).*

The limitations of stereotactic CNB seem to be more important when the indication for biopsy is indeterminate or suspicious microcalcifications. The risk for nonconcordance with radiography, underdiagnosing ADH in the presence of cancer, and missed invasion in DCIS is magnified when stereotactic CNBs are performed for microcalcifications.† The false-negative rate is significantly higher for calcifications.[84, 94, 112] Several studies have shown that the cancer miss rate is higher when no microcalcifications are found in the core specimens[3, 84, 94] and when fewer than six core biopsy specimens are taken.[18, 63, 86, 118]

Repeat biopsy must be considered with any stereotactic CNB that yields a benign diagnosis for calcifications highly suspicious for malignancy. Some investigators[8, 9, 40] recommend open wire localization biopsies for all Breast Imaging Reporting and Data System (BI-RADS) 5 lesions. In the hope of improving diagnostic accuracy, reducing false-negative rates, and reducing the rebiopsy rate of stereotactic CNBs, a vacuum-assisted needle biopsy was developed (Mammotome, Ethicon USA, Cincinnati, OH; Minimally Invasive Breast Biopsy [MIBB], United States Surgical Corporation, Norwalk, CT). These needles perform multiple vacuum-assisted biopsies in concentric directed circles through a single insertion point by stereotactic guidance. The technique has been well described.[24, 58, 90, 98] The individual 14-gauge vacuum-assisted needle biopsy device produced a specimen twice the size of a 14-gauge stereotactic CNB. The newer 11-gauge vacuum-assisted biopsies are 5.3-fold larger than are the 14-gauge CNBs.[10, 22] Escalation of individual and aggregate specimen size has improved the yield of calcifications in biopsy specimens and reduced the prevalence of specimen inadequacy and of radiographic discordance,[17, 90, 116] thereby reducing the rebiopsy rate.[90, 98, 116] The miss rate of cancer in 11-gauge vacuum-assisted biopsy specimens showing ADH ranges from 10.0% to 26.7%,[17, 90, 116, 136] with the exception of one study[23] reporting a 0% miss rate. The risk for missing invasive cancer in a vacuum-assisted biopsy showing DCIS has been reduced to 0% to 5%, although one study reported a 35% risk.[23, 90, 91, 136] The clearest advantage of vacuum-assisted biopsies over stereotactic CNBs is found in cases of microcalcification, in which CNBs are known to have the highest rebiopsy and false-negative rates.[90, 98, 116]

The literature shows that any diagnosis of ADH by stereotactic CNB or vacuum-assisted biopsy requires a repeat biopsy, preferably a large-tissue biopsy, to rule out malignancy.[17, 90, 116] Rebiopsy rates of 9%, 17%, and 23% have been reported for vacuum-assisted biopsy.[90, 116, 132] Patients should be informed that

---

*References 2, 3, 8, 9, 33, 46, 63, 79, 83, and 87.
†References 9, 18, 36, 47, 84, 99, 116, and 118.

they may have invasive cancer accompanying DCIS diagnosed by any needle-biopsy device and that the need for lymph node sampling or dissection is contingent on lumpectomy or mastectomy results.

The most recent evolution of image-guided breast biopsy devices is a stereotactic large CNB tool known as the Advanced Breast Biopsy Instrumentation (ABBI, United States Surgical Corporation) device. This device uses the same stereotactic technique as do needle-biopsy devices to direct an instrument that removes intact cylindrical specimens of 10-mm, 15-mm, or 20-mm diameter.[34, 35, 71, 72, 78, 121] A similar device (SiteSelect, Imagyn Medical Technologies, Newport Beach, CA) removes specimens of 15-mm diameter. These devices allow for intact removal of mammographic abnormalities for complete pathologic analysis of the lesion and margins, comparable with open excisional biopsy. In a multicenter study of 654 ABBI biopsies comprising the early experience of eight centers, specimens successfully were removed for biopsy in 99.7% of cases.[71] The yield of ADH was 5.4%, and the pathologists were confident in that diagnosis in all but 1 of 34 cases, which was an incisional biopsy with ADH at the margins. The overall rebiopsy rate was 0.4%, for one missed lesion, one inadequate specimen, and one case confirmed as ADH. No false-negative results occurred. The complication rate was 0.6%, comparable with multicenter series on stereotactic CNBs (0.2%)[112] and vacuum-assisted biopsies (0.14%).[64] Similar results have been reported in other studies of large CNBs.[35, 72, 95, 121] One series of 77 large CNBs reported a 4% complication rate (three hematomas) and one procedure-related technical failure.[81] A few series have inappropriately included digital radiography failures, pseudolesions, contraindicated lesions, and mistakes arising from inadequate training as technical failures of large CNBs.

The complication rates reported for large CNBs are comparable with individual series in the literature on vacuum-assisted breast biopsy, which reports 0% to 4% complication rates.[22, 23, 64, 99] The lesion miss rate with large CNB has been 0% to 2%,* the false-negative rate has been 0%,[81, 132] and the specificity and sensitivity have been 100% in most series.[34, 71, 122, 132] The incidence of ADH from the large CNB series has been 4% to 6%.[71, 72, 121, 122] Only one case of cancer found after rebiopsy of a large CNB diagnosed as ADH[81] and two cases of infiltrating ductal carcinoma underdiagnosed as DCIS[95] have been reported. The ratio of lesion size to cannula size was not stated for the three underdiagnosed lesions. The rebiopsy rate for large CNBs has been reported to be 0% to 1.3%.[34, 35, 71, 95, 122] Cost savings of up to $1000 have been reported for large CNBs compared with open wire localization techniques for a single procedure.[78] These cost savings are significant because the combined rebiopsy rate and lesion miss rate are equal to or less than the reported lesion miss rates for open wire localization biopsies. A large, single-institution study has compared a 15-month experience with stereotactic CNBs, vacuum-assisted procedures, large CNBs, and open wire localization techniques.[132] The sensitivity was higher for large CNBs than for the other minimal access procedures. The rebiopsy rate for large CNBs was 7.5%, which is the highest reported in the literature; however, rebiopsy rates were 25.7% for stereotactic CNBs and 23.2% for vacuum-assisted procedures. Sixty-four percent of cancers in the large CNB group had pathologically free margins compared with 50.9% of open wire localization biopsies. Of the available biopsy options, only large CNBs and open wire localization techniques permit accurate histologic assessment of margins and are approved by the US Food and Drug Administration for excisional breast biopsy.

---

*References 34, 35, 71, 72, 81, 122, and 132.

Sonography-guided procedures have quietly assumed a prominent role in minimal access breast biopsies. Nonpalpable mammographically detected breast lesions can be seen using sonography in approximately 55% of all cases: 88% of circumscribed densities, 80% of stellate lesions, 47% of asymmetric densities, and 9% of microcalcifications.[117] Articles describing FNA performed with sonographic guidance report a sensitivity of 65.0% to 89.3% and a specificity of 75.0% to 99.2%.[57, 73, 107, 108] Sonographic guidance also has been used successfully with CNBs.[112, 113, 119, 125] The cost-effectiveness of this procedure has been well documented, with a 39% decrease in the cost compared with open surgical biopsy.[88]

MINIMAL ACCESS SURGERY FOR BREAST CANCER TREATMENT

The National Surgical Adjuvant Breast and Bowel Project (NSABP) B-06 trial, published in 1985,[43] represented the first shift away from traditional mastectomies to breast conservation and lumpectomies in cases of invasive breast cancer. Later, the NSABP B-17 trial demonstrated that this was also possible with intraductal carcinoma.[44] Screening mammography programs and increased public awareness have resulted in a notable decrease in cancer size at presentation, with as many as 30% of lesions now being less than or equal to 1 cm.[26] Many cancers are nonpalpable, detected only by mammography or sonography. Lumpectomies performed on nonpalpable lesions require preoperative wire localizations. Controversy exists as to whether the care of these patients is improved if a diagnosis is first obtained with FNA or CNB. Success with a single-stage lumpectomy, combining the diagnostic with a successful therapeutic procedure so as to obtain negative margins in 161 (93.1%) of 173 cases,[70] has been reported. One (1.5%) of 66 patients first diagnosed with FNA had positive margins. Other surgeons have less success with this technique, with Velanovich et al[132] reporting positive margins in 50.9% of 520 wire localization breast biopsies. Yim et al[135] reported positive margins in 55% of 31 patients treated only with wire localization biopsy versus 0% of 21 patients having an initial diagnosis by stereotactic CNB. The radiologic literature reports success in obtaining negative margins in 57 (92%) of 62 patients first diagnosed by CNB versus 4 (95%) of 74 patients whose disease was revealed by surgical biopsy.[87] These investigators stress that a single surgical procedure was performed in 76 (84%) of 90 patients who were first diagnosed by CNB versus 31 (29%) of 107 patients who were diagnosed by open biopsy. They acknowledged that 5 (19%) of 26 patients diagnosed with DCIS by CNB had foci of invasive cancer at surgery.

Smaller cancers require the removal of less tissue while still obtaining adequate margins, resulting in a more cosmetically acceptable lumpectomy. This is sometimes difficult with needle localization techniques. Some reports have documented complete removal of mammographic lesions using image-guided techniques. Complete removal of mammographic lesions was demonstrated using vacuum-assisted devices, although residual cancer was identified on reexcision.[85] Margin adequacy cannot be assessed with this vacuum-assisted technique.[48] Large CNB ABBI demonstrates that a percentage of diagnostic biopsies performed with this technique have negative margins.[95, 132] Prospective clinical trials are needed to demonstrate therapeutic capability with these techniques.

Cryotherapy represents a minimal access, nonsurgical approach to breast cancer treatment. A probe is placed under sonographic guidance into the breast cancer, and the cancer is ablated with cryotherapy.[126] Cryotherapy seems to be effective if the tumors are less than 1 cm in diameter and are frozen to a temperature of $-40°C$. The cancers must be a sufficient distance from the skin and visible by sonography. Since 1968, this technique has been performed on more than 60 patients.[19] Only recently have clinical trials become practical. Patients with small, localized cancers are treated with cryotherapy. One week later, they undergo a standard lumpectomy. The tissue undergoes pathologic evaluation to ensure that no cancer cells remain.

Axillary node involvement is one of the most important prognostic factors in patients with breast cancer. Patients in the NSABP B-04 trial demonstrated a local axillary recurrence rate of 19% in the absence of surgical or radiotherapeutic treatment.[45] The 10-year relative survival rate of patients with Stage I and II breast cancer treated with breast conservation, axillary dissection, and radiation therapy is 94% for Stage I and 72% for Stage II versus 85% for Stage I when the axillary dissection is omitted.[13] This implies a therapeutic role for the axillary dissection.

The concept of a sentinel lymph node as the lymph node most likely to contain metastases seems valid. Sentinel lymph node analysis is a new minimal access procedure for staging the axilla in patients with breast cancer. The concept of a sentinel lymph node is based on the fact that areas of the skin and body have specific patterns of lymphatic drainage into regional nodal basins and specific lymph nodes within that basin. Cabanas[25] first reported clinical use of this concept in 1977 in the treatment of penile cancer. Morton et al[104] successfully used isosulfan blue dye to perform intraoperative lymphatic mapping in melanoma patients, reporting his results in 1992. Krag et al[77] reported on the use of technetium-labeled colloid to perform intraoperative lymphatic mapping of breast cancer patients in 1993. Successful use of isosulfan blue dye in the intraoperative mapping of breast cancer patients was reported by Guiliano et al in 1994[52] and again in 1997.[51] In 1996, surgeons from the H. Lee Moffitt Cancer Center reported on the combined use of radiolabeled colloid and lymphazurium blue to perform intraoperative breast cancer mapping.[1] Preprocedure lymphoscintigraphy with radionuclide increased the accuracy of axillary sentinel lymph node identification.[16] In 1998, Krag et al[76] reported lymphatic mapping in a multi-institutional study involving 443 patients. Hot spots were identified in 413 (93%) of 443 patients. The sensitivity was 89% and the specificity was 100%. The largest series to date is that reported by Cox et al.[30] Using lymphatic mapping and isosulfan blue, the sentinel lymph node was successfully identified in 440 (94%) of 466 patients.

Numerous studies report the rate of sentinel lymph node detection to be at least 92%.[96] False-negative rates, calculated as the number of noncancerous sentinel lymph nodes divided by the number of node-positive patients, range from 4% to 12%.[96] The rate of detection and the accuracy may depend on technique, which may include the use of preprocedure lymphoscintigraphy, filtered or unfiltered radionuclides, various vital blue dyes, and different gamma probes. The optimum time for radionuclide injections and for obtaining preprocedure lymphoscintigrams remains unclear, but usually ranges from 2 to 6 hours. Injection techniques differ, with most surgeons injecting around the tumor using a four-quadrant approach. Some surgeons inject directly into the tumor,[96] whereas others use a subdermal injection technique.[74, 133] Sentinel lymph node biopsies were initially performed only on patients whose diagnostic biopsies were obtained by FNA or CNB. Subsequent studies confirmed that the technique also could be used in patients who had been diagnosed with equal success by excisional biopsy. Cox et al[30] identified the sentinel lymph nodes in 216 (95.2%) of 227 patients diagnosed by excisional biopsy and in 180 (92.3%) of 195 patients diagnosed by FNA or CNB.[30] This accuracy may be less precise when larger excisional biopsies are performed at the time of diagnosis. In one recent report, a sentinel lymph node was identified in 70 (93%) of 75 patients, with 21 of these patients having positive axillary nodes. Four of these 21 patients had sentinel lymph nodes that were free of cancer, giving a false-negative rate of 19%. All of these patients had been diagnosed by prior large excisional biopsies.[42]

Surgeons working with Guiliano have published three articles on their experience with sentinel lymph node biopsy. These articles provide validity to the technique and may point to future applications. The accuracy of staging was examined in a study comparing 134 patients undergoing standard axillary dissection against 162 matched patients who underwent a sentinel lymph node biopsy followed by a standard axillary dissection.[50] Sentinel lymph nodes were examined using serial sectioning and immunohistochemical stains. Metastases were identified in the sentinel lymph nodes of 68 (38.2%) of 162 patients treated with this procedure. In contrast, only 39 (29.1%) of 134 patients treated with standard axillary dissection had metastases. Of patients with positive lymph nodes, 38.2% of the patients with sentinel lymph nodes and 10.3% of patients with standard axillary dissection had lymph node micrometastases (≤ 2 mm). The significance of micrometastases was confirmed in a second article,[28] which examined the rate of nonsentinel lymph node involvement in 157 patients with positive sentinel lymph nodes. The rate of nonsentinel lymph node involvement was only 7% in patients having sentinel lymph node micrometastases. This increased to 55% when the sentinel lymph node contained macrometastases. The presence of nonsentinel lymph node metastases also increased with increasing primary tumor size and in patients who had clinically palpable lymph nodes. The therapeutic effect of sentinel lymphadenectomy was evaluated in 142 patients with T1 breast cancer.[109] Fifteen (37.5%) of 40 T1 premenopausal patients and 20 (25.6%) of 78 T1 postmenopausal patients received recommendations for chemotherapy when the sentinel lymph node revealed axillary metastases. All 15 premenopausal and 6 postmenopausal patients received chemotherapy. The investigators believed that surgical axillary dissection was essential to proper breast cancer management and should not be abandoned.

PATHOLOGY

Stereotactic CNB provides a directed sampling, whereby the tissue removed, and thus the pathologic examination, is focused on a particular lesion of interest. Extraneous tissue, with minimal diagnostic utility, is not removed. Physicians should not focus too narrowly on microcalcifications because they may be located exclusively in benign breast tissue adjacent to a significant lesion.[68] Therefore, complete intact removal of a mammographic lesion and the immediately surrounding nonlesional tissue should yield the most accurate histologic evaluation.[132] Traditional wire localization open breast biopsy of nonpalpable lesions typically accomplishes this goal in 10% to 40% of cases,* but also, significant extraneous tissue is removed. On average, more extraneous tissue is excised for nonpalpable lesions than for palpable lesions.[14] Conversely, minimally invasive breast surgery may mean minimal tissue available for pathologic evaluation. Therefore, costs of a more limited pathologic evaluation must be outweighed by the benefits of newer, minimally invasive biopsies.

Among the most important histologic parameters to be assessed in patients

---

*References 12, 20, 53, 54, 56, 103, and 135.

with newly diagnosed breast cancer are the histologic type of tumor, the grade of the tumor, maximum tumor size, type and extent of DCIS, and the presence or absence of angiolymphatic invasion, in relation to the tumor. Despite its limitations, wire localized excisional breast biopsy is the gold standard with which newer techniques should be compared.

A patient and her physician initially may be interested only in a "positive" or "negative" result. For most patients, the presence of cancer can be determined; however, in women with breast cancer, relevant histologic information should be obtained at some point. A diagnostic procedure should not compromise later histologic evaluation. Despite the advent of numerous prognostic markers and other ancillary studies, histopathologic evaluation is the most informative and cost-effective method of analysis.[124]

Stereotactic FNA is no longer commonly performed in the United States since the advent of the CNB. Stereotactic FNA of the breast in general has been shown to have an acceptable degree of diagnostic accuracy (sensitivity, 68–100%; specificity, 82–100%).[7] Another significant advantage of FNA is the ability to quickly stain slides for a rapid diagnosis. FNA is also the least invasive of these procedures. Disadvantages include the difficulty of obtaining adequate material.[7, 120] Successful stereotactic FNA requires special training by surgeons who perform the FNA and pathologists who interpret the smears.

CNB offers advantages over FNA, including the ability to identify microcalcifications in specimen radiographs and in tissue sections. Because tissue fragments are obtained, additional confirmation of the presence of an invasive process can be documented, together with the histologic grade. Estrogen-receptor and progesterone-receptor studies can be performed in tissue sections from CNBs, with a 93% concordance for estrogen receptor and 69% for progesterone receptor compared with subsequent surgical excision.[138] Additional studies (e.g., of flow cytometry or oncogene status) also can be performed given sufficient tissue.

CNB, however, is a sampling technique with an inherent possibility of sampling error. CNB yields only a small percentage of a lesion for histologic examination. An underlying assumption is that a small sample of a lesion in a core is representative of the remainder of the lesion in the breast. This is not always true. Stereotactic CNB has been shown to have a sensitivity of 71% to 100% and specificity of 85% to 100%.[7] Philpotts et al[116] reported discordance rates of 13.7% for 14-gauge stereotactic CNBs that required subsequent surgical excisions. The most common discordances occur in cases of ADH and DCIS. ADH in a CNB is an indication for surgical excision, given that in as many as 50% of cases, in situ or invasive cancer is identified in the excised specimen. A similar phenomenon is observed in cases of DCIS in CNBs that are proven to contain invasive cancer in subsequent excision.[83, 87, 91] The opposite phenomenon also may occur in that no additional lesional tissue may be present in the excision at mastectomy, the diagnostic lesion having been seen only in the core sample. Sampling error also may affect the evaluation of angiolymphatic invasion, often a local phenomenon, and the presence and extent of DCIS in invasive cancer.

One of the great drawbacks of CNB is introduction of artifacts, including fragmentation of lesional tissue into many small pieces. Also, tumor size cannot be determined accurately on the basis of histologic examination of tumor in CNB specimens alone. A minimum tumor size might be estimated, but the authors have seen misinterpretation of these data result in a drastic underestimation of tumor size. An additional artifact introduced by CNB has been well documented in many organs, including breast. This is the displacement of carcinomatous epithelium into the fibrous needle tract. In cases of DCIS, this displacement can result in a mistaken impression of invasion.[91, 137]

Tissue specimens produced by vacuum-assisted techniques are similar to CNB specimens for histologic evaluation. They do, however, offer advantages over CNB, including a greater volume of tissue and larger individual tissue fragments.[22, 24] This increases diagnostic accuracy as has been shown by greater correlation between biopsy diagnoses and follow-up excisional results.[116] A significant rate of upgrading of ADH to DCIS[116] and DCIS to invasion[91, 136] still occurs, however. Some articles have estimated the rate of upgrading ADH to DCIS at 0% to 26.7% of cases.[23, 116] As with CNB, fragmentation of tissue occurs. Concerns also have been raised that biopsy with large-caliber needle cores results in a significant downstaging of cancer because often, a significant proportion of tumor is excised for diagnosis and only the residual tumor size is documented for staging purposes.[48, 85] Radiographic tumor size may be an acceptable substitute for pathologic examination, but well-known underestimation of tumor size occurs by radiographic techniques.[59, 85] Finally, epithelial displacement seems to be less common with the mammotome than with CNB, but it still occurs.[91]

Stereotactic excisional techniques, such as large CNB, offer the advantage of a single intact tissue specimen without fragmentation. These biopsies are equivalent to wire localization excisional biopsies,[35] with the added benefit of stereotactic targeting and removal of less tissue. Lesions less than 2 cm can be removed whole and intact by the largest ABBI cannula now available. Larger lesions are sampled generously without tissue fragmentation. Because small lesions can be removed within one complete tissue sample, evaluation of surgical margins is possible.[132]

Unfortunately, a 20-mm large-core ABBI cannula, the largest diameter now available, is too small to entirely remove many lesions. Margins are reported involved in 63.6% of large CNB.[132] The authors have found large CNBs to be the equivalent of wire localization excisional biopsies for full evaluation of all types of benign and malignant breast lesions.*

The sentinel lymph node biopsy offers new challenges for pathologists. Serial sectioning of lymph nodes removed during an axillary dissection and staining of these nodes with hematoxylin and eosin have resulted in increased detection of micrometastases ($\leq$ 2 mm).[96] The use of immunohistochemical stains also has increased the positive yield of occult metastases.[50, 115] Reverse transcriptase polymerase chain reaction analysis is sensitive in the detection of metastases.[100] Although these techniques provide a more accurate assessment of metastatic disease, most pathology departments do not have the resources to perform these tests on all lymph nodes obtained with a standard axillary dissection. The sentinel lymph node biopsy technique provides pathologists with a few appropriately identified nodes on which these tests may be performed. This allows for more accurate breast cancer staging and, therefore, treatment at the time of diagnosis.

SUMMARY

Minimal access procedures have great potential for providing patients with equal, if not superior, forms of breast cancer diagnosis and treatment. Many of these procedures are in a process of evolution. The reliability of each method

---

*References 34, 35, 71, 72, 78, 95, 120, 121, and 132.

probably depends heavily on the training, ability, and experience of the operator. Surgeons should be aware of the advantages and pitfalls of these techniques and exercise caution during the initial phases of their learning experience.

References

1. Albertini JJ, Lyman GH, Cox C, et al: Lymphatic mapping and sentinel node biopsy in the patient with breast cancer. JAMA 276:1818, 1996
2. Acheson MB, Patton RG, Howisey RL, et al: Histologic correlation of image-guided core biopsy with excisional biopsy of nonpalpable breast lesions. Arch Surg 132:815, 1997
3. Andreu FJ, Sentis M, Castaner E, et al: The impact of stereotactic large-core needle biopsy in the treatment of patients with nonpalpable breast lesions: A study of diagnostic accuracy in 510 consecutive cases. Eur Radiol 8:1468, 1998
4. Antley CM, Mooney EE, Layfield LJ: A comparison of accuracy rates between open biopsy, cutting-needle biopsy, and fine-needle aspiration biopsy of the breast: A 3-year experience. The Breast Journal 4:3, 1998
5. Azavedo E, Svane G, Auer G: Stereotactic fine-needle biopsy in 2594 mammographically detected non-palpable lesions. Lancet 1:1033, 1989
6. Ballo MS, Sneige N: Can core needle biopsy replace fine-needle aspiration cytology in diagnosis of palpable breast carcinoma: A comparison study of 124 women. Cancer 78:773, 1996
7. Bassett L, Winchester DP, Caplan RB, et al: Stereotactic core-needle biopsy of the breast: A report of the joint task force of the American College of Radiology, American College of Surgeons, and College of American Pathologists. CA Cancer J Clin 47:171, 1997
8. Bauer RL, Sung J, Eckhert KH, et al: Comparison of histologic diagnosis between stereotactic core needle biopsy and open surgical biopsy. Ann Surg Oncol 4:316, 1997
9. Berg WA: When is core breast biopsy or fine-needle aspiration not enough? Radiology 198:313, 1996
10. Berg WA, Krebs TL, Campassi C, et al: Evaluation of 14- and 11-gauge directional, vacuum-assisted biopsy probes and 14-gauge biopsy guns in a breast parenchymal model. Radiology 205:203, 1997
11. Berg WA, Ruben RH, Kymer D, et al: Lessons from mammographic-histopathologic correlation of large-core needle breast biopsy. Radiographics 16:1111, 1996
12. Bernstein JR: Role of stereotactic breast biopsy. Semin Surg Oncol 12:290, 1996
13. Bland KI, Scott-Conner CEH, Menck H, et al: Axillary dissection in breast-conserving surgery for Stage I and II breast cancer: A national cancer data base study of patterns of omission and implications for survival. J Am Coll Surg 188:586, 1999
14. Bleznak AD, Magaram D: Surgical biopsy techniques for mammographically detected abnormalities. The Breast Journal 4:426, 1998
15. Bolmgren J, Jacobson B, Nordenstrom B: Stereotaxic instrument for needle biopsy of the mamma. AJR Am J Roentgenol 129:121, 1977
16. Borgstein PJ, Pijpers R, Comans EF, et al: Sentinel lymph node biopsy in breast cancer: Guidelines and pitfalls of lymphoscintigraphy and gamma probe detection. J Am Coll Surg 186:275, 1998
17. Brem RF, Behrndt VS, Sanow L, et al: Atypical ductal hyperplasia: Histologic underestimation of carcinoma in tissue harvested from impalpable breast lesions using 11-gauge stereotactically guided directional vacuum-assisted biopsy. AJR Am J Roentgenol 172:1405, 1999
18. Brenner RJ, Fajardo L, Fisher PR: Percutaneous core biopsy of the breast: Effect of operator experience and number of samples on diagnostic accuracy. AJR Am J Roentgenol 166:341, 1996
19. Brown KS: In from the cold, cryotherapy gets a second look. J Natl Cancer Inst 90:351, 1998
20. Brown ML, Houn F, Sickles EA, et al: Screening mammography in community

practice: Positive predictive value of abnormal findings and yield of follow-up diagnostic procedures. AJR Am J Roentgenol 165:1373, 1995

21. Brown TA, Wall JW, Christensen ED, et al: Atypical hyperplasia in the era of stereotactic core needle biopsy. J Surg Oncol 67:168, 1998
22. Burbank F: Stereotactic breast biopsy: Comparison of 14- and 11-gauge mammotome probe performance and complication rates. Am Surg 63:988, 1997
23. Burbank F: Stereotactic breast biopsy of atypical ductal hyperplasia and ductal carcinoma in situ lesions: Improved accuracy with directional, vacuum-assisted biopsy. Radiology 202:843, 1997
24. Burbank F, Parker SH, Fogarty TJ: Stereotactic breast biopsy: Improved tissue harvesting with the mammotome. Am Surg 62:738, 1996
25. Cabanas RM: An approach for the treatment of penile carcinoma. Cancer 39:456, 1977
26. Cady B, Stone MD, Schuler JG, et al: The new era in breast cancer: Invasion, size and nodal involvement dramatically decreasing as a result of mammographic screening. Arch Surg 131:301, 1996
27. Cheung PS, Yan KW, Alagaratnam TT: The complementary role of fine needle aspiration cytology and Tru-Cut needle biopsy in the management of breast masses. Aust N Z J Surg 57:615, 1987
28. Chu KU, Turner RR, Hansen NM, et al: Do all patients with sentinel node metastasis from breast carcinoma need complete axillary node dissection? Ann Surg 229:536, 1999
29. Cote JF, Klijanienko J, Meunier M, et al: Stereotactic fine-needle aspiration cytology of nonpalpable breast lesions: Institut Curies' experience of 243 histologically correlated cases. Cancer Cytopathol 84:77, 1998
30. Cox CE, Pendas S, Cox JM, et al: Guidelines for sentinel lymph node biopsy and lymphatic mapping of patients with breast cancer. Ann Surg 5:645, 1998
31. Cross MJ, Evans WP, Peters GN: Stereotactic breast biopsy as an alternative to open excisional biopsy. Ann Surg Oncol 2:195, 1995
32. Cyriak D: Induced costs of low-cost screening mammography. Radiology 168:661, 1988
33. Dahlstrom E, Sutton S, Jain S: Histological precision of stereotactic core biopsy in diagnosis of malignant and premalignant breast lesions. Histopathology 28:537, 1996
34. Damascelli BD, Frigerio LF, Patelli G, et al: Stereotactic breast biopsy: En bloc excision of microcalcifications with a large-bore cannula device. AJR Am J Roentgenol 173:895, 1999
35. D'Angelo PC, Galliano DE, Rosemurgy AS: Stereotactic excisional breast biopsies utilizing the advanced breast biopsy instrumentation system. Am J Surg 174:297, 1997
36. Dershaw DD: Stereotactic biopsy: Advantages and limitations. The Breast Journal 3:215, 1997
37. Dershaw DD, Liberman L: Stereotactic breast biopsy: Indications and results. Oncology 12:907, 1998
38. Dershaw DD, Morris EA, Liberman L, et al: Nondiagnostic stereotaxic core breast biopsy: Results of rebiopsy. Radiology 198:323, 1996
39. Dowlatshahi K, Yaremko ML, Kluskens LF, et al: Nonpalpable breast lesions: Findings of stereotaxic needle-core biopsy and fine-needle aspiration cytology. Radiology 181:745, 1991
40. Elvecrog EL, Lechner MC, Nelson MT: Nonpalpable breast lesions: Correlation of stereotaxic large-core needle biopsy and surgical biopsy results. Radiology 188:453, 1993
41. Fajardo LL, DeAngelis GA: The role of stereotactic biopsy in abnormal mammograms. Surg Oncol Clin North Am 6:285, 1997
42. Feldman SM, Krag DN, McNally RK, et al: Limitation in gamma probe localization of the sentinel node in breast cancer patients with large excisional biopsy. J Am Coll Surg 188:248, 1999
43. Fisher B, Bauer M, Margolese R, et al: Five-year results of a randomized clinical trial comparing total mastectomy and segmental mastectomy with or without radiation in the treatment of breast cancer. N Engl J Med 312:665, 1985
44. Fisher B, Costantino J, Redmond C, et al: Lumpectomy compared with lumpectomy

and radiation therapy for the treatment of intraductal breast cancer. N Engl J Med 328:1581, 1993

45. Fisher B, Redmond C, Fisher ER, et al: Ten-year results of a randomized clinical trial comparing radical mastectomy and total mastectomy with or without radiation. N Engl J Med 312:674, 1985

46. Fuhrman GM, Cederborn GJ, Bolton JS, et al: Image-guided core-needle breast biopsy is an accurate technique to evaluate patients with nonpalpable imaging abnormalities. Ann Surg 227:932, 1998

47. Gadzala DE, Cederbom GJ, Bolton JS, et al: Appropriate management of atypical ductal hyperplasia diagnosed by stereotactic core needle breast biopsy. Ann Surg Oncol 4:283, 1997

48. Gajdos C, Levy M, Herman Z, et al: Complete removal of nonpalpable breast malignancies with a stereotactic percutaneous vacuum-assisted biopsy instrument. J Am Coll Surg 189:237, 1999

49. Gisvold JJ, Goellner JR, Grank CS, et al: Breast biopsy: A comparative study of stereotaxically guided core and excisional techniques. AJR Am J Roentgenol 16:815, 1994

50. Guiliano AE, Dale PS, Turner RR, et al: Improved axillary staging of breast cancer with sentinel lymphadenectomy. Ann Surg 222:394, 1995

51. Guiliano AE, Jones RC, Brennan M, et al: Sentinel lymphadenectomy in breast cancer. J Clin Oncol 15:2345, 1997

52. Guiliano AE, Kirgan DM, Guenther JM, et al: Lymphatic mapping and sentinel lymphadenectomy for breast cancer. Ann Surg 220:391, 1994

53. Hall FM: Technologic advances in breast imaging. Surg Oncol Clin North Am 6:403, 1997

54. Hall FM, Starella JM, Silverstone DZ, et al: Non-palpable breast lesions: Recommendations for biopsy based on suspicion of carcinoma at mammography. Radiology 167:353, 1988

55. Halsted WS: The results of operations for the cure of cancer of the breast performed at the Johns Hopkins Hospital from June 1889 to January 1894. Johns Hopkins Hospital Report 4:297, 1894–1895

56. Hasselgren PO, Hummel RP, Georgian-Smith D, et al: Breast biopsy with needle localization: Accuracy of specimen x-ray and management of missed lesions. Surgery 114:836, 1993

57. Hatada T, Aoki I, Okada K, et al: Usefulness of ultrasound-guided, fine-needle aspiration biopsy for palpable breast tumors. Arch Surg 131:1095, 1996

58. Heywang-Kobrunner SH, Schaumloffel U, Hofer H, et al: Minimally invasive stereotaxic vacuum core breast biopsy. Eur Radiol 8:377, 1998

59. Holland R, Hendricks JHCL, Verbeek ALM, et al: Extent, distribution, and mammographic/histological correlations of breast ductal carcinoma in situ. Lancet 335:519, 1990

60. Innes DJ, Feldman PS: Comparison of diagnostic results obtained by fine needle aspiration cytology and Tru-Cut or open biopsies. Acta Cytol 27:350, 1983

61. Israel PZ, Fine RE: Stereotactic needle biopsy for occult breast lesions: A minimally invasive alternative. Am Surg 61:87, 1995

62. Jackman RJ, Nowels KW, Rodriguez-Soto J, et al: Stereotactic, automated, large-core needle biopsy of nonpalpable breast lesions: False-negative and histologic underestimation rates after long-term follow-up. Radiology 210:799, 1999

63. Jackman RJ, Nowels KW, Shepard MJ, et al: Stereotaxic large-core needle biopsy of 450 nonpalpable breast lesions with surgical correlation in lesions with cancer or atypical hyperplasia. Radiology 193:91, 1994

64. Jackman RJ, Burbank F, Parker S, et al: Atypical ductal hyperplasia diagnosed at stereotactic breast biopsy: Improved reliability with 14-gauge, directional, vacuum-assisted biopsy. Radiology 204:485, 1997

65. Jackman RJ, Marzoni FA: Needle-localized breast biopsy: Why do we fail? Radiology 204:677, 1997

66. Jackson VP: Mammographically guided fine-needle aspiration cytology of nonpalpable breast lesions. Radiology 2:741, 1990

67. Jackson VP, Reynolds HE: Stereotaxic needle-core biopsy and fine-needle aspiration cytologic evaluation of nonpalpable breast lesions. Radiology 181:633, 1991
68. Johnson JM, Dalton RR, Wester SM, et al: Histological correlation of microcalcifications in breast biopsy specimens. Arch Surg 134:712, 1999
69. Jortay AM, Daled H, Faverly D: Contribution of hook-guided breast biopsy to the pathological diagnosis of mammographic lesions. Acta Chir Belg 99:26, 1999
70. Kearney TJ, Morrow M: Effect of reexcision on the success of breast-conserving surgery. Ann Surg Oncol 2:303, 1995
71. Kelley WE, Bailey R, Bertelsen C, et al: Stereotactic automated surgical biopsy using the ABBI biopsy device: A multicenter study. The Breast Journal 4:302, 1998
72. Kelley W, Melzig E, Knaysi G, et al: Stereotactic automated surgical biopsy of the breast with the A. B. B. I. device: Techniques and results. *In* 6th World Congress of Endoscopic Surgery. Rome, 1998, p 503
73. Klijanienko J, Cote JF, Thibault F, et al: Ultrasound-guided fine-needle aspiration cytology of nonpalpable breast lesions. Cancer Cytopathol 84:36, 1998
74. Klimberg VS, Rubio IT, Henry R, et al: Subareolar versus peritumoral injection for location of the sentinel lymph node. Ann Surg 229:860, 1999
75. Kline TS, Neal HS: Role of needle aspiration biopsy in diagnosis of carcinoma of the breast. Obstet Gynecol 1975:89, 1975
76. Krag D, Weaver D, Takamaru A, et al: The sentinel lymph node in breast cancer: A multicenter validation study. N Engl J Med 339:941, 1998
77. Krag DN, Weaver DL, Alex JC, et al: Surgical resection and radiolocalisation of the sentinel lymph node in breast cancer using a gamma probe. Surg Oncol 2:335, 1993
78. LaRaja RD, Saber AA, Sickles A: Early experience in the use of the advanced breast biopsy instrumentation: A report of one hundred twenty-seven patients. Surgery 125:380, 1999
79. Lee CH, Egglin TK, Philpotts L, et al: Cost-effectiveness of stereotactic core needle biopsy: Analysis by means of mammographic findings. Radiology 202:849, 1997
80. Lee CH, Philpotts LE, Horvath LJ, et al: Follow-up of breast lesions diagnosed as benign with stereotactic core-needle biopsy: Frequency of mammographic change and false-negative rate. Radiology 212:189, 1999
81. Leibman AJ, Frager D, Choi P: Experience with breast biopsy using the advanced breast biopsy instrumentation system. AJR Am J Roentgenol 172:1409, 1999
82. Liberman L, Cohen MA, Dershaw DD, et al: Atypical ductal hyperplasia diagnosed at stereotactic core biopsy of breast lesions: An indication for surgical biopsy. AJR Am J Roentgenol 164:1111, 1995
83. Liberman L, Dershaw DD, Rosen PP, et al: Stereotactic core biopsy of breast carcinoma: Accuracy at predicting invasion. Radiology 194:379, 1995
84. Liberman L, Dershaw DD, Glassman JR, et al: Analysis of cancers not diagnosed at stereotactic core breast biopsy. Radiology 203:151, 1997
85. Liberman L, Dershaw DD, Rosen PP, et al: Percutaneous removal of malignant mammographic lesions at stereotactic vacuum-assisted biopsy. Radiology 206:711, 1998
86. Liberman L, Dershaw DD, Rosen PP, et al: Stereotactic 14-gauge breast biopsy: How many core biopsy specimens are needed? Radiology 192:793, 1994
87. Liberman L, Fahs MC, Dershaw DD, et al: Impact of stereotaxic core breast biopsy on cost of diagnosis. Radiology 195:633, 1995
88. Liberman L, Feng TL, Dershaw D, et al: US-guided core breast biopsy: Use and cost-effectiveness. Radiology 208:717, 1998
89. Liberman L, LaTrenta LR, Dershaw CD, et al: Impact of core biopsy on the surgical management of impalpable breast cancer. AJR Am J Roentgenol 168:495, 1997
90. Liberman L, Smolkin JH, Dershaw DD, et al: Calcification retrieval of stereotactic, 11-gauge, directional, vacuum-assisted breast biopsy. Radiology 208:251, 1998
91. Liberman L, Vuolo M, Dershaw DD, et al: Epithelial displacement after stereotactic 11-gauge directional vacuum-assisted breast biopsy. AJR Am J Roentgenol 172:677, 1999
92. Lin PH, Clyde JC, Bates DM, et al: Accuracy of stereotactic core-needle breast biopsy in atypical ductal hyperplasia. Am J Surg 175:380, 1998

93. Lind DS, Minter R, Steinbach B, et al: Stereotactic core biopsy reduces the reexcision rate and the cost of mammographically detected cancer. J Surg Res 78:23, 1998
94. Mainiero MB, Philpotts LE, Lee CH, et al: Stereotaxic core needle biopsy of breast microcalcifications: Correlation of target accuracy and diagnosis with lesion size. Radiology 198:665, 1996
95. Matthews BD, Williams GB: Initial experience with the advanced breast biopsy instrumentation system. Am J Surg 177:97, 1999
96. McIntosh SA, Purushotham AD: Lymphatic mapping and sentinel node biopsy in breast cancer. Br J Surg 85:1347, 1998
97. Meyer JE, Eberlein TJ, Stomper PC, et al: Biopsy of occult breast lesions: Analysis of 1261 abnormalities. JAMA 263:2341, 1990
98. Meyer JE, Smith DN, DiPiro PJ, et al: Stereotactic breast biopsy of clustered microcalcifications with a directional, vacuum-assisted device. Radiology 204:575, 1997
99. Meyer JE, Smith DN, Lester SC, et al: Large-needle core biopsy: Nonmalignant breast abnormalities evaluated with surgical excision or repeat core biopsy. Radiology 206:717, 1998
100. Min CJ, Tafra L, Verbanac KM: Identification of superior markers for polymerase chain reaction detection of breast cancer metastases in sentinel lymph nodes. Cancer Res 58:4581, 1998
101. Mitnick JS, Vazquez MF, Pressman PI, et al: Stereotactic fine-needle aspiration biopsy for the evaluation of nonpalpable breast lesions: Report of an experience based on 2,988 cases. Ann Surg Oncol 3:185, 1996
102. Moore MM, Hargett CW, Hanks JB, et al: Association of breast cancer with the finding of atypical ductal hyperplasia at core breast biopsy. Ann Surg 223:726, 1997
103. Morrow M, Schmidt R, Cregger B, et al: Preoperative evaluation of abnormal mammographic findings to avoid unnecessary breast biopsies. Arch Surg 129:1091, 1994
104. Morton DL, Wen DR, Wong JH, et al: Technical details of intra-operative lymphatic mapping for early stage melanoma. Arch Surg 127:392, 1992
105. National Cancer Institute Conference: Final version: The uniform approach to fine-needle aspiration biopsy. Diagn Cytopathol 16:295, 1997
106. Nordenstrom B, Zajicek J: Stereotactic needle biopsy and preoperative indication of non-palpable mammary lesions. Acta Cytol 21:350, 1977
107. Ogawa Y, Kato Y, Nakata B, et al: Diagnostic potential and pitfalls of ultrasound-guided fine-needle aspiration cytology for breast lesions. Jpn J Surg 28:167, 1998
108. Okamoto H, Ogawara T, Inoue S, et al: Clinical management of nonpalpable or small breast masses by fine-needle aspiration biopsy (FNAB) under ultrasound guidance. J Surg Oncol 67:246, 1998
109. Ollila DW, Brennan MB, Guiliano AE: Therapeutic effect of sentinel lymphadenectomy in T1 breast cancer. Arch Surg 133:647, 1998
110. Oliver DJ, Frayne JR, Sterrett G: Stereotactic fine needle biopsy of the breast. Aust N Z J Surg 62:463, 1992
111. Orel SG, Kay N, Reynolds C, et al: BI-RADS categorization as a predictor of malignancy. Radiology 211:845, 1999
112. Parker SH, Burbank F, Jackman RJ, et al: Percutaneous large-core breast biopsy: A multi-institutional study. Radiology 193:359, 1994
113. Parker SH, Jobe WE, Dennis MA, et al: US-guided automated large-core breast biopsy. Radiology 187:507, 1993
114. Parker SH, Levin JD, Jobe WE, et al: Nonpalpable breast lesions: Stereotactic automated large-core biopsies. Radiology 180:403, 1991
115. Pendras S, Dauway E, Cox CE, et al: Sentinel node biopsy and cytokeratin staining for the accurate staging of 478 breast cancer patients. Am Surg 65:500, 1999
116. Philpotts LE, Shaheen NA, Carter S, et al: Comparison of rebiopsy rates after stereotactic core needle biopsy of the breast with 11-gauge vacuum suction probe versus 14-gauge needle and automatic gun. AJR Am J Roentgenol 172:683, 1999
117. Rissanen T, Pamilo M, Suramo I: Ultrasonography as a guidance method in the evaluation of mammographically detected nonpalpable breast lesions of suspected malignancy. Acta Radiol 39:292, 1998
118. Rich PM, Michell MJ, Humphreys S, et al: Stereotactic 14G core biopsy of non-

palpable breast cancer: What is the relationship between the number of core samples taken and the sensitivity for detection of malignancy? Clin Radiol 54:384, 1999

119. Roe SM, Matthews JA, Burns RP: Stereotactic and ultrasound core needle breast biopsy performed by surgeons. Am J Surg 174:699, 1997
120. Schmidt RA: Stereotactic breast biopsy. CA Cancer J Clin 44:172, 1994
121. Schwartzberg BS: Advanced breast biopsy instrumentation: The Denver experience. In 6th World Congress of Endoscopic Surgery. Rome, June 1998, p 513
122. Schwartzberg BS, Goates JJ, Keeler SA, et al: Use of advanced breast biopsy instrumentation while performing stereotactic breast biopsies: Review of 150 consecutive biopsies. J Am Coll Sug 191:9, 2000
123. Shapiro S, Benet W, Strax P, et al: Periodic Screening for Breast Cancer: The Health Insurance Plan Project and its Sequelae, 1963–1986. Baltimore, Johns Hopkins University Press, 1988
124. Simpson JF, Page DL: Prognostic value of histopathology in the breast: Semin Oncol 19:254, 1992
125. Staren ED: Ultrasound-guided biopsy of nonpalpable breast masses by surgeons. Ann Surg Oncol 3:476, 1996
126. Staren ED, Sabel MS, Gianakakis LM, et al: Cryosurgery of breast cancer. Arch Surg 132:28, 1997
127. Sterns EE: Changing emphasis in breast diagnosis: The surgeon's role in evaluating mammographic abnormalities. J Am Coll Surg 184:297, 1997
128. Tabar L: Control of breast cancer through screening mammography. Radiology 174:655, 1990
129. Tabar L, Farberg G, Chen HH, et al: Efficacy of breast cancer screening by age: New results from the Swedish two-county trial. Cancer 75:2507, 1995
130. Tocino I, Garcia BM, Carter D: Surgical biopsy findings in patients with atypical hyperplasia diagnosed by stereotaxic core needle biopsy. Ann Surg Oncol 3:483, 1996
131. Tomlinson J, Harvey J, Sterrett G: An audit of 267 consecutively excised mammographically detected breast lesions 1989–1993. Pathology 29:21, 1997
132. Velanovich V, Lewis FR, Nathanson SD: Comparison of mammographically guided breast biopsy techniques. Ann Surg 229:625, 1999
133. Veronesi U, Paganelli G, Galimberti V, et al: Sentinel-node biopsy to avoid axillary dissection in breast cancer with clinically negative lymph nodes. Lancet 349:1864, 1997
134. Wilkinson EJ, Masood S: Cytologic needle samplings of the breast: Techniques and end results. In Bland K, Copeland E III (eds): The Breast: Comprehensive Management of Benign and Malignant Disease. Philadelphia, WB Saunders, 1998, p 705
135. Yim JH, Barton P, Weber B, et al: Mammographically detected breast cancer: Benefits of stereotactic core versus wire localization. Ann Surg 223:688, 1996
136. Won B, Reynolds HE, Lazaridis CL, et al: Stereotactic biopsy of ductal carcinoma in situ of the breast using an 11-gauge vacuum-assisted device: Persistent underestimation of disease. AJR Am J Roentgenol 173:227, 1999
137. Youngsen BJ, Liberman L, Rosen PP: Displacement of carcinomatous epithelium in surgical breast specimens following stereotaxic core biopsy. Am J Clin Pathol 103:598, 1995
138. Zidan A, Christie-Brown JS, Preston D, et al: Oestrogen and progesterone receptor assessment in core biopsy specimens of breast carcinoma. J Clin Pathol 50:27, 1997

Address reprint requests to

Barbara S. Schwartzberg, MD
4500 East Ninth Avenue
Suite 710-S
Denver, CO 80220

MINIMALLY INVASIVE PARATHYROID SURGERY

James R. Howe, MD

Only a decade ago, it was anathema to most parathyroid surgeons not to perform bilateral exploration to evaluate all glands in each patient. Many things have changed in surgery during this time, however, and especially striking has been the trend toward less invasive procedures. In parathyroid surgery, several developments have allowed for a change in the traditional paradigm. One of these has been the advent of a more reliable preoperative imaging technique, sestamibi scanning. Another was the development of an intraoperative assay to confirm normalization of parathyroid hormone (PTH) after the removal of parathyroid glands. Others have used a hand-held gamma probe to help to localize the abnormal parathyroid glands, and some have applied videoendoscopic techniques to neck exploration. These factors have made more surgeons comfortable with unilateral exploration in most patients with primary hyperparathyroidism (HPT), which has allowed for smaller incisions, shorter operative times, and the use of monitored sedation instead of general anesthesia. The goal of this article is to review how each of these areas has evolved to bring about the current changes in the approach of many endocrine surgeons to the treatment of primary HPT.

RATIONALE FOR BILATERAL EXPLORATION

The success rate of experienced endocrine surgeons at curing primary HPT should exceed 95%.[29, 67] Most surgeons have advocated routine bilateral exploration and identification of all glands, although for some time, others have not endorsed this view, most notably Tibblin et al[60] and Wang.[65] The reason to perform bilateral exploration in all patients is that a subset of patients has multiglandular disease (MGD) caused by four-gland hyperplasia or multiple adenomas, which could be missed if not all glands are visualized. Surgeons

From the Department of Surgery, University of Iowa Health Care, Iowa City, Iowa cannot expect to be helped by pathologists intraoperatively to determine who has hyperplasia versus multiple adenomas. The roles of pathologists are only to confirm that the sample removed is parathyroid tissue and to report its weight to surgeons, which typically is the most useful piece of information in determining whether the gland is pathologically enlarged. Wang[64] found that the average weight of 645 normal parathyroid glands from 160 cadavers was 35 mg to 40 mg, with the largest being 78 mg.

Because most patients with primary HPT have single adenomas, at what point is it no longer justified to dissect both sides of the neck in all patients, exposing them to higher risk for recurrent laryngeal nerve injury, postoperative hypocalcemia, injury to normal parathyroid glands, and permanently altering the normal tissue planes in the central neck? The answer to this question has been almost a religious issue for many parathyroid surgeons, and individual surgeons must arrive at their own answer based on the available data. The incidence of MGD has varied widely in studies examining it, from as low as 7% in some series[1] to as high as 30%[53] in others (Table 1). No one would disagree that patients with hyperplasia should have bilateral exploration, so patients with multiple endocrine neoplasia (MEN) type 1 or 2A, familial HPT, and secondary HPT should not be considered as candidates for unilateral exploration. Therefore, the most important issue in this decision for parathyroid surgeons is the prevalence of multiple adenomas because, regardless of surgeons' enthusiasm for unilateral exploration, when two enlarged or normal glands are found on one side of the neck, surgeons are obligated to explore the contralateral side. The question then is, if one enlarged gland is removed from one side, then what is the risk for failure to cure HPT caused by a residual parathyroid adenoma?

This is not a simple question, for some would argue that double adenomas do not exist and that rather they are just another form of hyperplasia. This idea was proposed by Wang and Rieder,[66] who found no cases of double adenoma in 73 explorations for HPT. Part of the controversy comes from the fact that no good test exists to differentiate whether a gland is hyperplastic, adenomatous, or even normal, other than its weight. Harrison et al[24] reported that none of 16 patients diagnosed with adenomas and microscopic hyperplasia of the suppressed glands by a pathologist had recurred in 4 to 8 years of follow-up, suggesting that microscopic hyperplasia may not be clinically significant. Despite Wang's claims, most investigators agree that double adenomas exist but that their frequency in different series has varied considerably. Wells et al[70] found

Table 1. INCIDENCE OF HYPERPLASIA, SOLITARY, DOUBLE, AND TRIPLE ADENOMAS IN VARIOUS SERIES

Study	No. Patients	Solitary (%)	Double (%)	Triple (%)	Hyperplasia (%)
Wang[66]	73	90.4	0	—	8.2
Harness[23]	300	—	1.7	—	—
Bruining[5]	615	70.4	17.2	7.0	5.4
Verdonk[62]	1962	—	1.9	—	—
Russell[51]	500	78.0	3.2	—	14.8
Wells[70]	375	—	9.0	13.6	—
Attie[1]*	865	91.9	3.4	0.3	2.3
Tezelman[58]*	416	—	9.4	13.9	—
Denham[15]	6331	87	3.0	—	9

*May have been included in meta-analysis of Denham.[15]

that 9% of 375 patients who underwent surgery for primary HPT had double adenomas and that 14% had three adenomas; however, in this study, adenomas were defined as weighing more than 50 mg, and even though all enlarged glands were excised and normal glands sampled for biopsy at exploration, the high prevalence of triple adenomas and the extensive experience of the author with familial causes of HPT suggest that many of these cases could have represented hyperplasia. Tezelman et al[58] reviewed 416 patients presenting to University of California at San Francisco for primary HPT between 1982 and 1992 and found the prevalence of double adenoma to be 9% and that of hyperplasia, 14%. They defined adenomas as weighing more than 65 mg, measuring more than 7 mm in diameter, dark in color, and firmer than normal glands. In 865 patients on whom Attie et al[1] performed surgery for the treatment of primary HPT, 795 (92%) had solitary adenomas, 41 (5%) had multiple adenomas (29 patients with double adenomas, 4 with triple adenomas, and 8 lost to follow-up), 20 (2%) had hyperplasia, and 9 (1%) had carcinoma. In five patients with multiple adenomas, second adenomas developed 3 to 18 years after initial surgery (which had resulted in normocalcemia). Bruining et al[5] found solitary adenomas in 433 of 615 (70%) patients with primary HPT, double adenomas in 106 (17%), three enlarged glands in 43 (7%), and hyperplasia in 33 (5%). This group only removed grossly enlarged glands (> 50 mg). Russell and Edis[51] found that 380 of 500 (78%) patients who underwent surgery for the treatment of primary HPT had solitary adenomas; 16 (3%), double adenomas; 74 (15%), hyperplasia (defined as three or more enlarged glands); 2 (0.4%), carcinoma; and 27 (5%), normal glands. Verdonk and Edis[62] examined the records of 1962 patients who underwent surgery for the treatment of HPT at the Mayo Clinic and found 38 (2%) patients meeting the criteria for double adenomas: two enlarged glands with histologic evidence of hyperplasia, each weighing more than 70 mg, and identification of two normal-appearing glands. These criteria probably underestimated the prevalence of double adenomas, similar to Harness et al,[23] who found a 2% prevalence of double adenomas in 5 of 300 cases at the University of Michigan. Denham and Norman[15] performed a meta-analysis of 6331 patients with primary HPT (excluding familial cases) reported in the literature between 1987 and 1997 and found that 87% had single adenomas; 9%, four-gland hyperplasia; 3%, multiple adenomas; and less than 1%, cancer. Based on these larger studies, the prevalence of multiple adenomas seems to be 2% to 4%, so unilateral exploration with identification of both glands misses approximately 2% of cases (assuming all represented double adenomas, with a frequency of 3% and an equal risk [1%] for being ipsilateral or contralateral superior or inferior glands). The question surgeons face now is whether all patients with primary HPT should have bilateral exploration so that 2% do not have missed adenomas. Also, could the number of failed explorations be reduced by preoperative imaging studies?

STUDIES OF UNILATERAL EXPLORATION

When the best noninvasive parathyroid imaging tests had sensitivities of 60% to 70%, the call for bilateral exploration by most endocrine surgeons made good sense. It is hard to argue with the often-quoted success rate of 95% for bilateral exploration by an experienced endocrine surgeon, which is much higher than the success rates for most surgical diseases. Even before good preoperative imaging studies were available, however, several surgeons stepped forward and suggested that patients would benefit from unilateral exploration in terms of shorter operative time, reduced scarring, decreased morbidity, and an acceptably low risk for persistent or recurrent HPT (Table 2).

Roth et al[50] advocated unilateral exploration in 1975, recommending that the side to be explored be chosen based on palpation, esophagram, venography, or angiography. If an enlarged and normal gland were found on the initial side, then contralateral exploration was not carried out. After removal of the adenoma, a 0.1-cm to 0.2-cm biopsy specimen of the normal-appearing parathyroid gland was obtained. The danger of this technique would be cases of double adenoma, and the inability to diagnose hyperplasia based on such a small biopsy sample. The investigators recommended that intraoperative staining with Sudan black be performed by an experienced pathologist, which would show little staining in adenomas and hyperplasia and increased staining in suppressed normal glands caused by intracellular lipids. In cases in which two normal glands or two enlarged glands were present on the first side explored, the other side was explored. Of 108 patients explored in this fashion and thought to have adenoma, only two failed (had persistent hyperparathyroidism) after unilateral exploration and were later found to have hyperplasia.[65] Wang[68] believed that routine bilateral exploration for HPT would increase the risk, cost, and morbidity of the surgical treatment of HPT.

Tibblin et al[60] were the next group to recommend that solitary parathyroid adenomas be treated by unilateral parathyroidectomy in 1984, which they defined as removal of the adenoma and normal gland from one side. This technique depended on the complete removal of an entire macroscopically normal-appearing gland, which was stained intraoperatively with oil-red-O to rule out hyperplasia. Like Sudan black, oil-red-O stains fat, which is present intracellularly in normal chief cells but not in hyperfunctional ones. Because foci of nodular hyperplasia may be present within otherwise normal-appearing glands, the investigators believed that removal of an entire gland was essential to rule out hyperplasia. They studied 102 consecutive patients between 1977 and 1982, and no routine localization procedures were used. Forty-three patients (42%) were able to have unilateral parathyroidectomy on the first side explored, forty-five (44%) had unilateral parathyroidectomy but bilateral exploration, and 14 (14%) had atypical procedures performed. Those having unilateral exploration had a lower prevalence of postoperative hypocalcemia, and no patients in the series developed hypercalcemia with a minimum of 1 year of follow-up. A high prevalence of supernumerary glands was found (7%), which the investigators

Table 2. RESULTS OF UNILATERAL EXPLORATION FOR HYPERPARATHYROIDISM (PRE-99MTc SESTAMIBI ERA)

Study	No. Patients	Imaging	Unilateral Exploration (%)	Operative Time (min)	Cure Rate (%)
Tibblin[60]	102	None	43	—	100
Worsey[71]	371	None	34	69 Unilateral 92 Bilateral	99 Unilateral 93 Bilateral
Lucas[31]	36	US	53	65 Unilateral 84 Bilateral	—
Russell[52]	90	Tl/Tc	53	71 Unilateral 97 Bilateral	100
Robertson[49]	89	Tl/Tc or US	64	65 Unilateral 113 Bilateral	94

US = ultrasonography; Tl/Tc = thallium-201/technetium-99m.

believed was caused by the more meticulous dissection performed in these patients. They advocated unilateral parathyroidectomy with intraoperative oil-red-O staining as the procedure of choice for primary HPT caused by single adenoma and stated that they saw no cases of double adenoma using this technique in 250 patients. They believed the incidence of double adenoma to be less than 1% and that, if such a gland were missed on the unexplored side, then the difficulty of re-exploration on that side would be similar to that of the primary exploration.

Worsey et al[71] reported their results with 371 patients with sporadic primary HPT who underwent surgery between 1977 and 1992, in whom no preoperative imaging studies were routinely obtained.[71] Unilateral exploration was possible only in 125 (33.6%) patients, and the success rate of unilateral exploration was 99.2% versus 93.1% for bilateral exploration. The mean operative time was 69.4 minutes for unilateral exploration (range, 40–185 min), which was significantly shorter than the 91.8 minutes for bilateral exploration (range, 50–170 min; $P <$ 0.001). The investigators declared that selective unilateral exploration for primary HPT was safe and successful, even during this era of poor preoperative localization studies, as long as an approach of finding one normal and one enlarged gland was adopted.

The problem with the techniques as described earlier was that the choice of which side to explore initially was essentially random, which meant that more than half of patients would not receive unilateral exploration. The next wave was to attempt to guide unilateral exploration by preoperative imaging. Lucas et al[31] reviewed their experience with 75 patients who underwent surgery between 1979 and 1988. All patients who underwent surgery before 1985 had bilateral exploration ($n = 39$; group 1), whereas a selective approach based on the results of sonography was used for the 36 patients who underwent surgery between 1985 and 1988 (group 2). In group 1, 35 patients had adenomas and underwent biopsy of one or two normal glands, whereas 4 patients had hyperplasia and 3.5 glands underwent resection. Ten patients had transient hypocalcemia, none had permanent hypocalcemia or nerve injuries, and one had persistent hypercalcemia. In group 2, 32 patients had single adenomas, 1 had a double adenoma, and 3 had hyperplasia. Nineteen patients (53%) had unilateral exploration carried out because sonography demonstrated a probable adenoma in which the abnormal gland was removed and the normal gland was sampled for biopsy. The other 17 patients had bilateral exploration. In three patients, transient hypocalcemia developed (two from bilateral exploration), and two patients had temporary recurrent nerve paresis (both of whom had bilateral exploration). The mean operative time for those with unilateral exploration was 65.1 minutes (range, 45–95 min) and for bilateral exploration was 84.1 minutes (range, 50–165 min). None of the 19 patients having unilateral exploration had persistent hypercalcemia. On the basis of this experience, the investigators changed their approach to unilateral exploration for cases of adenoma diagnosed by sonography, with biopsy of the normal gland on the side of the adenoma to rule out hyperplasia.

Russell et al[52] used a similar approach based on thallium-201/technetium-99m (^{201}Tl/^{99m}Tc) subtraction scans on 90 consecutive patients with HPT between 1985 and 1988, none of whom had been previously explored. Bilateral exploration was carried out if the scan was nonlocalizing, more than one area of increased uptake was present, two enlarged glands were encountered on the same side, or the patient was thought to have familial HPT or multiple endocrine neoplasia. Unilateral exploration was performed in 48 patients, all of whom had adenomas, and the ipsilateral gland was identified in 85% of these cases. Of these patients, the scans correctly identified the location of the gland in 31;

lateralized the gland in 12; and in 5, the scan was negative but the gland was found on the first side explored (and the ipsilateral gland was normal). All patients had resolution of their hypercalcemia postoperatively, with no recurrences at a mean follow-up of 16.8 months. In the bilateral exploration group, 19 patients had negative scans, 14 had increased uptake on the wrong side of the neck. In 8 patients, the scans were correct, but bilateral exploration was carried out anyway, and 1 patient was suspected of having familial HPT. In the bilateral exploration group, adenomas were found in 33 patients, hyperplasia in 3, and the glands seemed normal in 6. Hypercalcemia resolved in 36 of 42 patients after bilateral explorations. They demonstrated a reduced mean operative time for patients having unilateral exploration (71 min for unilateral versus 97 min for bilateral; $P < 0.001$), without a higher risk for recurrent or persistent hypercalcemia, but still only 53% of patients had unilateral exploration. Similar results were reported in the study by Robertson et al,[49] in which 57 of 89 patients (64%) had unilateral exploration with a mean operative time of 65 minutes versus 113 minutes for bilateral exploration ($P = 0.081$). Recurrent hypercalcemia was seen in 3.5% of patients explored unilaterally (2 of 57 versus 3 of 42 for bilateral). Vogel et al[63] found that 46 of 77 patients (60%) having preoperative sonography could be explored unilaterally, with a mean operative time of 77 minutes compared with 98 to 106 minutes for bilateral exploration. The prevalence of postoperative hypocalcemia was decreased significantly in the unilateral group (22% versus 45% for bilateral; $P = 0.028$).

Tibblin et al[59] attempted to determine whether the results of unilateral exploration for solitary adenomas were acceptable by comparing the results obtained from five centers of expertise in parathyroid surgery in Europe and the United States. With a minimum of 5 years of follow-up, 96% of patients having unilateral exploration ($n = 50$) were normocalcemic at follow-up, 2% were hypercalcemic, and 2% were hypocalcemic. In the bilateral exploration group ($n = 222$), 89% of patients were normocalcemic, 5% were hypercalcemic, and 6% were hypocalcemic. The investigators concluded that unilateral exploration for solitary adenoma did not result in a higher level of persistent or recurrent hypercalcemia. Tibblin et al[61] also surveyed the approach to solitary adenoma used in 53 surgical departments from 14 nations in 1987. Only nine centers (17%) advocated unilateral exploration, and this approach was not favored by any of the 19 departments from North America. The most common procedure routinely performed was bilateral exploration with incisional biopsy of one or two normal glands (31%), followed by bilateral exploration and no biopsy of normal glands (21%), then bilateral exploration and biopsy of three normal glands (17%).

Duh et al[17] used a mathematic model to determine the risk for missing parathyroid tumors by adopting a unilateral approach at exploration, defined as the intent to perform unilateral exploration that could be modified based on the intraoperative findings. The prevalence of double adenoma was the primary determinant of the risk for leaving an adenoma on the unexplored side. With a preoperative imaging test with 90% sensitivity, and assuming a 14% prevalence of hyperplasia, 4% double adenoma, 1% triple adenoma, and 1% carcinoma, they calculated that 69% of patients would be able to undergo unilateral exploration, with a 1% risk for missing an adenoma on the unexplored side.

To summarize these studies, by the early 1990s, groups with an interest in unilateral exploration had shown that it could be performed with an acceptably low rate of recurrent or persistent HPT but that it was still not favored by most parathyroid surgeons. Although the biggest concern with using this approach has been the possibility of missing multiple adenomas and consequent persistent disease, this has not translated into higher rates of postoperative hypercalcemia in patients having unilateral exploration. The problem with unilateral exploration has been that 30% to 50% of eligible patients have bilateral exploration, even after preoperative localization studies, so the adoption of unilateral exploration by many surgeons would depend on improvements in parathyroid imaging.

SESTAMIBI SCANNING

In 1989, Coakley et al[13] reported that a new agent used for cardiac imaging, 99mTc sestamibi (MIBI), was avidly taken up by parathyroid tissue. O'Doherty et al[45] examined the utility of this isotope in patients with HPT by comparing preoperative 123I subtraction from 201Tl with subtraction from MIBI. Forty patients had adenomas at exploration, and 15 had hyperplasia (8 caused by secondary HPT). The abnormal glands were correctly localized by MIBI in 39 of 40 patients with adenomas (98%), versus 37 (93%) for thallium imaging. A false-negative MIBI scan occurred in a patient with a 2-g adenoma at the right lower aspect of the thyroid. In the patients with hyperplasia, 32 of 60 glands were seen by MIBI, and the investigators stated that the sensitivity of MIBI in hyperplasia was 55% versus 48% for 201Tl. This article also examined the uptake of these radioisotopes in parathyroid and thyroid tissue. 201Tl and MIBI were given to 13 patients with adenomas and 7 patients with hyperplasia in the surgical suite before the parathyroid glands were removed, and samples of parathyroid and thyroid tissue were saved for analysis from each patient. The uptake of thallium was greater than that of MIBI in parathyroid adenomas, hyperplastic glands, and thyroid tissue, but the ratio per gram of parathyroid versus thyroid tissue was higher for MIBI. Uptake of radioisotopes increased with the weight of the parathyroid glands, and the smallest gland found by imaging in this series was 194 mg. They calculated that the difference in MIBI activity between parathyroid and thyroid tissue was greatest at 15 to 28 minutes after administration, and that the dose of radiation to patients was approximately 10-fold less using MIBI than 201Tl. The investigators concluded that MIBI was superior to thallium for imaging of parathyroid tissue. The mechanism of increased uptake of MIBI in parathyroid and cardiac tissues has been postulated to be caused by increased numbers of mitochondria, where MIBI seems to be concentrated in animal studies.[46]

Taillifer et al[56] performed preoperative MIBI scanning in 23 patients with HPT (8 also underwent technetium or thallium scanning), 21 patients with adenomas found at surgery and 2 patients with hyperplasia. Nineteen adenomas were accurately localized by the MIBI scan and ranged in weight from 0.15 g to 8.0 g (mean, 1.6 g). One patient's MIBI scan showed increased uptake in the right lower neck, but a 175-mg adenoma was found in the right upper neck. Another patient had two areas of increased uptake; the less intense area proved to be a 400-mg adenoma, whereas the higher region of uptake was a 2 cm × 1.5 cm follicular adenoma of the thyroid. Of the two patients with hyperplasia, both scans were interpreted as normal. This study revealed two of the deficiencies of MIBI imaging, increased uptake in thyroid adenomas, and poor uptake in cases of hyperplasia.

Wei et al[68] evaluated 30 patients (23 with primary HPT, 3 with secondary HPT, and 4 with tertiary HPT) by MIBI/99mTc pertechnetate subtraction. Solitary adenomas were found at surgery in 13 patients and were found by imaging in 12 patients, with a mean weight of 960 mg (range, 0.2–3.0 g). The one adenoma not seen on MIBI weighed 0.2 g and was nonectopic. Ten patients with primary

HPT had hyperplasia, one of whom had glands removed previously, with the residual gland seen on MIBI scanning and successfully removed. The nine other patients had subtotal parathyroidectomy, with three having no glands seen on scan and the other six with bilateral uptake consistent with hyperplasia. In seven patients with secondary or tertiary HPT, five had bilateral uptake, and two had undergone surgery previously and the residual abnormal glands were identified by MIBI scanning. The investigators believed that MIBI and ^{99m}Tc subtraction scanning was faster and easier than was subtraction with ^{123}I, with similar results.[10] They also demonstrated that MIBI imaging might be more valuable than suggested by Taillifer et al[56] for identifying hyperplasia.

Geatti et al[21] performed MIBI/^{99m}Tc subtraction, ^{201}Tl/^{99m}Tc subtraction, sonography, and CT on 42 patients who subsequently underwent surgery for HPT. The sensitivity was highest for MIBI/^{99m}Tc subtraction (95%), followed by ^{201}Tl/^{99m}Tc subtraction (86%), CT (83%), and sonography (81%). Thirty-eight patients (90.5%) had solitary adenomas, one patient had two adenomas, and one patient had three adenomas, which were all seen on the MIBI scans. One false-negative study occurred in a patient with a cystic parathyroid gland. The images from the MIBI scans more clearly defined the adenomas than the ^{201}Tl/^{99m}Tc scans, with a 10-fold to 20-fold decrease in the radiation dose to patients. The investigators concluded that MIBI was the tracer of choice for parathyroid scintigraphy.

Hindie et al[25] prospectively studied 30 patients with HPT by MIBI/^{123}I subtraction, all of whom had sonography and 14 of whom had ^{201}Tl/^{99m}Tc subtraction scanning performed previously. Twenty-seven patients were found to have adenomas at surgery (range, 0.125–6.54 g), and 26 adenomas were detected by MIBI imaging. Two mediastinal glands were identified, and the one adenoma not found on MIBI weighed 126 mg. Three patients had parathyroid hyperplasia, two in whom MIBI demonstrated two areas of increased uptake, and one in whom one area of increased uptake was found. Ten patients had nodular thyroids, and in seven patients, the nodules had increased uptake of MIBI. [123]I subtraction helped in these cases, in which two nodules were determined to be functional; four were cold nodules; and in one, the thyroid nodule was misinterpreted as being a parathyroid. The investigators concluded that MIBI was better than was sonography or ^{201}Tl scanning.

Borley et al[4] reported their results of preoperative MIBI/^{123}I subtraction scanning in 48 patients, of whom 8 had secondary HPT. Of 36 patients found to have solitary adenomas at exploration, 35 had preoperative MIBI scans that correctly identified the abnormal parathyroid, whereas the other patient had two foci of uptake found to be a parathyroid adenoma on one side and a thyroid adenoma on the other at exploration. One scan in a patient with secondary HPT was inconclusive, but the patient had four-gland hyperplasia, and a patient with a normal MIBI scan who underwent exploration was found to have four normal glands. Ten patients had more than one gland seen on scan and found at surgery. The investigators concluded that this imaging modality was sufficiently reliable that unilateral exploration could be performed on patients predicted to have adenomas on the basis of the preoperative scan.

McHenry et al[35] prospectively studied dual-phase MIBI scanning (imaging at 10–15 min and 2–4 h after MIBI administration) with or without single photon emission CT (SPECT) or ^{123}I subtraction in 124 patients with HPT (118 primary, 4 secondary, 2 tertiary), 14 of whom had undergone previous exploration. At surgery, single adenomas were found in 95 patients, and double adenomas in 5; hyperplasia in 14; carcinoma in 1; and no abnormality in 9. In patients with single adenomas, 70 of 95 (74%) were detected by MIBI, whereas only 6 of 14 (43%) patients with hyperplasia and 1 of 5 (20%) with double adenomas had accurate preoperative imaging. Eight of 9 patients with no abnormality had false-positive MIBI scans, with tracer uptake in areas where no abnormal parathyroid tissue was found. Of 124 patients, 17 had false-positive scans, all of which showed uptake in the neck. In 6 patients with a single adenoma, the false-positive results were caused by thyroid disease in 5 and an enlarged lymph node in 1; however, 29 patients had nodular thyroid glands. Four of six ectopic mediastinal glands were identified by MIBI scanning. The investigators concluded that the low sensitivity of the MIBI scan in patients with MGD would preclude unilateral exploration in HPT.

Light et al[30] prospectively compared dual-phase MIBI without thyroid subtraction with high-resolution sonography in 16 patients with primary HPT, 4 with secondary HPT, and 1 with tertiary HPT. MIBI scanning was superior to sonography in parathyroid adenoma, with a sensitivity of 87% versus 57%, respectively. The smallest gland imaged by MIBI was 150 mg. In 6 patients with parathyroid hyperplasia, MIBI detected 11 of 25 (44%) glands, and 2 or more abnormal glands were seen in 5 patients (versus 24% of glands detected by sonography in 3 of 6 patients). MIBI successfully localized a mediastinal adenoma. The investigators concluded that dual-phase scanning is more sensitive than is sonography for HPT, that thyroid subtraction is unnecessary, and that MIBI and sonography are not good localization procedures for parathyroid hyperplasia.

Malhotra et al[32] retrospectively reviewed their experience with preoperative MIBI imaging in 32 patients with primary and 12 patients with secondary HPT. All 26 patients found to have single adenomas had been identified by MIBI scanning, but in two cases, additional faint areas of uptake were seen by MIBI that were not found to be parathyroids at surgery (i.e., false-positives). The smallest adenoma found was 80 mg, and the average weight was 2.42 g (range, 0.8–15.0 g). Ten of 18 patients with hyperplasia had scans positive for MGD, from whom 36 of 69 (52%) glands were removed at surgery and were seen on MIBI. In the patients with hyperplasia, 3 patients had no parathyroids seen on MIBI; 5 had one gland; 4 had two (bilateral); 1 had three; and in 5 patients, all 4 glands were seen. Reporting of sensitivity can be misleading in cases of parathyroid hyperplasia. To be clinically useful, the MIBI scan should demonstrate at least two foci of increased uptake, and although this could represent a double adenoma, hyperplasia would be more likely, and the surgeon would be compelled to identify all four glands. Using this as the definition, Malholtra et al[32] found the sensitivity of MIBI to be 56% in hyperplasia. They also examined seven patients undergoing reoperative parathyroid surgery, and the scan correctly identified the location of abnormal parathyroid glands in five, of which three were ectopic (two mediastinal, one carotid sheath). False-positive results were obtained in the other two patients. The investigators concluded that MIBI scanning was superior to other noninvasive procedures, equivalent to the combination of angiography and selective venous catheterization, and recommended its use in all patients before exploration for hyperparathyroidism.

Martin et al[33] reviewed their experience with 63 patients having dual-phase MIBI scanning preceding parathyroidectomy, of whom 50 patients had adenomas found at surgery, 11 had hyperplasia, and 2 had normal parathyroids. Forty-one of 50 patients with adenomas had accurate localization, with two false-positive results. In hyperplasia, 9 of 11 patients had positive scans, but only 9 of 29 glands were identified, so few cases would have met the more stringent criteria of a scan positive for hyperplasia as discussed earlier. The investigators believed that the results that they obtained in patients with hyperplasia justified bilateral exploration in all patients.

Table 3. RESULTS OF ^{99m}Tc SESTAMIBI SCANNING IN PATIENTS WITH HYPERPARATHYROIDISM

Study	Adenoma		Hyperplasia	
	Accurate Localization	Sensitivity (%)	Negative or Diffuse Uptake	Sensitivity (%)
O'Doherty[45]	39/40	97.5	8/15	55.0
Taillifer[56]	19/21	90.5	0/2	0
Casas[10]	15/17	88.2	5/5	100.0
Wei[68]	12/13	92.3	6/9	66.7
Geatti[21]	40/42	95.2	—	—
Hindie[25]	26/27	96.3	2/3	66.7
Borley[4]	35/36	97.2	10/11	90.9
McHenry[35]	70/95	73.7	6/14	42.9
Light[30]	13/15	86.7	5/6	83.3
Malhotra[32]	26/26	100.0	10/18	55.5
Martin[33]	41/50	82.0	9/11	81.8
Carter[8]	11/13	84.6	0/3	0

Carter et al[8] performed MIBI imaging of 16 patients with primary HPT, 13 whom were found to have adenomas and 3 of whom had parathyroid hyperplasia. Ten patients had single adenomas identified by MIBI scanning, as did 1 patient with a double adenoma. One patient had multiple sites of uptake in the neck and a mediastinal gland (seen on retrospective review). One patient had increased uptake consistent with adenoma, but this was not found at surgery. The latter two patients also had nodular thyroid glands at exploration. All three patients with parathyroid hyperplasia had negative scans, and the investigators believed that a negative scan was a strong predictor of MGD, which was helpful for preoperative education and planning of the procedures. The investigators also thought that preoperative MIBI scanning would be helpful to inexperienced parathyroid surgeons.

These studies are summarized in Table 3 and demonstrate sensitivity rates of 80% to 100% for parathyroid adenomas and 0% to 100% for hyperplasia. One interpretation of these results is that, if the scan shows a single focus of uptake, then unilateral exploration is likely to be successful, whereas if no areas or multiple areas of increased uptake are seen, then one should plan on bilateral exploration. In a meta-analysis of 784 patients having preoperative sestamibi scans prior to exploration for primary HPT, Denham and Norman[15] calculated the sensitivity of MIBI to be 91% and the specificity, 99%. They found no significant difference between dual-phase versus subtraction techniques. They determined that MIBI scanning was cost-effective for all patients when it allowed for 51% of patients with solitary adenomas to have unilateral exploration. Scans were not recommended in patients with MEN, familial HPT, secondary HPT, or tertiary HPT because all of these patients warrant bilateral exploration.

UNILATERAL EXPLORATION AFTER SESTAMIBI IMAGING

Although MIBI has been available for parathyroid imaging for a decade, few reports of the results of unilateral exploration after using MIBI for preoperative imaging have been published (Table 4). Takami[57] reported on his experience with 33 patients treated between 1995 and 1996 who were thought to have

Table 4. STUDIES OF UNILATERAL EXPLORATION FOR HYPERPARATHYROIDISM AFTER ^{99m}Tc SESTAMIBI SCANNING

Study	No. Patients	MIBI Success	Surgical Success	OR Time (unilateral; min)	Cure Rate (%)
Takami[57]	33	33 (100%)	31* (94%)	41	100
Gupta[22]	35	21 (60%)	20 (95%)	49	—
Norman[42]	25	18 (72%)	18 (100%)	49	100 (6-mo follow-up)

*Two mediastinal adenomas.

a solitary adenoma by MIBI/^{99m}Tc subtraction. All patients also underwent sonography, and some underwent CT. Parathyroidectomy was successful by limited neck dissection in all but two patients, who were found to have mediastinal adenomas. The mean operative time for these 31 patients was 41 minutes, and with limited follow-up, the cure rate was 100%.

Gupta et al[22] performed preoperative, dual-phase MIBI scanning on 35 consecutive patients and found that 21 patients had a solitary focus of increased uptake, whereas 14 did not localize with MIBI. Those with localization had unilateral exploration performed (with removal of the adenoma and biopsy of the normal gland), whereas those who did not had bilateral exploration. Of the 21 patients having unilateral exploration, in 1, surgery was converted to bilateral exploration because an adenoma was not found on that side. Twenty patients had accurate localization and were normocalcemic at follow-up. In 14 patients having planned bilateral exploration, 9 were found to have adenomas not seen on the scans, 1 had bilateral adenomas, 3 had hyperplasia, and 1 had four normal glands. The mean operative time for unilateral exploration was 49 minutes ($\pm$ 21 min) versus 103 minutes ($\pm$ 45 min) for bilateral exploration, and the sensitivity of MIBI scanning was calculated to be 70%. The investigators believed that patients likely to benefit from unilateral exploration reasonably could be selected based on preoperative MIBI scanning, which would result in shorter operative time, less risk for nerve injury and hypoparathyroidism, and leaving one side of the neck undisturbed.

In 25 patients who underwent MIBI imaging, Norman et al[42] performed MIBI-directed unilateral explorations in 18 consecutive patients in whom a solitary adenoma was suggested by the scanning. They found adenomas on the correct side in all patients, and all were normocalcemic with at least 6 months of follow-up. Compared with 25 patients who had bilateral exploration performed at the same institution, the investigators found a significantly reduced operative time (49 min versus 127 min; $P < 0.001$), incision length (3.0 cm versus 9.6 cm; $P < 0.001$), and hospital stay (15.2 versus 29.6 h; $P < 0.01$). They believed that the key to this procedure was a high-quality scan, such as that obtained using SPECT, and that the quality of scans seen from different institutions was highly variable.

One study that concluded no benefit exists to preoperative MIBI scanning was that of Shen et al.[53] They retrospectively reviewed their experience with 40 patients who had MIBI scanning (29 at outside institutions) before bilateral exploration for primary HPT at the University of California at San Francisco. They found that 27 patients would have had unilateral and 13 bilateral explorations based on the scans and intraoperative findings, and that 4 (10%) would have failed because of missing a second adenoma on the contralateral side. They did not believe that the benefit of more patients having unilateral exploration justified the expense ($800 per patient) of imaging everybody, but interestingly, they performed preoperative ultrasound in all of these patients. The problems with this study were that the sensitivity of MIBI was approximately 20% less than in most other reports, most scans were performed at outside hospitals, the rate of MGD (30%) was higher than in most series, and the investigators' preference for bilateral exploration is well known.

Some of the benefits of MIBI-directed unilateral exploration were calculated by Denham and Norman,[15] who reviewed the average operative times in 15 studies reporting bilateral exploration for primary HPT and determined the mean to be 109.3 minutes (range, 87–180 min). In three studies using MIBI-directed unilateral exploration, the mean was 1 hour less (mean, 49 min). They determined the cost of standard bilateral exploration to be $1773 versus $1123 (including MIBI scan) for unilateral exploration with the patient under outpatient local anesthesia.

INTRAOPERATIVE PARATHYROID HORMONE ASSAY

The studies mentioned earlier show that, despite the enthusiasm of some groups for using MIBI scanning to direct unilateral localization, many patients still require bilateral exploration. If an intraoperative method existed to accurately predict that the HPT would be cured after removing a parathyroid gland(s), then additional patients might be spared bilateral exploration. The first attempt at this was the measurement of cyclic adenosine monophosphate (cAMP) in the urine as proposed in 1978 by Spiegel et al,[55] but this was impractical because it required a mean of 100 minutes after excision of an adenoma to see a measurable decrease. The development of a radioimmunoassay specific for intact PTH (iPTH) then allowed for modification of the standard 24-hour assay that could be performed intraoperatively. Nussbaum et al[44] studied 12 patients with HPT who had preoperative sonography, of whom 8 had unilateral exploration and 4 had bilateral exploration. These 12 patients had resection of an adenoma and biopsy of the ipsilateral gland, and PTH samples were drawn from the internal jugular vein before, 15 minutes after, and 30 minutes after ligation of the parathyroid blood supply. Plasma was incubated with beads coated with radiolabeled anti-PTH (1–34) and anti-PTH (39–84) at 37°C for 15 minutes, then washed, and the amount of radiolabeled antibody released was measured. PTH levels decreased rapidly after resection of the adenoma, and its plasma half-life was found to be less than 5 minutes. In all patients with an adenoma resected, the PTH level decreased to less than 40% of pre-excision values within 15 minutes. All patients remained normocalcemic within a 2-month follow-up interval. The investigators advocated the use of this assay to determine whether resection of an adenoma was successful at unilateral exploration or whether bilateral exploration should be carried out to look for hyperplasia or double adenoma.

Davies et al[14] attempted to further study the kinetics of PTH after resection of abnormal parathyroid glands. They measured PTH levels from a vein in the foot at numerous intervals before and after excision of the glands. They studied six patients with solitary adenomas—two with primary hyperplasia, one with double adenoma, and three with secondary HPT (one with a hyperfunctioning autograft). They used an immunochemiluminescence assay with antibodies to the (1–34) and (44–68) portions of the PTH molecule, with a 1-hour incubation time. They calculated the half-life of iPTH in those with solitary adenomas to be 3.3 minutes and, in three patients with MGD, 2.9, 3.0, and 7.1 minutes after subtotal parathyroidectomy. In patients with primary HPT, iPTH levels were at their lowest 1 to 3 hours after surgery and recovered to normal levels within 40 hours.

Chapuis et al[12] evaluated intraoperative measurement of iPTH in 45 patients between 1989 and 1991. All patients had preoperative sonography suggestive of a single adenoma, no multinodular goiter or history of familial HPT and agreed to exploration under local anesthesia. Patients were given 100 mg hydroxyzine orally 30 minutes before infiltration of the skin with 1% Xylocaine and then were explored through a 2.5-cm to 3.5-cm incision. At unilateral exploration, adenomas were removed and normal glands sampled by biopsy. Urinary cAMP was collected in 35 patients, and serum iPTH was measured in 25 patients before incision and at intervals 5 to 90 minutes after excision of the adenoma. Forty-two patients had unilateral exploration under local anesthesia. In 3 patients, persistent elevation of PTH level occurred, and 2 underwent immediate bilateral exploration under general anesthesia, of whom one had a subtotal resection of four-gland hyperplasia and the other had only three normal glands that were identified and remained hypercalcemic at follow-up. The third patient would not consent to contralateral exploration at the time, but was explored 6 months later, when a second adenoma was removed from the other side. iPTH values decreased into the normal range within 15 to 30 minutes after excision of the adenoma, and the assay required 45 to 60 minutes to complete. Urinary cAMP levels decreased to normal 60 to 90 minutes after removal of the adenoma and required 60-80 minutes to run the assay. All 42 patients with an appropriate decrease in PTH or cAMP level were normocalcemic at 2 to 24 months of follow-up, and the operative time ranged from 15 to 55 minutes. Conclusions drawn from the study were that unilateral exploration is feasible with the patient under local anesthesia and that normalization of cAMP or PTH was an excellent predictor of cure. Serum PTH levels decreased more quickly than did the urinary cAMP levels and did not necessitate a catheter, and the results were available more quickly.

These investigators[11] published a follow-up of this work in 1996, with a total of 200 patients undergoing unilateral exploration under local anesthesia. Of 175 patients with intraoperative iPTH measurement, 156 (89%) had a significant decrease in PTH levels, whereas 17 patients (10%) did not, and technical failure of the assay occurred in 2 patients. Thirteen of 17 patients without adequate decrease in iPTH levels had bilateral exploration, and 11 patients became normo-calcemic postoperatively. In 188 patients with adequate follow-up (minimum, 1–6 mo; 179 patients with unilateral exploration and 9 converted to bilateral), the rate of persistent HPT was 4% (8 patients) and recurrent HPT was 1% (2 patients).

Irvin et al[26] studied intraoperative PTH in 61 patients who underwent 63 explorations for HPT (51 with primary HPT, 4 with secondary HPT, 2 with MEN-1, 4 with familial hyperparathyroidism, and 2 with metastatic parathyroid carcinoma; 22% were reoperations). Blood was drawn from the ipsilateral jugular vein or a peripheral vein before neck incision, just before excision of parathy-roids, then at 10 minutes after excision. The assays were carried out in the surgical suite with a turnaround time of 8 to 12 minutes. If the levels did not decrease at 10 minutes, they were rechecked at 20 minutes. The serum samples also were assayed using the standard 24-hour incubation time for comparison purposes. Criteria for a positive test were determined from 27 patients with primary HPT who were rendered normocalcemic postoperatively. They deter-mined that a 54% decrease at 10 minutes after excision constituted a positive test. Several patients did not have an adequate decrease in iPTH until 20 to 30 minutes, and the investigators believed this was because of manipulation of the other glands after excision of the adenoma. Their 12-minute turnaround assay had a sensitivity of 96%, specificity of 100%, and positive predictive value of 97%. Three false-positive results were found, one in a patient with metastatic carcinoma, and in two with familial HPT, all of whom had recurrent or persistent disease despite an appropriate decrease in intraoperative PTH levels. Three other patients with familial HPT did not have a decrease in intraoperative PTH level, one with metastatic cancer who had residual disease, and another with a tracheostomy that mandated only a unilateral exploration, which was unsuccessful in the identification of an adenoma. The investigators concluded that their shortened assay correlated well with the standard assay and accurately predicted surgical success in 43 patients. They believed that this technique could allow for unilateral exploration, shorten operative times, and improve the success rate of parathyroidectomy.

PREOPERATIVE SESTAMIBI SCANNING AND INTRAOPERATIVE PARATHYROID HORMONE MEASUREMENT

The development of an intraoperative assay for iPTH seemed to be a major step forward in predicting whether HPT would be cured after removal of a single enlarged gland (studies summarized in Table 5). Sofferman et al[54] performed preoperative sonography and MIBI scanning in 80 patients with primary HPT and coupled this with intraoperative iPTH assays in 40 patients with primary and secondary HPT treated between 1995 and 1998. Five adenomas were ectopic, and 89% of scans were found to be accurate after exploration. In patients with intraoperative iPTH measurement, 31 had adenomas, 6 had secondary HPT, and 3 had hyperplasia. Samples were measured before excision and 15 minutes after excision, with 6 patients requiring an additional sample being studied because the serum iPTH level did not decrease to normal levels after excision of the gland(s). Three of these patients had adenomas, and the investigators believed that manipulation of the gland and measurement of the iPTH level too early were the reasons for the elevated postexcision level, which

Table 5. STUDIES OF INTRAOPERATIVE INTACT PARATHYROID HORMONE MEASUREMENT IN HPT

Study	No. Patients	Solitary MGD	Unilateral Expl./ Bilateral Expl.	Turnaround Time (min)	Cure Rate (%)
Nussbaum[44]	12	12/0	8/4	—	100 (2-mo follow-up)
Chapuis[11]	173*	—	160/13	—	94 (1–6-mo follow-up)
Irvin[26]	61†	—	—	8–12	90
Sofferman[54]	40‡	31/9	—	20	100
Carty[9]	67	58/9	42/25	10–14	99 (6-mo follow-up)
Irvin[27]	18	18/0	—	12	89

*Two patients with technical failure of assay removed.
†51 primary HPT, 4 secondary HPT, 2 MEN-1, 4 familial HPT, 2 carcinoma.
‡Had preoperative MIBI scans; five glands were ectopic.
§Had preoperative MIBI scans; two glands were ectopic and could not be removed through cervical incision.

decreased to normal on the second or third assay. Two of the other patients had secondary HPT, and the third had hyperplasia. All 40 patients eventually had significant decreases in their iPTH levels, 32 into the normal range, and all were eucalcemic at follow-up. Although unilateral exploration was planned in patients with unequivocal evidence of a solitary adenoma, the number of patients who had unilateral exploration performed was not given. The average turnaround time from sending the sample to receiving results was 20 minutes, and the cost per assay was $169. The investigators described modifying the use of the standard assay reagents provided by Nichols Diagnostics (San Juan Capistrano, CA), which usually costs $1000 per patient. They believed that the benefit of intraoperative PTH testing was not necessarily a decrease in the operative time, but rather being sure that they had cured the HPT at the end of surgery. With PTH sampling, no frozen sections were required, and by extending the reagents in the PTH assay kit, significant savings could be achieved.

Carty et al[9] compared two operative strategies in 128 patients, with method A being their standard unilateral exploration for patients presenting between 1993 and 1994 (61 patients; using the method as described earlier by Worsey et al[71]). Since 1995, method B was used (67 patients), which consisted of intraoperative iPTH measurement and preoperative SPECT MIBI imaging in half of the patients. The sensitivity of SPECT MIBI was 93% for adenomas and 61% for hyperplasia (80.9% overall in 34 patients). In the absence of a localizing scan, intraoperative palpation was carried out to determine the first side to be explored, and by default, the right side was explored first if no enlarged glands were palpated. The iPTH testing was performed pre-excision and at 15 minutes after excision of the parathyroid gland(s), with turnaround times of 10 to 14 minutes. In 63 of 67 patients (94%), the postexcision iPTH level decreased by more than 50% and into the normal range, and all 63 of the patients were normocalcemic with a minimum of 6 months of follow-up. Three patients underwent bilateral exploration for continued iPTH elevation, which normalized after excision of additional glands, while one patient had persistent hypercalcemia. Unilateral exploration was possible in 63% of patients in group B, versus 41% in group A. In both groups, 87% of patients had adenomas; 4%, double adenomas; and 9%, hyperplasia. This translated into a slightly shorter mean operative time (96 versus 108 minutes, $P = $ NS), length of stay (1.1 versus 1.9 d, $P \leq 0.01$), and cost ($3325 versus $3636, $P = $ NS). The investigators concluded that method B could be performed safely, cost-effectively, and with a higher rate of unilateral exploration than could method A.

Irvin et al[27] described 18 patients with primary HPT having intraoperative iPTH monitoring, all of whom had had preoperative dual-phase MIBI scans. All scans were considered positive, with two showing ectopic mediastinal glands. Patients underwent unilateral exploration under general anesthesia, with quick iPTH assays performed before tumor excision and 5, 10, and 20 minutes after excision. The turnaround time for the assay was 12 minutes, and a 50% decrease after excision was taken as predictive of postoperative normocalcemia. Normal glands were not sought out or sampled for biopsy after an adenoma had been removed. All 16 patients with MIBI localization to the neck had adenomas removed and were normocalcemic postoperatively. One patient had a scan suggesting a superior adenoma, but this was found in the ipsilateral, inferior position. Three patients did not have a 50% decrease in iPTH level, one of which was a false-negative with just a 36% decrease. Another had a 32% decrease after removal of tissue determined to be a lymph node, and later at exploration the adenoma was found, which resulted in a 63% decrease. One patient had a delayed decrease in PTH at 5 minutes after excision but had a 70% decrease at

10 minutes. The mean operative time was 36 minutes (range, 13–120 min). Cervical exploration was unsuccessful for removing the mediastinal parathyroid adenomas seen in two patients. The investigators concluded that their approach of preoperative MIBI scanning and intraoperative PTH was cost-effective through decreasing the mean operative time (average surgical suite charge savings of $1000, plus the possibility of same-day discharge), including the $600 cost of MIBI scanning (but the cost of the quick PTH assay was not given). They stressed that the immunochemiluminescence method that they used allowed for a 6-month shelf life for their kits, which was much longer than the immunoradiometric method previously used, and that a good correlation was found between their quick and 24-hour iPTH assays.

RADIO-GUIDED PARATHYROIDECTOMY

Martinez et al[34] were the first to describe taking advantage intraoperatively of the fact that MIBI is avidly taken up by the parathyroid glands. Patients were given a dose of MIBI preoperatively and then were explored bilaterally. The radioactivity of the parathyroid glands and surrounding tissue was measured with a hand-held gamma probe (Neoprobe Corp., Columbus, OH). They described three patients with positive preoperative MIBI scans who were redosed with MIBI before surgery and had abnormal glands identified at surgery. The first had an ectopic adenoma just inferior to the aortic arch, with significantly higher counts at 3 or 4 hours after MIBI (2-mCi dose) than the background. The second patient had her 200-mg gland identified 6 hours after MIBI (0.4-mCi dose), but no audible counts were evident and no increase in counts over that of the background was noted. The third patient had secondary HPT, and at 3 or 4 hours after MIBI (1-mCi dose), three of four glands had increased counts over the background. In general, the counts were approximately 50% higher than the adjacent tissues, which is much less than that usually seen in sentinel node mapping for melanoma. The investigators concluded that exploration should be carried out before 6 hours after injection and that a dose of 1 mCi to 2 mCi of MIBI before surgery should be used.

Gallowitsch et al[20] used a gamma probe (C-Trak, Care Wise Inc., Morgan Hill, CA) intraoperatively in 11 patients with primary and 1 with secondary HPT. All patients had preoperative MIBI or tetrafosmin scans and sonography. Nine of 12 patients had positive scans, and in 11 of 12 patients, the glands could be identified with the gamma probe. The one false-negative result was from a gland 28 mm in diameter. The parathyroid tumor–to–background ratio ranged from 0.92 to 2.95 in situ, with a mean of 1.87. The investigators concluded that this approach was feasible and might be especially useful for ectopic adenomas.

Bonjer et al reported their experience with using the hand-held gamma probe during parathyroid explorations in 1997[3] and updated their experience in 1998.[2] In the latter article, they compared the results in 62 patients having radioguided parathyroid exploration to 60 patients without using the probe, between 1995 and 1997, from Rotterdam and Lille. In the former group, 32 patients had primary HPT; 4, secondary HPT; 25, recurrent or persistent HPT; and 1, MEN-1 (the group explored without the probe was not significantly different). MIBI scans were performed in 42 of the 62 radio-guided surgery patients. In explorations using the probe, 370 MBq of MIBI was given 1 hour before surgery, then the radioactivity was measured in four quadrants of the neck below the platysma with a 10-mm probe (Tecprobe 2000, Stratec, Roosendaal, The Netherlands). The middle thyroid vein was divided and the thyroid was retracted, and measurements were taken from the thyroid, thymus, esophageal region, superior mediastinum, thymus, and carotid sheath. Solitary adenomas were found in 49 of 62 patients. Ten had MGD, and in three patients, parathyroid tumors were not found. Twenty-three patients in this group had ectopic tumors, and seven required sternotomy. The gamma probe identified 80% of the tumors found at the initial exploration for HPT, with two false-positives in patients with thyroid nodules and six false-negatives (with glands ranging from 100–700 mg, one of which was retroesophageal, and another in the aortopulmonary window). Only 14 of 22 (64%) glands were found in patients with MGD at first exploration. Solitary adenomas were found in 22 of 25 patients having re-explorations, and 20 were found using the probe (two false-negative glands were found in normal positions and weighed 180 mg and 200 mg). The complication rates in those undergoing radio-guided surgery were not significantly different from those without, and 95% and 97% of patients were euparathyroid after exploration in each group, respectively. The investigators believed that 60 minutes after isotope administration was the optimal time for exploration and that, although it did not lead to improvements in outcomes in primary parathyroid surgery, it was useful in the reoperative situation. The ratio of radioactivity in the excised parathyroids to the background ranged from 1.2 to 5.1, with a mean of 2.0. They suggested that, if a parathyroid tumor could not be found intraoperatively during conventional exploration, then MIBI could be given and the probe used at that time.

Norman et al[41] selected 15 patients in whom MIBI scanning demonstrated a solitary adenoma and took them to the surgical suite within 2.5 ($\pm$ 0.1) hours of the scan. They were explored through a 2-cm to 3-cm transverse incision, and after raising platysmal flaps, an 11-mm hand-held gamma probe (Neoprobe Corp., Dublin, OH) was used to measure the radioactivity in all four quadrants. Dissection was directed toward the areas of highest counts, and the enlarged gland was identified and removed. If the radioactivity in the neck was similar in all four quadrants, then no attempt was made to identify normal glands. Five patients were explored under general anesthesia, then the subsequent 10 under local anesthesia and intravenous sedation with propofol. One patient required bilateral exploration for what proved to be hyperplasia after removal of the presumed adenoma did not result in a significant decrease in postexcision counts. The average incision size was 2.4 cm ($\pm$ 0.2), and the mean operative time was 48 minutes ($\pm$ 2.1). Patients who underwent surgery under local anesthesia were discharged home within 2.4 hours ($\pm$ 0.2) of surgery. By selecting only patients with quality scans demonstrating a solitary adenoma, patients with potentially false-negative MIBI scans were not candidates for the procedure. Use of the gamma probe helped to eliminate the possibility of inaccurate or false-positive scans, and the requirement of equilibration of all four quadrants of the neck before ceasing the exploration was used to avoid leaving additional hyperfunctioning glands. In general, the ex vivo counts of the excised gland ($\approx$ 1500 counts/s) were greater than 20% (mean, 32%) of the background of the neck, and thyroid nodules, fat, and lymph nodes never exceeded 3% of this level (usually $\approx$ 110 counts/s; mean, 1.8% of background). The level of radioactivity found in parathyroid glands using this technique is much less than that with sentinel node mapping for melanoma, in which the isotope is injected directly into the skin as opposed to intravenously in the former procedure, so no special handling of specimens was required in terms of radiation safety. The investigators stated that MIBI scans at their institution were of high quality and allowed for this approach in 84% of their patients. In a follow-up letter, Norman[39] later reported having performed this procedure on 200 patients with a mean operative time of 23 minutes, with 97% of patients being discharged home within 2 hours of surgery.

Norman and Denham[43] also used this technique in patients undergoing re-exploration for primary HPT. Twenty-four patients with HPT and previous exploration for primary HPT or thyroid lobectomy had MIBI scans performed between 1997 and 1998. One patient had a mediastinal adenoma near the right atrium, and two had negative scans and were excluded. The other 21 patients were explored using the technique described earlier, except that MIBI scans were obtained ahead of time, patients were redosed with MIBI the morning of surgery, and early images were repeated. Patients with increased uptake in the neck were given 0.125 mg/d of levothyroxine for 8 weeks preoperatively to suppress the background radioactivity. SPECT imaging was no longer used because equivalent information could be obtained with right and left anterior oblique views with less expense. Four patients seemed to have intrathyroidal increased uptake, and in these patients, sonography was performed for confirmation. Eighteen patients had local anesthesia, three had general anesthesia, and incisions ranged from 3 cm to 4 cm in length. Dissection was carried out through the midline or by a lateral approach for the deeper lesions, with dissections between the sternocleidomastoid and strap muscles. The gamma probe was then used to guide the dissection. All 21 patients explored were found to have a single adenoma, and all were normocalcemic at follow-up. The mean operative time was 44 minutes (± 5 min; range, 19–109 min), and 16 patients were discharged home within 2 hours of surgery. All patients were discharged home and instructed to take 2 g/d of calcium and calcitriol for 1 week, and no complications were noted. This study demonstrated that minimally invasive, radio-guided parathyroidectomy also could be highly successful in this group of challenging patients. Interestingly, only 1 of 24 patients referred had hyperplasia. The investigators pointed out that timing surgery to within 3 hours of MIBI injection was critical to the success of surgery.

Moore et al[38] studied 48 consecutive patients with nonfamilial primary HPT who underwent preoperative dual-phase MIBI or tetrafosmin scanning and unilateral exploration when appropriate, with intraoperative measurement of PTH. Patients found to have solitary adenomas underwent outpatient exploration, in which unilateral exploration was carried out. When the abnormal gland was found, a blood sample was drawn from the ipsilateral jugular vein, then the adenoma was removed, and a second iPTH sample was drawn 10 minutes after excision. Then the normal gland was searched for and sampled for biopsy. If the adenoma could not be found in the predicted location, then a gamma probe was used to define the site of the adenoma (patients were dosed with 10 mCi MIBI 2 hours before planned exploration). After exploration, 41 (85%) patients were found to have solitary adenomas; 6 (13%), double adenomas; and 1 (2%), hyperplasia. Thirty-two (67%) patients had successful unilateral exploration, whereas 16 had bilateral exploration. MIBI scanning was performed in 46 patients; in 32 patients, the findings were compatible with a single adenoma, and 4 patients had bilateral foci of increased uptake. Interestingly, of the 32 patients with a unilateral focus seen on the MIBI scan, only 27 (85%) were found to be correct at surgery. In three of these patients, the adenomas were found on the opposite side of the neck, and two patients were found to have double adenomas. Sixteen patients had unilateral exploration planned but bilateral exploration carried out, seven because the iPTH levels did not decrease by 50% within 10 minutes of removal of a presumed solitary adenoma. Five of these patients had double adenomas, and two had slow metabolism of PTH. Five other patients had bilateral exploration because of erroneous localization studies (two MIBI scans showed bilateral disease when it was unilateral, three showed uptake on the wrong side of the neck). Two other patients had negative MIBI scans (one had a single, and the other, double adenomas), and two required bilateral exposure to find the localized gland. In 31 patients, the gamma probe was used but was only found to be useful in 4 cases (but not critically important). The mean time of surgery was 60 minutes for unilateral (range, 35–88 min) and 93 minutes (range, 50–140 min) in bilateral cases. They found a sensitivity of 71% and positive predictive value of 90% for MIBI scanning, and it was especially poor in detecting MGD. MGD was found only through the intraoperative iPTH assays, and the 13% rate of double adenomas was higher than in most series. They concluded that, even with a perfect test for preoperative localization, and in this series MIBI scanning was not, only 85% of cases could have had unilateral exploration because of the prevalence of MGD.

Flynn et al[18] reported their experience with minimally invasive, radio-guided parathyroidectomy, in which they selected 39 patients with biochemical evidence of HPT (three having reoperations) and preoperative localization by MIBI suggesting a solitary adenoma. Patients were redosed with MIBI on the day of surgery and were given intravenous methylene blue intraoperatively under general anesthesia, and the gamma probe was used to guide the exploration. Intraoperative iPTH levels were performed at 5 and 10 minutes after the resection of the adenoma. In 36 patients having their first exploration, 32 were found to have single adenomas, 2 had double adenomas, and 2 had hyperplasia. Nine patients had bilateral exploration, two because iPTH remained elevated, and two had a delayed decrease in iPTH. All patients were rendered normocalcemic, and two temporary recurrent nerve injuries occurred. The estimated cost of this approach was $7451 (including PTH testing and an extra MIBI dose) versus $8416 for standard exploration. Studies of radio-guided parathyroidectomy are summarized in Table 6.

LOCAL ANESTHESIA AND OUTPATIENT PARATHYROIDECTOMY

Pyrtek et al[48] showed that parathyroid exploration could be carried out under local anesthesia with reasonable results. They described 29 patients thought to be at high risk for general anesthesia who underwent surgery be-

Table 6. STUDIES OF RADIO-GUIDED PARATHYROIDECTOMY

Study	No. Patients	Solitary/ MGD	Unilateral Expl./ Bilateral Expl.	Probe Success (%)	Cure Rate (%)
Martinez[34]	3	2/1	—	67	—
Gallowitsch[20]	12	—	—	92	—
Bonjer[2]	62	49/10*	—	80	95
Norman[41]	15	15/0	14/1	100	—
Norman[43]	24†	21/0	21/0	100	—
Flynn[18]	39	32/6‡	30/9	—	100

*No parathyroid tumors were found in two patients; 23 glands were ectopic, 7 required sternotomy.
†All reoperations; two excluded due to negative MIBI scans; one patient had a mediastinal gland.
‡Three patients were reoperations.

tween 1982 and 1986. Preoperative localization studies included sonography and $^{201}Tl/^{99m}Tc$ subtraction and CT in some cases. The patients were given intravenous sedation, and 0.5% lidocaine–0.5% bupivacaine was used for local anesthesia. Incisions were made along the anterior border of the sternocleidomastoid muscle, and parathyroid glands were identified from a lateral approach. The mean operative time was 115 minutes (range, 1–4 h), and 23 of 29 cases resulted in normocalcemia. In the six patients with failure, three had incorrect localization studies (two patients became normocalcemic after contralateral exploration), one had an incorrect diagnosis of parathyroid adenoma on frozen section (which proved to be a thyroid nodule), one had too much tissue left behind after reoperation for hyperplasia, and one patient had a large thyroid extending into the mediastinum not allowing for mobilization of the gland from the lateral approach. The investigators concluded that surgery was safe in these high-risk patients and that those with MGD that were not cured by unilateral exploration were candidates for contralateral exploration under local anesthesia.

Ditkoff et al[16] retrospectively reviewed their results with parathyroid exploration under local anesthesia between 1987 and 1996. During this period, 49 patients who requested local anesthesia had parathyroid exploration carried out using 0.5% lidocaine–0.25% bupivacaine cervical plexus or field block with intravenous sedation. Eleven patients had preoperative localization procedures, which were not routinely performed. All four glands were searched for at each exploration, in which 46 patients were found to have a single adenoma and 3 had hyperplasia. No nerve injuries occurred, but one patient underwent reoperation for postoperative hemorrhage, and one patient had to be converted to general anesthesia. Eighty-two percent of patients surveyed believed that surgery was equal to or less painful than having a tooth filled, and 95% stated they would choose to have local anesthesia again. The mean length of stay was 1.4 days (versus 1.6 d for those explored under general anesthesia), 47% underwent surgery on an outpatient basis, and patients returned to work within an average of 6 days (versus 8 d for general anesthesia). The mean operative times were similar to those seen for patients who underwent surgery under general anesthesia, which was 56 minutes for single adenomas (range, 18–100 min), and 65 minutes for multiple gland parathyroidectomy (range, 45–85 min). All patients were eucalcemic postoperatively, and the authors believed that the most important predictors of success for surgery with local anesthesia were a surgeon experienced in parathyroid surgery and cervical plexus block.

Irvin et al[28] offered outpatient parathyroidectomy to 57 patients, who were explored under general anesthesia after preoperative MIBI scans. Explorations were directed by preoperative MIBI scans and were terminated if intraoperative iPTH assays showed a decrease of more than 50%. Of these patients, 42 (74%) were discharged the day of surgery as planned, and 15 (26%) were admitted for overnight stay. One of those admitted had a hematoma requiring drainage; 3 had nausea, urinary retention, or migraine; and 11 were admitted because of prolonged surgical procedures. One patient experienced a recurrent laryngeal nerve injury. The authors believed that their approach of preoperative scanning and intraoperative iPTH testing allowed for decreased surgical times and same-day discharge, even when general anesthesia was used. The largest series of neck exploration for primary HPT under local anesthesia was 200 patients described by Chapuis et al[11] (studies summarized in Table 7), and no untoward effects of this approach were reported. Norman et al[42, 43] also have shown the benefits of local anesthesia in primary explorations and reoperations for HPT in terms of cost savings and earlier discharge.

Table 7. STUDIES OF LOCAL ANESTHESIA OR OUTPATIENT PARATHYROIDECTOMY

Study	No. Patients	Solitary/ MGD	Local	Outpatient	Unilateral Expl./ Bilateral Expl.	Operative Time (min)	Cure Rate (%)
Pyrtek[48]	29	—	Yes	—	29/0	115	79
Ditkoff[16]	49	46/3	Yes	No	0/49	56–65	100
Irvin[28]	57	—	No	Yes (74%)	—	—	—
Chapuis[11]	200	—	Yes	—	179/9	—	95 (1–6-mo follow-up)
Norman[39]	~200	—	Yes	Yes	—	23	—

ENDOSCOPIC PARATHYROIDECTOMY

Because of advances in miniaturization of laparoendoscopic instruments, several investigators have explored the utility of applying these technologies toward endoscopic parathyroidectomy (Table 8). The first report of endoscopic removal of a parathyroid tumor was by Prinz et al[47] in 1994. They reported a series of four patients with persistent HPT after neck exploration who were found to have mediastinal parathyroid glands on follow-up imaging studies. Patients were placed in the right lateral decubitus position, and a 10-mm thoracoscopic port was placed in the sixth intercostal space in the left midaxillary line, a 5-mm port in the third to fourth intercostal space at the anterior axillary line, and a third port in the fifth to sixth intercostal space. The mediastinal parathyroid glands in all our patients were inferior to the level of the aortic arch, one being adjacent to the main pulmonary artery, another in the aortopulmonary window, one just inferior to the aortic arch, and the other to the left of the ascending aortic arch. Essential to this technique was preoperative localization of the gland, and based on this experience, the investigators thought that identification of mediastinal glands would be difficult through the thoracoscope without these studies. With accurate localization, however, the glands were identified and removed in a mean operative time of 3.25 hours (range, 2–4 h). Three of the four patients had supernumerary glands, none experienced major morbidities, and one developed recurrent HPT 9 months later. The investigators showed that this procedure was safe, effective, and may replace median sternotomy as the treatment of choice for removal of mediastinal parathyroid glands.

Wei et al[69] explored a man with three previous failed neck explorations after

Table 8. STUDIES OF ENDOSCOPIC PARATHYROIDECTOMY

Study	No. Patients	Site	Comment	Operative Time	Success Rate (%)
Prinz[47]	4	Mediastinum	Right lateral decubitis	3.25 h	75
Wei[69]	1	Mediastinum	Subxiphoid	—	—
Gagner[19]	1	Neck	3.5 glands	5 h	—
Brunt[7]	5	Neck	Cadavers	69 min	—
Yeung[72, 73]	4	Neck	All adenomas	120–150 min	75
Norman[40]	4	Neck	All adenomas	—	75
Miccoli[36, 37]	39	Neck	All adenomas	65 min	100

a MIBI scan demonstrated an anterior mediastinal gland. They made a 4-cm subxiphoid incision, dissected the pericardial fat pad from the underside of the sternum, and placed a 10-mm cannula and laparoscope through this incision. A second 5-mm trocar was placed 6 cm to the left, through which the thymus and pleura were dissected from the sternum. Insufflation of carbon dioxide gas was performed to 5 to 10 mm Hg but was no longer needed when the anterior mediastinum had been dissected because the heart and great vessels fell posteriorly. They made a 5-cm incision just superior to the sternal notch and developed a plane behind the manubrium. A 1.6-g adenoma was found along the right internal mammary vein, and the patient became normocalcemic postoperatively. A mediastinal drainage tube was placed, and the patient was discharged on postoperative day 3.

The first report of endoscopic removal of parathyroid glands in the neck came from Gagner[19] in 1996. In a patient with familial hypercalcemia, the neck was explored using four 5-mm ports placed posterior to the platysma muscle, approximately 1 cm superior to the clavicle and sternal notch. The neck was insufflated to 15 mm Hg, and the anterior and lateral aspects of the thyroid gland and trachea were dissected. All four parathyroid glands were identified, and a 3.5 gland excision was performed. The procedure required 5 hours to complete, and was complicated by hypercarbia intraoperatively (controlled by hyperventilation) and postoperatively by subcutaneous emphysema extending from the scrotum to the eyelids. This resolved after 3 days, and the patient was rendered normocalcemic. Gagner[19] suggested that one advantage of this procedure was the 15-fold to 20-fold magnification using the videoscope, which might result in fewer injuries to the recurrent laryngeal nerve.

Brunt et al[7] tried to develop a technique for videoendoscopic parathyroidectomy in the laboratory using dogs and human cadavers. They found that carbon dioxide insufflation to pressures of more than 9 mm Hg led to radiographically detectable pneumomediastinum and that pressures of 15 to 20 mm Hg caused significant subcutaneous emphysema and pneumomediastinum, so they abandoned insufflation and instead used an external lift device. They made a 2.0-cm to 2.5-cm incision low in the neck, bluntly dissected inferiorly to the pretracheal space, then distended a modified hernia balloon to 300 mL to create a working space. The lift device was used to suspend the incision, a 12-mm camera port was placed in the incision, and additional 5-mm ports were placed in the supraclavicular position under direct vision. In five cadavers, they were able to remove four glands from two subjects, three glands from two subjects, and found only two glands in another subject. The other two glands in the latter subject were identified at open exploration and were thought to have been displaced by the balloon dissector. In one subject with three glands found endoscopically, a superior gland was found at open exploration. The mean operative time was 68.8 minutes ($\pm$ 38.2; range, 45–135 min). The investigators concluded that a gasless endoscopic approach was safer than using insufflation, that an ultrasonic dissector was better than cautery, and that this technique would have a limited role for ectopic glands or MGD. Brunt[6] later reported that he successfully performed their technique in two living patients but believed that significant difficulties occurred with the procedure.

Yeung[72] and Yeung and Ng[73] described performing endoscopic parathyroidectomy and hemithyroidectomy with patients under general anesthesia. Insufflation was achieved through a port placed through an 11-mm incision superior to the sternal notch after developing a plane between the sternocleidomastoid muscles. A 5-mm trocar was placed along the medial border of the sternocleidomastoid muscles several centimeters superior to the level of the first incision. Four patients with primary HPT were explored by this technique after having sonography, neck CT, thallium–technetium subtraction, and MIBI scanning performed, all confirming a solitary adenoma. The technique was successful in three of four patients, with one patient requiring open exploration for a gland firmly adherent to the esophagus. These surgeries ranged from 120 to 150 minutes, and the adenomas weighed between 0.84 g and 3.75 g. The investigators concluded that larger prospective studies were necessary to thoroughly evaluate this procedure versus the open approach.

Norman and Albrink[40] first performed parathyroidectomy and thyroidectomy in four dogs to work out technical details, then used the technique on four patients whose MIBI scans were highly suggestive of a single adenoma. They made a 1.5-cm transverse incision lateral to the midline and 1 cm superior to the head of the clavicle. Dissection was carried out to the thyroid gland in the midline, and the space anterior to the thyroid was opened bluntly. A 2-mm camera port was placed just inferior to this incision, and a green retractor then was placed in the original incision and the skin closed around it with a running nylon suture. Two or three additional ports then were placed under direct vision after insufflation to 8 mm Hg. At the end of surgery, the incision was extended to 3.5 cm to remove the adenoma and check hemostasis. In these four patients, the adenoma was found in three but could not be identified in the fourth despite accurate preoperative imaging. This gland was in the tracheoesophageal groove and was found on opening. Normal ipsilateral glands were identified in only one of these four patients, which was more technically difficult than adenomas because they tended to be posterior to the thyroid rather than lateral to it. No patients had significant postoperative subcutaneous emphysema, and all recovered well. The investigators concluded that the limited exposure with the videoscopic technique did not enhance parathyroidectomy. Norman[39] later reported that the major drawback of this procedure was a small working space, which could easily be obscured by even 1 mL of blood.

Miccoli et al[36, 37] have published the largest series of endoscopic parathyroidectomy, which described 39 patients with sporadic HPT and no previous history of surgery, and in whom imaging suggested a single adenoma and no goiter (sonography was performed in all patients, and MIBI, in some patients). Their approach was described as gasless, although insufflation of carbon dioxide was performed temporarily at the start of surgery to create a working space in the neck. They made a 15-mm incision at the sternal notch, incised the midline so that a 12-mm trocar could be placed on the side of the adenoma, then insufflated to 12 mm Hg for 3 or 4 minutes. They then placed a 5-mm camera through this incision, which was held open with conventional retractors. Two-millimeter forceps and scissors were then used for the dissection, one through the incision, and the other through a small supraclavicular incision. After excision of the gland, intraoperative plasma iPTH levels were measured to confirm removal of the adenoma. They successfully removed adenomas in all 39 cases by virtue of a decrease of more than 50% in iPTH levels, and at a mean follow-up of 7 months, no patients had recurrent hypercalcemia or elevated PTH levels. The mean operative time was 65.1 minutes ($\pm$ 27.8; range, 30–180 min). The investigators concluded that the procedure was safe and effective for selected patients with primary HPT and that more than 60% of patients in their experience were candidates.

SUMMARY

The traditional algorithm of mandatory bilateral exploration continues to make sense for patients with familial forms of HPT (MEN-1, MEN-2A, familial

HPT) and secondary HPT. In patients with solitary adenomas, this approach remains the gold standard but may result in a higher risk for postoperative hypocalcemia, may increase the risk associated with future neck explorations, and may not result in a significantly higher cure rate. Preoperative imaging studies are important for determining whether patients are candidates for unilateral exploration, and MIBI scanning represents a step forward in noninvasive imaging; however, surgeons at most hospitals may not find this imaging modality to be as accurate as that reported from a few select centers. Some surgeons believe that reliance on these preoperative studies results in parathyroid surgery being performed by surgeons with less experience and that patient care ultimately will suffer as a result. Whether this is true remains to be seen, but patients and insurance companies are driving changes in practice toward unilateral exploration for solitary adenomas.

If preoperative imaging studies show a single, intense focus of uptake on

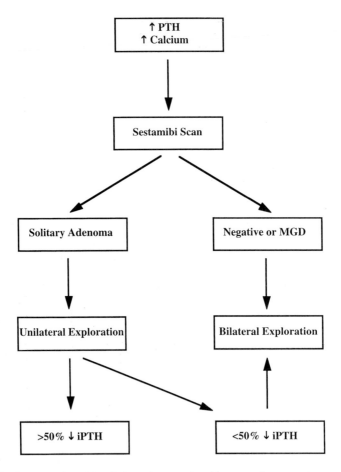

Figure 1. Algorithm for minimally invasive parathyroidectomy. Some surgeons substitute radio-guided exploration for intraoperative iPTH measurement, and others may use both techniques. MGD = multiglandular disease; iPTH = intact serum parathyroid hormone.

MIBI scan, then the literature reviewed would support that these patients can undergo unilateral exploration safely (Fig. 1). The author's practice is to remove the enlarged gland, then identify, record the size of, and sample by biopsy the ipsilateral normal parathyroid gland. These steps are important to confirm that the gland was found and that no evidence of hyperplasia or double adenoma is present. Quick intraoperative PTH testing is a valuable method for confirming that surgery is curative, but the author has not used it thus far because of its expense and technical demands. Although a few investigators have found the gamma probe to be useful for intraoperative localization of the parathyroid glands, this has not been the author's experience. Even when exploration is undertaken within 1.5 to 3.0 hours of MIBI injection, and with the probe lying on top of adenomas weighing more than 1 g, the author has found little difference in the counts between the adenoma and the adjacent thyroid and has not found the probe to be useful to direct dissection in the neck; however, the author has used the standard probe for lymphatic mapping, which has retrograde collimation. Norman (personal communication, 2000) recommends using a probe with forward collimation, which has an expanded view and is more useful for differentiating hot areas, such as the thyroid, from hotter ones, such as a parathyroid adenoma. Whether the probe is used or not, when the adenoma has been localized by a MIBI scan, it usually is dissected easily through a 3-cm incision. Because the other side of the neck is left undisturbed, in the unlikely situation in which a contralateral adenoma that was not seen on the MIBI scan is found during workup for persistent hypercalcemia, then exploration of that side would not be complicated by previous dissection. Patients rarely develop symptomatic hypocalcemia after unilateral exploration and can go home the same day, even if they have undergone exploration under general anesthesia.

ACKNOWLEDGMENT

The author thanks Nelson Gurll, MD, for reviewing the manuscript.

References

1. Attie JN, Bock G, Auguste LJ: Multiple parathyroid adenomas: Report of thirty-three cases. Surgery 108:1014, 1990
2. Bonjer HJ, Bruining HA, Pols HA, et al: 2-Methoxyisobutylisonitrile probe during parathyroid surgery: Tool or gadget? World J Surg 22:507, 1998
3. Bonjer HJ, Bruining HA, Pols HA, et al: Intraoperative nuclear guidance in benign hyperparathyroidism and parathyroid cancer. Eur J Nucl Med 24:246, 1997
4. Borley NR, Collins RE, O'Doherty M, et al: Technetium-99m sestamibi parathyroid localization is accurate enough for scan-directed unilateral neck exploration. Br J Surg 83:989, 1996
5. Bruining HA, van Houten H, Juttmann JR, et al: Original scientific reports: Results of operative treatment of 615 patients with primary hyperparathyroidism. World J Surg 5:85, 1981
6. Brunt LM: Reply: Endoscopic versus radioguided parathyroidectomy. Surgery 124:119, 1998
7. Brunt LM, Jones DB, Wu JS, et al: Experimental development of an endoscopic approach to neck exploration and parathyroidectomy. Surgery 122:893, 1997
8. Carter WB, Sarfati MR, Fox KA, et al: Preoperative detection of sporadic parathyroid adenomas using technetium-99m-sestamibi: What role in clinical practice? Am Surg 63:317, 1997
9. Carty SE, Worsey J, Virji MA, et al: Concise parathyroidectomy: The impact of preoper-

ative SPECT ^{99m}Tc sestamibi scanning and intraoperative quick parathormone assay. Surgery 122:1107, 1997
10. Casas AT, Burke GJ, Sathyanarayana, et al: Prospective comparison of technetium-99m-sestamibi/iodine-123 radionuclide scan versus high-resolution ultrasonography for the preoperative localization of abnormal parathyroid glands in patients with previously unoperated primary hyperparathyroidism. Am J Surg 166:369, 1993
11. Chapuis Y, Fulla Y, Bonnichon P, et al: Values of ultrasonography, sestamibi scintigraphy, and intraoperative measurement of 1-84 PTH for unilateral neck exploration of primary hyperparathyroidism. World J Surg 20:835, 1996
12. Chapuis Y, Icard P, Fulla Y, et al: Parathyroid adenomectomy under local anesthesia with intra-operative monitoring of UcAMP and/or 1-84 PTH. World J Surg 16:570, 1992
13. Coakley AJ, Kettle AG, Wells CP, et al: ^{99m}Tc sestamibi: A new agent for parathyroid imaging. Nucl Med Commun 10:791, 1989
14. Davies C, Demeure MJ, St. John A, et al: Study of intact (1-84) parathyroid hormone secretion in patients undergoing parathyroidectomy. World J Surg 14:355, 1990
15. Denham DW, Norman J: Cost-effectiveness of preoperative sestamibi scan for primary hyperparathyroidism is dependent solely upon the surgeon's choice of operative procedure. J Am Coll Surg 186:293, 1998
16. Ditkoff BA, Chabot J, Feind C, et al: Parathyroid surgery using monitored anesthesia care as an alternative to general anesthesia. Am J Surg 172:698, 1996
17. Duh QY, Uden P, Clark OH: Unilateral neck exploration for primary hyperparathyroidism: Analysis of a controversy using a mathematical model. World J Surg 16:654, 1992
18. Flynn MB, Bumpous JM, Scill K, et al: Minimally invasive radioguided parathyroidectomy. J Am Coll Surg 191:24, 2000
19. Gagner M: Endoscopic subtotal parathyroidectomy in patients with primary hyperparathyroidism. Br J Surg 83:875, 1996
20. Gallowitsch HJ, Fellinger J, Kresnik E, et al: Preoperative scintigraphic and intraoperative scintimetric localization of parathyroid adenoma with cationic Tc-99m complexes and a hand-held gamma-probe. Nuklearmedizin 36:13, 1997
21. Geatti O, Shapiro B, Orsolon PG, et al: Localization of parathyroid enlargement: Experience with technetium-99m methoxyisobutylisonitrile and thallium-201 scintigraphy, ultrasonography and computed tomography. Eur J Nucl Med 21:17, 1994
22. Gupta VK, Yeh KA, Burke GJ, et al: Technetium-99m sestamibi localized solitary parathyroid adenoma as an indication for limited unilateral surgical exploration. Am J Surg 176:409, 1998
23. Harness JK, Ramsburg SR, Nishiyama RH, et al: Multiple adenomas of the parathyroids: Do they exist? Arch Surg 114:468, 1979
24. Harrison TS, Duarte B, Reitz RE, et al: Primary hyperparathyroidism: Four- to eight-year postoperative follow-up demonstrating persistent functional insignificance of microscopic parathyroid hyperplasia and decreased autonomy of parathyroid hormone release. Ann Surg 194:429, 1981
25. Hindie E, Melliere D, Simon D, et al: Primary hyperparathyroidism: Is technetium 99m sestamibi/iodine-123 subtraction scanning the best procedure to locate enlarged glands before surgery? J Clin Endocrinol Metab 80:302, 1995
26. Irvin GL, Dembrow VD, Prudhomme DL: Clinical usefulness of an intraoperative "quick parathyroid hormone" assay. Surgery 114:1019, 1993
27. Irvin GL, Prudhomme DL, Deriso GT, et al: A new approach to parathyroidectomy. Ann Surg 219:574, 1994
28. Irvin GL, Sfakianakis G, Yeung L, et al: Ambulatory parathyroidectomy for primary hyperparathyroidism. Arch Surg 131:1074, 1996
29. Kaplan EL, Yashiro T, Salti G: Primary hyperparathyroidism in the 1990s. Choice of surgical procedures for this disease. Ann Surg 215:300, 1992
30. Light VL, McHenry CR, Jarjoura D, et al: Prospective comparison of dual-phase technetium-99m-sestamibi scintigraphy and high resolution ultrasonography in the evaluation of abnormal parathyroid glands. Am Surg 62:562, 1996
31. Lucas RJ, Welsh RJ, Glover JL: Unilateral neck exploration for primary hyperparathyroidism. Arch Surg 125:982, 1990

32. Malhotra A, Silver CE, Deshpande V, et al: Preoperative parathyroid localization with sestamibi. Am J Surg 172:637, 1996
33. Martin D, Rosen IB, Ichise M: Evaluation of single isotope technetium-99m-sestamibi in localization efficiency for hyperparathyroidism. Am J Surg 172:633, 1996
34. Martinez DA, King DR, Romshe C, et al: Intraoperative identification of parathyroid gland pathology: A new approach. J Pediatr Surg 30:1306, 1995
35. McHenry CR, Lee K, Saadey J, et al: Parathyroid localization with technetium-99m sestamibi: A prospective evaluation. J Am Coll Surg 183:25, 1996
36. Miccoli P, Bendinelli C, Conte M, et al: Endoscopic parathyroidectomy by a gasless approach. J Laparoendosc Adv Surg Tech A 8:189, 1998
37. Miccoli P, Bendinelli C, Vignali E, et al: Endoscopic parathyroidectomy: Report of an initial experience. Surgery 124:1077, 1998
38. Moore FD, Mannting F, Tanasijevic M: Intrinsic limitations to unilateral parathyroid exploration. Ann Surg 230:382, 1999
39. Norman J: Endoscopic versus radioguided parathyroidectomy [letter; comment]. Surgery 124:118, 1998
40. Norman J, Albrink MH: Minimally invasive videoscopic parathyroidectomy: A feasibility study in dogs and humans. J Laparoendosc Adv Surg Tech A 7:301, 1997
41. Norman J, Chheda H: Minimally invasive parathyroidectomy facilitated by intraoperative nuclear mapping. Surgery 122:998, 1997
42. Norman J, Chheda H, Farrell C: Minimally invasive parathyroidectomy for primary hyperparathyroidism: Decreasing operative time and potential complications while improving cosmetic results. Am Surg 64:391, 1998
43. Norman J, Denham D: Minimally invasive radioguided parathyroidectomy in the reoperative neck. Surgery 124:1088, 1998
44. Nussbaum SR, Thompson AR, Hutcheson KA, et al: Intraoperative measurement of parathyroid hormone in the surgical management of hyperparathyroidism. Surgery 104:1121, 1988
45. O'Doherty MJ, Kettle AG, Wells P, et al: Parathyroid imaging with technetium-99m sestamibi: Preoperative localization and tissue uptake studies. J Nucl Med 33:313, 1992
46. Piwnica-Worms D, Kronauge JF, Chiu ML: Uptake and retention of hexakis (2-methoxyisobutyl isonitrile) technetium(I) in cultured chick myocardial cells: Mitochondrial and plasma membrane potential dependence. Circulation 82:1826, 1990
47. Prinz RA, Lonchyna V, Carnaille B, et al: Thoracoscopic excision of enlarged mediastinal parathyroid glands. Surgery 116:999, 1994
48. Pyrtek LJ, Belkin M, Bartus S, et al: Parathyroid gland exploration with local anesthesia in elderly and high-risk patients. Arch Surg 123:614, 1988
49. Robertson GS, Johnson PR, Bolia A, et al: Long-term results of unilateral neck exploration for preoperatively localized nonfamilial parathyroid adenomas. Am J Surg 172:311, 1996
50. Roth SI, Wang CA, Potts JT Jr: The team approach to primary hyperparathyroidism. Hum Pathol 6:645, 1975
51. Russell CF, Edis AJ: Surgery for primary hyperparathyroidism: Experience with 500 consecutive cases and evaluation of the role of surgery in the asymptomatic patient. Br J Surg 69:244, 1982
52. Russell CF, Laird JD, Ferguson WR: Scan-directed unilateral cervical exploration for parathyroid adenoma: A legitimate approach? World J Surg 14:406, 1990
53. Shen W, Sabanci U, Morita ET, et al: Sestamibi scanning is inadequate for directing unilateral neck exploration for first-time parathyroidectomy. Arch Surg 132:969, 1997
54. Sofferman RA, Standage J, Tang ME: Minimal-access parathyroid surgery using intraoperative parathyroid hormone assay. Laryngoscope 108:1497, 1998
55. Spiegel AM, Marx SJ, Brennan MF, et al: Urinary cAMP excretion during surgery: An index of successful parathyroidectomy in patients with primary hyperparathyroidism. J Clin Endocrinol Metab 47:537, 1978
56. Taillefer R, Boucher Y, Potvin C, et al: Detection and localization of parathyroid adenomas in patients with hyperparathyroidism using a single radionuclide imaging procedure with technetium-99m-sestamibi (double-phase study). J Nucl Med 33:1801, 1992

57. Takami H: Surgical management of hyperparathyroidism in view of a reliable parathyroid adenoma localization test. Surgery 122:120, 1997
58. Tezelman S, Shen W, Shaver JK, et al: Double parathyroid adenomas: Clinical and biochemical characteristics before and after parathyroidectomy. Ann Surg 218:300, 1993
59. Tibblin S, Bizard JP, Bondeson AG, et al: Primary hyperparathyroidism due to solitary adenoma: A comparative multicentre study of early and long-term results of different surgical regimens. Eur J Surg 157:511, 1991
60. Tibblin S, Bondeson AG, Bondeson L, et al: Surgical strategy in hyperparathyroidism due to solitary adenoma. Ann Surg 200:776, 1984
61. Tibblin S, Bondeson AG, Uden P: Current trends in the surgical treatment of solitary parathyroid adenoma: A questionnaire study from 53 surgical departments in 14 countries. Eur J Surg 157:103, 1991
62. Verdonk CA, Edis AJ: Parathyroid "double adenomas": Fact or fiction? Surgery 90:523, 1981
63. Vogel LM, Lucas R, Czako P: Unilateral parathyroid exploration. Am Surg 64:693, 1998
64. Wang C: The anatomic basis of parathyroid surgery. Ann Surg 183:271, 1976
65. Wang CA: Surgery of hyperparathyroidism: a conservative approach. J Surg Oncol 16:225, 1981
66. Wang CA, Rieder SV: A density test for the intraoperative differentiation of parathyroid hyperplasia from neoplasia. Ann Surg 187:63, 1978
67. Weber CJ, Sewell CW, McGarity WC: Persistent and recurrent sporadic primary hyperparathyroidism: Histopathology, complications, and results of reoperation. Surgery 116:991, 1994
68. Wei JP, Burke GJ, Mansberger AR Jr: Preoperative imaging of abnormal parathyroid glands in patients with hyperparathyroid disease using combination Tc-99m-pertechnetate and Tc-99m-sestamibi radionuclide scans. Ann Surg 219:568, 1994
69. Wei JP, Gadacz TR, Weisner LF, et al: The subxiphoid laparoscopic approach for resection of mediastinal parathyroid adenoma after successful localization with Tc-99m-sestamibi radionuclide scan. Surg Laparosc Endosc 5:402, 1995
70. Wells SA Jr, Leight GS, Hensley M, et al: Hyperparathyroidism associated with the enlargement of two or three parathyroid glands. Ann Surg 202:533, 1985
71. Worsey MJ, Carty SE, Watson CG: Success of unilateral neck exploration for sporadic primary hyperparathyroidism. Surgery 114:1024, 1993
72. Yeung GH: Endoscopic surgery of the neck: A new frontier. Surg Laparosc Endosc 8:227, 1998
73. Yeung GH, Ng JW: The technique of endoscopic exploration for parathyroid adenoma of the neck. Aust N Z J Surg 68:147, 1998

Address reprint requests to

James R. Howe, MD
Department of Surgery
University of Iowa College of Medicine
200 Hawkins Drive
Iowa City, IA 52242–1086

e-mail: james-howe@uiowa.edu

LAPAROSCOPIC APPROACH TO ADRENAL AND ENDOCRINE PANCREATIC TUMORS

Christopher D. Raeburn, MD, and Robert C. McIntyre, Jr, MD

The adrenal gland lends itself well to laparoscopic removal because it is small, and adrenal tumors are most often benign. The open approach to the adrenal gland typically requires a large incision to expose a small working space with its resultant postoperative morbidity. Similarly, most endocrine tumors of the pancreas are small and benign or are slow-growing malignancies. These tumors usually can be removed by enucleation or distal pancreatectomy. Proper application of minimally invasive surgery for adrenal and endocrine pancreatic tumors must take into account expertise in endocrine and laparoscopic surgery. One without the other may lead to unfavorable outcomes. The first report of laparoscopic adrenalectomy in the literature was by Gagner et al[15] in 1992. Since then, multiple reports have demonstrated a decreased hospital stay, narcotics requirement, blood loss, and recovery time, and overall increased patient satisfaction.[6, 17, 28, 36] Laparoscopic adrenalectomy rapidly has become the procedure of choice for most surgeons. Because pancreatic endocrine tumors are rare, evidence to support the use of minimally invasive approaches comes from case reports and small series.[9, 11, 18]

LAPAROSCOPIC ADRENALECTOMY

Adrenalectomy may be performed through an open or laparoscopic approach, including (1) laparoscopic lateral or anterior transabdominal approach for most adrenal tumors, (2) laparoscopic posterior approach for small tumors or bilateral adrenalectomy, and (3) open anterior transabdominal or thoracoabdominal incision for large tumors (>10 cm) or cancer with likely local invasion.[3, 6, 17, 25, 29, 36, 40] The transperitoneal lateral approach first described by Gagner et al[15]

From the Department of Surgery, University of Colorado Health Sciences Center (CDR, RCM); and the Department of Surgery, Veterans Affairs Hospital (RCM), Denver, Colorado is most commonly used because it provides a large working space. Patient positioning helps to retract organs by gravity; however, if bilateral adrenalectomy is required, it necessitates repositioning the patient. The transperitoneal anterior laparoscopic approach provides a conventional view of the anatomy and allows for bilateral adrenalectomy without repositioning the patient. It requires additional ports for retraction and has been associated with increased operative times compared with the lateral approach.[6] An endoscopic posterior retroperitoneal approach may be used to avoid entering the peritoneal cavity altogether and may be preferred for patients with previous abdominal surgery and for obese patients.[6, 13, 25, 40] The retroperitoneal approach also may be beneficial for bilateral adrenalectomy. A drawback to this approach, however, is the limited working space, making it difficult for the extraction of large tumors.[6, 13, 25] Another difficulty with this approach is controlling bleeding from the vena cava if it occurs.[25] The open approach still may be preferred for large (>10 cm) tumors that may be locally invasive malignancies.

Indications

Patients are referred for surgical evaluation for an incidental adrenal mass, a functioning benign tumor, or a large mass suspicious for malignancy. Indications for laparoscopic adrenalectomy vary little from that of open adrenalectomy. Barresi and Prinz[3] list six indications for laparoscopic adrenalectomy: (1) Cushing's syndrome caused a benign cortisol-producing adenoma, (2) Cushing's disease that has not improved with other forms of therapy (e.g., bilateral adrenalectomy), (3) aldosterone-producing adenoma (i.e., Conn's syndrome), (4) benign adrenal pheochromocytoma, (5) nonfunctioning adenomas or incidentalomas that meet accepted criteria for adrenalectomy (size >4 cm at presentation or growth on follow-up), and (6) benign lesions that are symptomatic. In a series of 100 laparoscopic adrenalectomies by Gagner et al,[17] 25% were for pheochromocytoma; 21%, for aldosteronoma; 20%, for nonfunctioning adenoma; 13%, for cortisol-producing adenoma; 8%, for Cushing's disease; 3%, for carcinoma; and 10%, for other reasons. A few relative contraindications to the laparoscopic approach exist,[17] including coagulopathy, previous surgery or trauma in the direct vicinity of the adrenal gland, a large right hepatic lobe, and diaphragmatic hernia.[3, 17, 40] Of note, however, is the potential benefit of the posterior retroperitoneal endoscopic approach in some of these settings because it avoids entering the peritoneal cavity altogether, so tissue planes may be preserved.[6, 13, 25]

Preoperative Diagnostic Evaluation

Determination whether an incidentaloma is a functioning tumor is important because virtually all functioning tumors should be excised. Approximately 0.3% to 5.0% of all CT scans of the abdomen performed for nonadrenal reasons show incidental adrenal lesions.[2, 4, 5, 19, 24, 30, 34] The evaluation of such patients should include a thorough history and physical examination. Biochemical workup should focus on the history and physical examination; however, a few simple tests can be done to assess adrenal function. The laboratory evaluation of patients includes a serum potassium level and a 24-hour urine collection for metanephrines, vanillylmandelic acid, 17-hydroxycorticosteroids, and free cortisol. If the tumor is nonfunctional at evaluation, repeat CT is done within 6 months. Resection is recommended for tumors of more than 4 cm at baseline or for growth on follow-up evaluation.

Hypertensive patients who are hypokalemic and not on diuretic therapy suggest primary hyperaldosteronism (0.05–2.0% of hypertensive patients). Patients with an aldosterone-producing adenoma have an elevated plasma aldosterone (PA) level with a decreased plasma renin activity (PRA). Diuretic, β-blockade, and angiotensin-converting enzyme inhibitor therapy should be discontinued for 2 weeks before testing. Prazosin can be used for hypertension. Patients should consume 150 mEq/d sodium and be given potassium supplements to keep the potassium level at more than 3.5 mEq/L. A liberal sodium diet should suppress PA. A PA–PRA ratio of more than 20 suggests primary hyperaldosteronism. Some endocrinologists prefer the saline load test instead of a high-salt diet; however, 12% of patients with primary hyperaldosteronism have a PA–PRA ratio of less than 20. In these cases, a 24-hour urine aldosterone level of more than 20 μg/d suggests primary hyperaldosteronism. If a patient has hyperaldosteronism, bilateral adrenal hyperplasia (i.e., idiopathic hyperaldosteronism) must be ruled out before surgery. High-quality CT commonly does so, but iodocholesterol scintigraphy or adrenal vein sampling should be performed to resolve remaining questions.

Excess glucocorticoid secretion may be caused by Cushing's disease (i.e., pituitary adenoma), ectopic adrenocorticotropic hormone (ACTH) production, adrenal adenoma, adrenal carcinoma, or macronodular adrenal hyperplasia. Patients with glucocorticoid-producing adrenal adenoma or adrenal carcinoma should undergo resection. Rarely, patients with pituitary adenoma or ectopic ACTH production require bilateral adrenalectomy for failure to control excess production through pituitary or primary tumor resection. Glucocorticoid-producing adrenal tumor results in an elevated urinary free cortisol and 17-hydroxycorticosteroid level. An alternative screening test is the 1-mg overnight dexamethasone suppression test. If a patient has Cushing's syndrome, the next step is to determine whether the patient has ACTH-dependent disease (pituitary, 70%; ectopic, 15%) or ACTH-independent disease (adrenal tumor, 15%). A normal or slightly elevated ACTH level suggests pituitary disease, whereas a markedly elevated level is usually of ectopic origin (i.e., lung cancer). Suppressed levels of ACTH suggest an adrenal source. CT differentiates an adrenal tumor from macronodular adrenal hyperplasia.

The classic presentation of pheochromocytoma (incidence, 1–2/100,000 adults per year) occurs in only one third of patients. Other presentations include a normotensive patient with episodic hypertension or chronic hypertension without symptomatic episodes. Urinary collection for metanephrines, normetanephrines, vanillylmandelic acid, and fractionated catecholamines constitutes an appropriate evaluation. Diagnostic accuracy can be increased by measurement of plasma catecholamines drawn from an indwelling venous catheter with the patient at rest. When the biochemical diagnosis is confirmed, CT or magnetic resonance imaging is used to localize the tumor. Scintigraphy with [131]iodobenzylguanidine may reveal multiple tumors or unsuspected metastasis.

Androgen-producing adrenal tumors are rare but suggested by virilization. These patients should have a 24-hour urine collection for 17-ketosteroids and plasma testosterone and dehydroepiandrosterone levels determined.

Adrenocortical carcinoma is a rare malignancy that is suspected in patients with tumors of more than 6 cm, an elevated urinary 17-ketosteroid level, evidence of local invasion, or distant metastasis. Metastatic disease to the adrenal gland includes lung, breast, stomach, pancreas, colon, kidney, melanoma, and lymphoma. Fine-needle aspiration of adrenal lesions typically is unhelpful because it is difficult to distinguish adenoma from well-differentiated carcinoma on cytology.[34] In patients with a known nonadrenal malignancy, however, fine-needle aspiration may be useful in determining whether an adrenal lesion is malignant and, thus, amenable to resection[7, 8]; however, pheochromocytoma must be ruled out first to avoid fatal complications.[8]

Perioperative Considerations

Physicians must correct metabolic abnormalities (e.g., hypokalemia, metabolic alkalosis, and hyperglycemia) and control hypertension before surgery. Patients with Cushing's syndrome can be treated with ketoconazole or the antiglucocorticoid agent RU 486. After surgery, patients with Cushing's syndrome require glucocorticoid replacement to prevent postoperative adrenal insufficiency. Patients with an aldosterone-producing adenoma should be treated with spironolactone. Patients with pheochromocytoma require α-antagonists (e.g., phenoxybenzamine, prazosin, or doxazosin) to control hypertension. If a patient is tachycardic after blood pressure control, β-blockade is indicated. Patients with suspected adrenal malignancy should undergo evaluation for metastatic disease.

Technique

Transperitoneal Lateral Adrenalectomy

For left adrenalectomy, the patient is positioned in the right lateral decubitus position. An axillary roll and kidney rest are placed, and the table is then flexed so that the patient's left side is extended to open up the space between the costal margin and the iliac crest (Fig. 1). The surgeon stands on the right side of the table, facing the patient, and the patient is rotated slightly away from the surgeon. After prep and drape, the patient's abdomen is insufflated by Veress needle or open laparoscopy technique approximately 2 cm inferior to the costal margin in the anterior axillary line. A 10-cm port is placed at this site, and a 0° or 30° angled laparoscope is placed into the abdomen. Two additional ports then are placed under direct vision at least 5 cm from the first. One port is placed subcostally at the midclavicular line, and the other is placed posteriorly just anterior to the 11th or 12th rib. Laparoscopic sonography is a useful adjunct to identify the adrenal gland and its tumor in patients with a small tumor or generous amount of adipose tissue. It also may identify the vascular anatomy of the gland before dissection.[3, 17, 20] The camera is then switched to the most anterior port, and dissection is begun by mobilizing the splenic flexure and left colon. This dissection is accomplished by laparoscopic shears or Harmonic Scalpel (Ethicon Endo-surgery, Cincinnati, OH). The spleen is mobilized by taking down its lateral attachments in the same manner. As the spleen is mobilized, gravity should help it to fall medially to expose the left kidney and adrenal lying within Gerota's fascia. At this point, an additional port can be placed as needed at the costovertebral angle just superior to the kidney for additional retraction of the spleen, kidney, or surrounding fat. Next, the patient is placed into a reverse Trendelenburg position to assist with exposure, and then dissection of the adrenal gland is begun. Starting laterally, the adrenal gland is dissected free from the adjacent perinephric fat using electrocautery shears or the Harmonic Scalpel. Caution is exercised to avoid tearing the delicate capsule

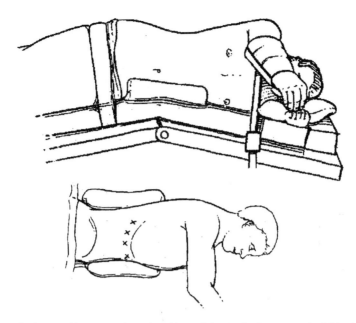

Figure 1. Patient positions seen from the side and the top for laparoscopic right adrenalectomy. X = port placements. (*From* Duh QY, Siperstein AE, Clark OH, et al: Laparoscopic adrenalectomy. Comparison of the lateral and posterior approaches. Arch Surg 131(8):870–875, 1996; with permission.)

of the adrenal gland by grasping the surrounding fat instead of the gland. Ideally, the adrenal vein should be isolated and ligated early during surgery to prevent injuring it during mobilization of the rest of the gland; however, in some cases, the size of the tumor prohibits ligation of the vein until the superior and medial sides of the gland are mobilized. When ligating the left adrenal vein, it is not necessary to trace its course to the junction with the left renal vein; however, it must be observed to enter the substance of the gland. The vein is usually approximately 1 cm in diameter and can be controlled by placing clips and then transecting it with scissors (Fig. 2). If not already done, the medial and superior portions of the gland are dissected from the perinephric fat. Most of the arteries to the adrenal gland are small and can be controlled with electrocautery or the Harmonic Scalpel; however, branches from the inferior phrenic artery can be significant and, when identified, should be ligated with clips. When the adrenal gland has been completely dissected from its bed, it is placed into a bag and removed through one of the two anterior port sites. Drainage of the area is not required routinely. The fascia at each of the 10-mm port sites is closed with a single absorbable suture, and the skin is closed with a subcuticular stitch.

For laparoscopic right adrenalectomy, the patient is positioned in the same manner as described earlier for left adrenalectomy, but with the left side down. Four ports usually are required on the right side and can be placed approximately 2 cm inferior to the costal margin in the anterior, midaxillary, and posterior axillary lines, with the fourth in the midclavicular line. A fan-shaped retractor is placed in the most medial port to retract the liver, and the laparoscope usually is placed by the second-most medial port. Dissection is begun by

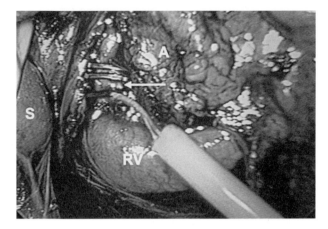

Figure 2. Left adrenal vein *(arrows)* about to be transected after clipping. A = adrenal; RV = renal vein; S = spleen.

taking down the lateral attachments of the liver so that the right lobe can be mobilized and retracted. Dissection of the adrenal gland is begun as described for left adrenalectomy. The dissection should proceed from lateral to medial and should start on the superior surface. As the dissection proceeds medially, the inferior vena cava is retracted gently medially with a blunt probe to expose its junction with the right adrenal vein, which is often short and broad (Fig. 3). Two or three clips should be left on the vena cava side. Rarely, the right adrenal vein must be ligated with an endovascular stapler. When the gland has been completely dissected free, it is removed, and surgery is completed as described for left adrenalectomy.

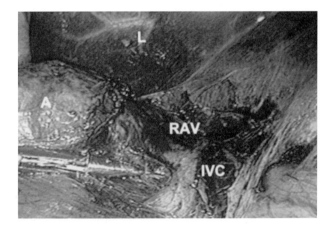

Figure 3. Dissection of the right adrenal vein. A = adrenal; RAV = right adrenal vein; IVC = inferior vena cava; L = liver.

Transperitoneal Anterior Adrenalectomy

With the anterior approach, the patient is positioned supine, and insufflation of the abdomen is achieved with the Veress needle or an open technique at the umbilicus. Two 10-mm ports are placed in the midline above the umbilicus, and two additional ports are placed in the midclavicular and anterior axillary lines 3 cm or 4 cm inferior to the costal margin on the side of the tumor. The patient can then be placed in the reverse Trendelenburg position and rotated into a hemilateral position so that the side undergoing surgery is up. For left adrenalectomy, the left colon is taken down from the splenic flexure to the sigmoid and is then retracted medially to reveal the left kidney and adrenal gland. The left renal vein is identified, and its superior border is dissected until the left adrenal vein is identified and clipped as described for the lateral approach (see Fig. 2). The adrenal gland then is removed by a circumferential dissection, with any larger vessels being clipped. The gland is removed and surgery completed as described for the lateral approach. For right adrenalectomy by the anterior transperitoneal approach, the hepatic flexure must be mobilized by taking down the hepatocolic ligament and its lateral peritoneal attachments so that it can be reflected to expose the upper pole of the right kidney, adrenal gland, and inferior vena cava. The lateral border of the inferior vena cava is traced until the right adrenal vein is identified, dissected carefully, and ligated as described for the lateral approach. The gland then is removed by dissecting it free of the surrounding adipose tissue.

Endoscopic Retroperitoneal Approach

For the endoscopic retroperitoneal approach, the patient is placed in a prone jackknife position, and the surgeon stands on the side of the patient from which the adrenal gland is to be removed. An incision is made inferior or lateral to the 12th rib, and blunt and balloon dissection is used to create the retroperitoneal space. A standard laparoscopic port then can be placed by this incision. Two or three additional laparoscopic ports then are placed under direct vision into this working space along a curve that is formed from the tips of the 11th and 12th ribs and the subcostal margin of the 10th rib. The ports should be separated from each other by at least 4 cm. Retraction of the kidney downward opens up the retroperitoneal space, and dissection is performed by the two most lateral ports with the camera in the medial one. Initial dissection is similar for both adrenal glands and is begun on the superior and lateral surfaces, proceeding medially and anteriorly by electrocautery, Harmonic Scalpel, or endoclips as necessary. As the adrenal veins are encountered, they are ligated as described for the lateral approach. When the adrenal gland has been completely dissected free of surrounding tissues, it is removed, and surgery is completed as described earlier.

Outcome

No randomized, controlled trials have compared laparoscopic with open adrenalectomy. It is unlikely one will be completed because of multiple series demonstrating the safety of the laparoscopic technique. Several small, retrospective comparisons of the two techniques have been published. The largest such study was published by Thompson et al,[36] who performed a matched, case-control study comparing 50 patients undergoing laparoscopic adrenalectomy with 50 patients undergoing open posterior adrenalectomy at a similar time. They found the operative time to be significantly longer for laparoscopic adrenalectomy than for open posterior adrenalectomy (167 min versus 127 min). The overall rate of conversion to open technique was 12%; however, a significant learning curve was found. The conversion rate for the last 43 procedures decreased to 4.5%. Laparoscopic adrenalectomy also was associated with a significant decrease in mean hospital stay (3.1 d versus 5.7 d), postoperative pain, and late morbidity (0% versus 54%).

Numerous other series confirm these results.* Overall, the reported mean operative time required for unilateral laparoscopic adrenalectomy varies from 116 minutes to 295 minutes compared with that for open adrenalectomy, from 79 minutes to 174 minutes. The mean operative time for endoscopic retroperitoneal approach ranges from 118 minutes to 150 minutes for unilateral adrenalectomy.[25, 39] Experience leads to a decrease in operative times, however.[17, 28, 35, 36] Overall, the conversion rate ranges from 0% to 14% but decreases with surgeon experience. Estimated blood loss is uniformly less with the laparoscopic compared with the open approach for adrenalectomy, ranging from 40 mL to 270 mL versus 172 mL to 408 mL, respectively. The decrease in postoperative narcotic requirements associated with laparoscopic adrenalectomy is uniform in all studies. Laparoscopic adrenalectomy is associated with a decreased length of stay. Overall, length of stay for laparoscopic adrenalectomy is significantly shorter than that for open adrenalectomy, with ranges of 1.7 days to 5 days versus 5.4 days to 9 days, respectively.

Complications associated with laparoscopic adrenalectomy are usually minor, such as port site bleeding, hematoma, subcutaneous emphysema, urinary tract infections, and deep venous thrombosis. Rarely, more severe complications occur, such as significant bleeding secondary to vena cava injury or solid-organ injuries caused by retraction or trocar insertion. Overall, intraoperative and early complication rates seem to be similar among the two procedures, ranging from 0% to 15% for the laparoscopic technique and 5% to 20% for open adrenalectomy; however, long-term morbidity is avoided with the laparoscopic approach because this technique avoids many of the wound complications, such as chronic pain, numbness, and muscle laxity that are associated with open adrenalectomy.[12, 21, 36]

ENDOCRINE TUMORS OF THE PANCREAS

Minimally invasive surgical techniques have multiple applications in pancreatic surgery, including staging, resection, and palliation of benign or malignant tumors, and pancreatic drainage procedures.[27, 38] Endocrine tumors are usually benign or slow-growing malignancies, and treatment strategies must address two goals: (1) control excess hormone production and (2) the tumor process; however, localization of these tumors may present a formidable challenge to plan for a minimally invasive approach. Selection of the specific surgical procedure for an endocrine tumor of the pancreas depends on several factors, including the functional nature of the tumor, the predilection for malignancy, whether it is sporadic or a part of the multiple endocrine neoplasia (MEN) syndrome, location and size, and relationship to major vascular structures and the pancreatic duct. Most benign pancreatic endocrine tumors are amenable to local resection or enucleation. A few such tumors require a formal anatomic resection.

---

*References 6, 12, 13, 17, 21, 25, 29, 32, 33, 35, and 36.

Specific Endocrine Tumors of the Pancreas

The most common endocrine tumor of the pancreas is insulinoma (incidence, 1/1 million population per year). It is usually a small, benign tumor (90%), so it rarely necessitates more than enucleation even if the tumor is close to the pancreatic duct. These tumors are evenly distributed throughout the pancreas. Enucleation for insulinoma in the tail of the pancreas is acceptable, but distal pancreatectomy is usually the preferred technique. The rare finding of local infiltration suggests malignancy (10%) and mandates a formal resection in the form of a pancreaticoduodenectomy or distal pancreatectomy. Blind distal pancreatectomy is not recommended in patients when a tumor cannot be found at surgery. Neuroglycopenic symptoms include headache, visual disturbance, lightheadedness, somnolence, and coma. Other symptoms include palpitations, diaphoresis, and hunger. Patients typically gain weight as they eat to control the symptoms. The diagnosis is established by a supervised, 72-hour fast. When the patient develops symptoms, the glucose, insulin, C peptide, and proinsulin levels are measured.[31] A diagnosis of insulinoma is made when the symptomatic patient has a glucose level of less than 40 mg/dL, an insulin level of more than 5 μU/mL, a proinsulin level of more than 25%, and a C peptide level of more than 1.25 ng/mL. Factitious hypoglycemia from insulin injection or oral hypoglycemic use must be ruled out by examining for insulin antibodies and screening for sulfonylureas.

In contrast to insulinoma, most gastrinomas (incidence, 1/2 million population per year) are malignant (70%). Patients without metastatic disease at diagnosis are candidates for curative resection.[1, 14, 22, 26] Sporadic gastrinomas are usually solitary tumors. Most (80%) are within the gastrinoma triangle, which includes the head and uncinate process of the pancreas (20–50%), duodenum (30–50%), and lymphatics (20–30%); however, 10% of gastrinomas may be within the body or tail of the pancreas. A gastrinoma in the head or uncinate process may be enucleated; however, resection should be done for local infiltration when no evidence of metastasis is present. A gastrinoma in the body or tail of the pancreas should be treated by distal pancreatectomy because of the probable malignant nature of the tumor.

Patients with gastrinoma typically present with refractory or complicated peptic ulcer disease (PUD). Recurrent PUD after adequate treatment (i.e., medical or surgical therapy) is an indication for an evaluation for gastrinoma. Other indications for a workup include PUD associated with hyperparathyroidism, a pediatric patient with acute PUD, and ulcers in unusual locations (e.g., the jejunum). Other manifestations include abdominal pain, diarrhea, steatorrhea, and malabsorption and malnutrition. Evaluation begins with a measurement of the fasting serum gastrin level. Omeprazole therapy must be discontinued for at least 3 days before obtaining the level; however, histamine receptor blockade can be continued. A fasting gastrin level of more than 1000 pg/mL is diagnostic, and a level of less than 100 pg/mL essentially rules out the diagnosis. Gastric analysis is useful to exclude achlorhydria. Patients with untreated gastrinoma and no history of surgery have a basal acid output level of more than 15 mEq/h and a basal acid output to maximal acid output ratio of less than 0.6. In patients with previous vagotomy or gastric resection, basal acid output level is more than 5 mEq/h. In the absence of a definitive fasting gastrin level, a secretin or calcium provocative test differentiates patients with gastrinoma from those with other causes of hypergastrinemia (e.g., pernicious anemia, G-cell hyperplasia, atrophic gastritis, omeprazole, or H_2 receptor antagonists). Secretin is given at a dose of 2 U/kg intravenously, and gastrin levels are performed at baseline, then at 2, 5, 10, 15, and 30 minutes. An increase of the gastrin level of more than 200 pg/mL over baseline is diagnostic of gastrinoma. Antacid therapy can be continued for secretin-provocative testing. Preoperative care should include confirmation of the biochemical diagnosis, exclusion of a family history of MEN, screening for pituitary and parathyroid disease, localization procedures, and optimization of the patient's acid-secretion control and nutritional status.

Other endocrine tumors of the pancreas include vasoactive intestinal polypeptide-secreting tumor (VIPoma; incidence, 1/10 million population per year), glucagonoma (incidence, 1/20 million population per year), somatostatinoma, and nonfunctioning islet cell tumors. Glucagonoma is a rare malignant islet cell tumor characterized by necrolytic migratory erythema, weight loss, type 2 diabetes mellitus, and cachexia. These patients have elevated plasma levels of glucagon (>500 pg/mL). Octreotide can provide symptomatic improvement. The VIPoma also is called *watery diarrhea, hypokalemia,* and *achlorhydria,* or the *Verner-Morrison syndrome.* These patients present with abdominal cramping, weakness, flushing, 5 L to 10 L of stool per day, and dehydration and electrolyte disturbances. The diagnosis is made when the fasting VIP level is more than 500 pg/mL in the presence of a secretory diarrhea. Other islet cell tumors are exceptional.

The exact proportion of patients with endocrine tumors that are sporadic versus part of MEN varies greatly among series but approximates 20% to 30%. Pancreatic islet cell tumors are the second most common abnormality (80%), behind hyperparathyroidism (90%), in patients with MEN. The most common islet cell tumor is gastrinoma (two thirds of pancreatic endocrine tumors associated with MEN-1), followed by insulinoma and glucagonoma, but any cell type can occur in patients with MEN. Patients with MEN and gastrinoma usually have multiple tumors, and surgical exploration in this setting is controversial. Acid hypersecretion can be controlled with proton pump inhibition. Surgical cure is the exception in MEN patients with gastrinoma, and data showing that surgery alters the natural history of the disease are lacking. In the absence of metastatic disease, most investigators recommend exploration,[23, 37] which includes enucleation of tumors in the head or uncinate process, duodenotomy, resection of enlarged lymph nodes, and distal pancreatectomy. Like patients with gastrinoma, patients with insulinoma in the setting of MEN typically have multicentric disease. Distal pancreatectomy with enucleation of lesions in the head or uncinate process is preferred.

Localization Studies

Preoperative localization of the tumor is essential for minimally invasive therapy. Islet cell tumors are classified as (1) insulinoma and (2) all others.[41] Localization of tumors, excluding insulinoma, is most accurately achieved by endoscopic sonography or somatostatin receptor scintigraphy. Endoscopic sonography has the highest resolution but is operator dependent. Somatostatin receptor scintigraphy has a high degree of sensitivity in tumors excluding insulinoma. CT has a high degree of accuracy for the detection of metastasis but is usually poor for the detection of the primary tumor. Intraoperative sonography is useful for insulinoma. Selective arterial stimulation with hepatic venous sampling using calcium or secretin can identify the region of the pancreas containing gastrinoma or insulinoma and has largely replaced portal venous sampling.

Technique

Laparoscopic surgery for endocrine pancreatic tumor resection could include enucleation, distal pancreatectomy, or pancreaticoduodenectomy. Pancreaticoduodenectomy is far more difficult than are the other two techniques and has been attempted by only a few surgeons. Little evidence shows that a laparoscopic technique has clear benefit over conventional surgery, and safety concerns likely limit this approach to a few, select surgical teams.[16]

The laparoscopic approach to islet cell tumors should proceed in an orderly fashion.[10] Laparoscopy is performed with the patient under general anesthesia. The patient is supine on the surgical table, with the surgeon on the right side of the pancreas. Pneumoperitoneum is accomplished with a Veress needle or by open laparoscopy. Initially, four ports are placed to allow for staging of the tumor (Fig. 4). An exploration of the peritoneal cavity is performed to exclude peritoneal spread. A 30° laparoscope assists with adequate visualization. The patient then is placed in the reverse Trendelenburg position with 10° of left lateral tilt. The anterior and posterior surfaces of both lobes of the liver are inspected for evidence of metastatic disease. Correct positioning of the 30° laparoscope allows for inspection of the foramen of Winslow for enlarged periportal lymph nodes. The greater curve of the stomach is grasped and lifted, allowing the surgeon to open the gastrocolic ligament. The Harmonic Scapel assists with rapid, bloodless exposure of the pancreas. Adhesions from the posterior surface of the stomach to the pancreas are taken down to allow for full exposure. The window in the gastrocolic ligament must be wide. A Kocher maneuver is done to allow for a full view of the proximal duodenum and

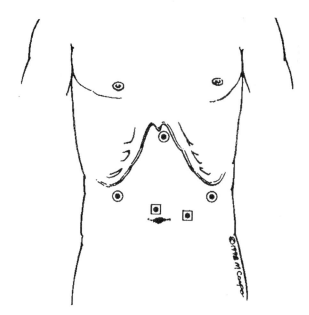

Figure 4. Five-millimeter (*circles*) and 10-mm (*squares*) port placement for laparoscopic exploration of the pancreas. (*From* Park A, Schwartz R, Tandan V, et al: Laparoscopic pancreatic surgery. Am J Surg 177(2):158–163, 1999; with permission.)

peripancreatic lymph nodes. When exposure has been achieved, superficial tumors can be visualized to confirm the preoperative localization. A 7.5-MHz laparoscopic sonography probe is used to inspect all areas of the pancreas if the tumor is not seen on inspection. When the tumor has been localized, it can be enucleated from the surrounding pancreas, or a distal pancreatectomy with or without splenic preservation is performed.

Distal pancreatic resection can be performed with the patient in the supine position. A wedge can be placed under the patient to elevate the left side. The patient is secured to the table to avoid movement with shift in the table position. Access to the abdomen is gained through multiple upper abdominal cannulas (Fig. 4). The laparoscope is placed through an umbilical port. Exposure of the distal pancreas is done as described earlier by opening the gastrocolic attachments. Retractors are placed to elevate the stomach and depress the colon. The surgical table can be placed into the reverse Trendelenburg, with the left side up to enhance exposure. Laparoscopic sonography of the distal pancreas then can be performed to locate the tumor. Mobilization of the pancreas is begun by incising along the inferior border of the pancreas. A combination of blunt and sonographic dissection is used to help to mobilize the distal pancreas. If necessary, the dissection is carried distal to the spleen, and the splenic attachments to the diaphragm, colon, kidney, and pancreas are divided, which allows for full mobilization of the distal pancreas. Enucleation of a lesion can be done with a sonographic cavitation device. The tumor can be placed into an endoscopic bag for removal from the peritoneal cavity. If formal resection is required, the tail of the pancreas is dissected free of the splenic artery and vein (Fig. 5). A laparoscopic stapling device is placed across the distal pancreas proximal to the tumor (Fig. 6). The staple line can be oversewn to reinforce closure of the pancreatic duct.

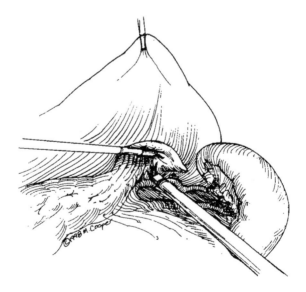

Figure 5. Dissection of the tail of the pancreas away from the splenic artery and vein. (*From* Park A, Schwartz R, Tandan V, et al: Laparoscopic pancreatic surgery. Am J Surg 177(2):158–163, 1999; with permission.)

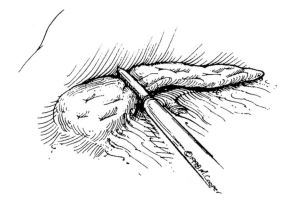

Figure 6. Laparoscopic stapling of the distal pancreas. (*From* Park A, Schwartz R, Tandan V, et al: Laparoscopic pancreatic surgery. Am J Surg 177(2):158–163, 1999; with permission.)

Outcome

Evidence in favor of laparoscopic surgery for treatment of pancreatic endocrine tumor comes from small series and case reports.[9, 11, 18, 38] The largest experience is by Gagner et al,[16] who reported on 10 Whipple procedures, 9 distal pancreatectomies, and 4 endocrine tumor enucleations. Of these, eight distal pancreatectomies were for islet cell tumors. The conversion rate for distal pancreatectomy or enucleation was 36%, and the mean operative time was 4.5 hours for laparoscopic distal pancreatectomy and 3 hours for laparoscopic enucleation. The mean hospital stay was 5 days and 4 days, respectively. All of the Whipple procedures were done for cancer. In this group, the rate of conversion to an open procedure was 40%. The average operative time was 8.5 hours, and the mean hospital stay was 22.3 days, so the benefit of a laparoscopic approach seems less obvious.

SUMMARY

Laparoscopic adrenalectomy quickly has become the procedure of choice for benign adrenal lesions because it results in less pain, shorter hospital stay, comparable safety, and more patient satisfaction overall. The laparoscopic approach requires advanced laparoscopic surgical skills. Surgeons should be familiar with these techniques and the open approaches before attempting this procedure. When first learning the technique, small left-sided lesions are likely the easiest, and a more experienced surgeon should be present for the initial few cases; however, at this point, the laparoscopic approach to pancreatic endocrine tumors does not have a clear benefit, and it should be considered primarily investigational without clearly established benefits.

References

1. Alexander HR, Bartlett DL, Venzon DJ, et al: Analysis of factors associated with long-term (five or more years) cure in patients undergoing operation for Zollinger-Ellison syndrome. Surgery 124:1160–1166, 1998

2. Angeli A, Osella G, Ali A, et al: Adrenal incidentaloma: An overview of clinical and epidemiological data from the National Italian Study Group. Horm Res 47:279–283, 1997
3. Barresi RV, Prinz RA: Laparoscopic adrenalectomy. Arch Surg 134:212–217, 1999
4. Barry MK, van Heerden JA, Farley DR, et al: Can adrenal incidentalomas be safely observed? World J Surg 22:599–604, 1998
5. Barzon L, Scaroni C, Sonino N, et al: Risk factors and long-term follow-up of adrenal incidentalomas. J Clin Endocrinol Metab 84:520–526, 1999
6. Brunt LM, Doherty GM, Norton JA, et al: Laparoscopic adrenalectomy compared to open adrenalectomy for benign adrenal neoplasms. J Am Coll Surg 183:1–10, 1996
7. Candel AG, Gattuso P, Reyes CV, et al: Fine-needle aspiration biopsy of adrenal masses in patients with extraadrenal malignancy. Surgery 114:1132–1137, 1993
8. Casola G, Nicolet V, vanSonnenberg E, et al: Unsuspected pheochromocytoma: Risk of blood-pressure alterations during percutaneous adrenal biopsy. Radiology 159:733–735, 1986
9. Chapuis Y, Bigourdan JM, Massault PP, et al: Videolaparoscopic excision of insulinoma: A study of 5 cases. Chirurgie 123:461–467, 1998
10. Conlon KC, Dougherty E, Klimstra DS, et al: The value of minimal access surgery in the staging of patients with potentially resectable peripancreatic malignancy. Ann Surg 223:134–140, 1996
11. Dexter SP, Martin IG, Leindler L, et al: Laparoscopic enucleation of a solitary pancreatic insulinoma. Surg Endosc 13:406–408, 1999
12. Dudley NE, Harrison BJ: Comparison of open posterior versus transperitoneal laparoscopic adrenalectomy. Br J Surg 86:656–660, 1999
13. Duh QY, Siperstein AE, Clark OH, et al: Laparoscopic adrenalectomy: Comparison of the lateral and posterior approaches. Arch Surg 131:870–876, 1996
14. Fraker DL, Norton JA, Alexander HR, et al: Surgery in Zollinger-Ellison syndrome alters the natural history of gastrinoma. Ann Surg 220:320–330, 1994
15. Gagner M, Lacroix A, Bolte E: Laparoscopic adrenalectomy in Cushing's syndrome and pheochromocytoma. N Engl J Med 327:1033, 1992
16. Gagner M, Pomp A: Laparoscopic pancreatic resection: Is it worthwhile? J Gastrointest Surg 1:20–26, 1997
17. Gagner M, Pomp A, Heniford BT, et al: Laparoscopic adrenalectomy: Lessons learned from 100 consecutive procedures. Ann Surg 226:238–247, 1997
18. Gagner M, Pomp A, Herrera MF: Early experience with laparoscopic resections of islet cell tumors. Surgery 120:1051–1054, 1996
19. Graham DJ, McHenry CR: The adrenal incidentaloma: Guidelines for evaluation and recommendations for management. Surg Oncol Clin North Am 7:749–764, 1998
20. Heniford BT, Lannitti DA, Hale J, et al: The role of intraoperative ultrasonography during laparoscopic adrenalectomy. Surgery 122:1068–1074, 1997
21. Imai T, Kikumori T, Ohiwa M, et al: A case-controlled study of laparoscopic compared with open lateral adrenalectomy. Am J Surg 178:50–54, 1999
22. Jensen RT, Fraker DL: Zollinger-Ellison syndrome: Advances in treatment of gastric hypersecretion and the gastrinoma. JAMA 271:1429–1435, 1994
23. MacFarlane MP, Fraker DL, Alexander HR, et al: Prospective study of surgical resection of duodenal and pancreatic gastrinomas in multiple endocrine neoplasia type 1. Surgery 118:973–980, 1995
24. Mantero F, Masini AM, Opocher G, et al: Adrenal incidentaloma: An overview of hormonal data from the National Italian Study Group. Horm Res 47:284–289, 1997
25. Mercan S, Seven R, Ozarmagan S, et al: Endoscopic retroperitoneal adrenalectomy. Surgery 118:1071–1076, 1995
26. Norton JA, Fraker DL, Alexander HR, et al: Surgery to cure the Zollinger-Ellison syndrome. N Engl J Med 341:635–644, 1999
27. Park A, Schwartz R, Tandan V, et al: Laparoscopic pancreatic surgery. Am J Surg 177:158–163, 1999
28. Prinz RA: A comparison of laparoscopic and open adrenalectomies. Arch Surg 130:489–494, 1995
29. Prinz RA: Laparoscopic adrenalectomy. J Am Coll Surg 183:71–73, 1996

30. Ross NS, Aron DC: Hormonal evaluation of the patient with an incidentally discovered adrenal mass. N Engl J Med 323:1401–1405, 1990
31. Service FJ: Hypoglycemic disorders. N Engl J Med 332:1144–1152, 1995
32. Shen WT, Lim RC, Siperstein AE, et al: Laparoscopic vs open adrenalectomy for the treatment of primary hyperaldosteronism. Arch Surg 134:628–632, 1999
33. Smith CD, Weber CJ, Amerson JR: Laparoscopic adrenalectomy: New gold standard. World J Surg 23:389–396, 1999
34. Staren ED, Prinz RA: Selection of patients with adrenal incidentalomas for operation. Surg Clin North Am 75:499–509, 1995
35. Takeda M, Go H, Imai T, et al: Laparoscopic adrenalectomy for primary aldosteronism: Report of initial ten cases. Surgery 115:621–625, 1994
36. Thompson GB, Grant CS, van Heerden JA, et al: Laparoscopic versus open posterior adrenalectomy: A case-control study of 100 patients. Surgery 122:1132–1136, 1997
37. Thompson NW: Management of pancreatic endocrine tumors in patients with multiple endocrine neoplasia type 1. Surg Oncol Clin North Am 7:881–891, 1998
38. Underwood RA, Soper NJ: Current status of laparoscopic surgery of the pancreas. J Hepatobiliary Pancreat Surg 6:154–164, 1999
39. Walz MK, Peitgen K, Saller B, et al: Subtotal adrenalectomy by the posterior retroperitoneoscopic approach. World J Surg 22:621–627, 1998
40. Wells SA, Merke DP, Cutler GB Jr, et al: Therapeutic controversy: The role of laparoscopic surgery in adrenal disease. J Clin Endocrinol Metab 83:3041–3049, 1998
41. Wiedenmann B, Jensen RT, Mignon M, et al: Preoperative diagnosis and surgical management of neuroendocrine gastroenteropancreatic tumors: General recommendations by a consensus workshop. World J Surg 22:309–318, 1998

Address reprint requests to

Robert C. McIntyre, Jr, MD
Department of Surgery
The University of Colorado Health Sciences Center
4200 East Ninth Avenue
Box C313
Denver, CO 80262

e-mail: robert.mcintyre@uchsc.edu

ADVANCED LAPAROSCOPIC GYNECOLOGIC SURGERY

G. Rodney Meeks, MD

Laparoscopic sterilization was the breakthrough procedure that showed the utility of surgical laparoscopy. Next, laparoscopy made an impact on gynecologic surgery by reducing the need for laparotomy in treatment of endometriosis, pelvic adhesions, and ectopic pregnancy. The technical feasibility of performing hysterectomy with laparoscopic assistance was first shown in 1989 by Reich et al,[38] who used electrocautery to perform a hysterectomy with laparoscopic assistance in a woman who had endometriosis and severe pelvic adhesions. In 1990, Nezhat et al[28] described a second case of laparoscopically assisted hysterectomy but used miniaturized staples. In 1993, a laparoscopic colposuspension technique to correct urinary incontinence was described.[22] Laparoscopic techniques to correct pelvic organ prolapse also have been described.[19, 23, 29, 46]

Expansion of the types of procedures done with laparoscopic assistance has been made possible by improvements in video endoscopy. Xenon vapor bulbs, which provide excellent illumination; the three-chip camera, which separates red, green, and blue colors; and the high-definition monitor, which significantly enhances image quality, are a few of the major developments. An array of laparoscopic surgical instruments has allowed surgeons to perform ever-more sophisticated procedures endoscopically. Laparoscopy, fueled by broadened indications and refinement of surgical technique, has become the most commonly performed surgery in the United States.

PREPARING THE PATIENT FOR LAPAROSCOPIC GYNECOLOGIC SURGERY

Patient Positioning

Just as with traditional laparotomy, proper positioning ensures adequate exposure for surgery and minimizes pressure on skin, nerves, bony prominences,

From the Department of Obstetrics and Gynecology, University of Mississippi Medical Center, Jackson, Mississippi and joints. Unique to gynecologic surgery is the need for access to the perineum and vagina. Because lithotomy allows for exposure to these areas, it is the most commonly used surgical position. Low and high lithotomy may be instituted. The patient's buttocks should be positioned at the edge of the surgical table. Leg supports with boot stirrups, such as Allen Universal stirrups (Allen Medical Systems, Mayfield, OH), which can be adjusted during the procedure without contaminating the surgical field, are a great convenience. The legs should be flexed at the knee and the feet secured in boot stirrups. Compression of the calves should be alleviated during positioning. If one envisions the patient standing on her feet, this would mimic the position of the feet in the stirrups. The thighs should be flexed so that the knees are positioned slightly superior to the iliac crest, which prevents the knees from blocking the surgical field. The thighs are abducted sufficiently to allow access to the lower abdominal quadrants and to allow an assistant to stand comfortably between them (Fig. 1). This position maximizes the surgeon's space and mobility of the instruments. When additional perineal exposure is needed to complete a procedure through the vagina or to repair the posterior vaginal compartment and perineal body, the legs can be shifted to the high lithotomy position.

A surgical table that accommodates the patient's arms being at the sides or in the traditional extended position allows the surgeon to be positioned as comfortably as possible at the surgical table. After the patient is satisfactorily positioned, she can be prepped with antiseptic solution in a traditional fashion from the upper abdomen to the perineum, including the vagina and rectum. A urethral catheter is inserted. Lastly, placing the patient in the Trendelenburg position after the trocars are placed helps to keep the bowel out of the pelvis.

Vaginal Manipulators

Even subtle changes in uterine or vaginal position may make dissection and suturing easier by optimizing the angles for the laparoscopic instruments. Uter-

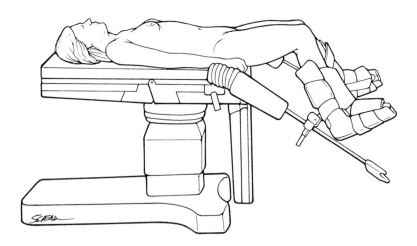

Figure 1. Patient positioning. The patient is positioned with universal stirrups. The thigh is flexed slightly so that the knees are slightly higher than the pubic symphysis and abducted approximately 45° from the midline.

ine manipulators are effective for elevating the uterus, which places tissue on tension. They also allow the uterus to be manipulated from side to side, which optimizes exposure of the broad ligament, the uterine vessels, and the uterosacral cardinal ligament complex. Some of the more popular uterine manipulators are the olive-tipped (R. Wolf, Vernon Hills, IL), Hasson (Aesculap, San Francisco, CA), and HUMI (Cooper Surgical, Shelton, CT) cannulas and the Hulka (R. Wolf, Vervon Hills, IL) tenaculum. A moistened sponge attached to a sponge forceps can be helpful in distending the anterior vaginal fornix and posterior cul-de-sac. Distending the anterior vaginal fornix makes creation of the bladder flap easier because the tissue planes are placed on tension and helps to identify the attachment of the vagina to the cervix, where the anterior colpotomy is made. Distending the posterior cul-de-sac helps with the identification of the rectovaginal septum and creation of the posterior colpotomy. The position of the rectum can be defined by placing a rectal probe. Clearly delineating these structures may reduce the risk for rectal trauma.

Correction of pelvic organ prolapse requires that the apex of the vagina be elevated in the pelvis. Placement of a Lucite (Miltex, Lake Success, NY) cylinder or metal rectal sizer into the vagina accomplishes this maneuver nicely. Also, the surgeon's fingers can be used to manipulate the vagina to better expose the supporting fascia of the vagina and to better position the vagina for suturing and knot tying. A rectal probe is helpful during prolapse surgery involving the cul-de-sac.

Trocars

Trocars provide various sites of entry into the abdominal cavity. Some combination of 5-mm and 10-mm trocars usually is needed for adequate exposure to accomplish the surgical procedure. Occasionally, a 12- to 15-mm port is needed. The first trocar usually is inserted at the umbilicus, which is the thinnest portion of the abdominal wall. A 5-mm or 10-mm trocar can be inserted as needed to accommodate a lens; however, with a 5-mm lens, the camera port can be changed to use any of the trocar sites. The primary trocar may be inserted directly or after establishment of pneumoperitoneum. One technique does not seem to have an advantage over the other.

For most laparoscopic procedures, a minimum of three trocar ports must be inserted, but a fourth or fifth ancillary port (or even more) may be needed based on the needs of the patient. Often, one port is placed in a midline suprapubic position. Caution must be exercised to avoid bladder injury by inserting the suprapubic port at least 5 cm superior to the pubic symphysis. Lateral ports must avoid the epigastric vessels. Localization of the epigastric vessels can be achieved by transillumination to see the course of vessels in the abdominal wall. Direct visualization of the vessels as they run just posterior to the surface of the peritoneum is possible with the laparoscope. The trocars can be inserted in a manner to avoid these vessels. Lower abdominal trocars are placed approximately 1 cm to 2 cm superior to the pubic rami and lateral to the epigastric vessels. Midabdominal trocars should be inserted lateral to the border of the rectus abdominis muscle (Fig. 2). Using these sites provides adequate access to the pelvis while providing protection to the major abdominal wall vasculature.

SURGICAL LAPAROSCOPIC PROCEDURES

For the most part, a patient is prepared for surgery as described earlier without regard to the specific procedure that she will undergo. The first step for

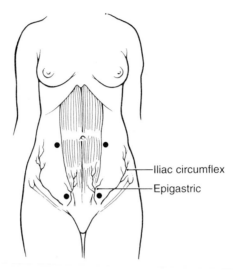

Figure 2. Abdominal wall anatomy. Trocar sites are located to avoid the epigastric and circumflex iliac vessels.

all procedures is a thorough inspection of the abdomen and pelvis. The anatomy should be defined. Recognized trauma should be repaired, and significant adhesions should be lysed before surgery.

HYSTERECTOMY

Approximately 75% of hysterectomies are performed by the abdominal route, whereas 25% are performed by the vaginal route.[49] The percentage of vaginal hysterectomies has decreased over the past decade. Historically, patients who have a history of pelvic adhesions, chronic pain, pelvic inflammatory disease, or prior surgery or an adnexal mass are candidates to have hysterectomy performed by the abdominal route. Laparoscopy enables the surgeon to evaluate a patient with one or more of these contraindications before determining the route of hysterectomy. No absolute indications for laparoscopically assisted vaginal hysterectomy (LAVH) exist, and preoperative selection criteria are still evolving. Unfortunately, few studies have addressed candidacy for routes of hysterectomy. Available studies provide only minimal information regarding the decision-making process for selection of the route of hysterectomy.[17]

In 1990, Kovac et al[16] assessed a group of women believed to be candidates for abdominal hysterectomy because of a contraindication to vaginal hysterectomy. They wanted to determine whether laparoscopy performed immediately before hysterectomy could be used to alter the planned route of hysterectomy. Of this group of women, 91% underwent vaginal hysterectomy without complications. They concluded that laparoscopy may allow more hysterectomies to be performed by the vaginal route by eliminating some of the reasons that hysterectomies are traditionally performed abdominally; however, no portion of the hysterectomy was completed with laparoscopy. Although Kovac et al used the laparoscope only to inspect the pelvis, others[20, 28, 38, 40] have advocated total laparoscopic hysterectomy.

LAVH does not define a single technique. A classification system to define the portion of the hysterectomy done during the laparoscopy may be helpful. Unfortunately, consensus has not been reached regarding a universal classification system to define the extent to which laparoscopy is used for LAVH. One proposed classification system with five levels of LAVH includes:

Level 0: Laparoscopy is used to inspect the pelvis, but no portion of the hysterectomy is done.

Level I: Laparoscopy is used up to but excluding the uterine arteries, which may include adhesiolysis and ligation of the ovarian vessels.

Level II: The ovarian vessels are transected.

Level III: At least a portion of the uterosacral cardinal ligament complex is dissected through the laparoscope.

Level IV: The entire uterosacral cardinal ligament complex is taken through the laparoscope and anterior or posterior colpotomy incisions are created. Total laparoscopic hysterectomy is included.

A classification system for LAVH may allow for communication among surgeons and collection of meaningful data. Data collection also may allow for critical analysis of benefits and risks of this alternative, analysis of data among institutions, and facilitation of education in a stepwise fashion.

INDICATIONS FOR LAPAROSCOPICALLY ASSISTED VAGINAL HYSTERECTOMY

The indications for hysterectomy must not be confused with indications for route of hysterectomy. This discussion centers on the route of hysterectomy. Some of the indications for laparoscopic hysterectomy include:

Documented endometriosis
Known pelvic adhesions
Cystic adnexal mass with indications for hysterectomy
Prior major pelvic surgery
Inadequate bony pelvis
Inadequate mobility of the uterus
Stage I endometrial cancer

Documented endometriosis has been an indication for abdominal hysterectomy to assess the extent of the lesions, lyse adhesions, destroy endometriotic implants, and remove the ovaries. Abdominal hysterectomy also was favored because the extent of disease could not be predicted. LAVH allows the surgeon to address these issues. LAVH may be especially good for stage III and stage IV endometriosis, which may be associated with extensive adhesions and endometriomas.[11]

Cystic adnexal masses have been addressed with abdominal hysterectomy because of the need to assess the remainder of the abdomen and possibly obtain biopsy specimens from other tissues; however, most masses are not malignant; therefore, excision of the cyst or entire ovary is adequate therapy. Both can be done with laproscopic assistance. The mass can be well visualized with laparoscopy, and the laparoscopic approach may be especially appropriate if the adnexal structures require extensive dissection before removal.[34] When the adnexal mass has been excised, it can be sent for pathologic evaluation. If evaluation reveals a malignant tumor, the laparoscopic approach should be converted to laparotomy with appropriate staging. LAVH is not always indicated when oophorectomy is necessary because Sheth[41] was able to remove 94% of ovaries by the vaginal route when indicated.

One indication for abdominal hysterectomy is prior surgery, primarily because of the concern for adhesions; however, Coulum and Pratt[10] demonstrated that prior surgery did not preclude vaginal hysterectomy. Even patients who had previous uterine suspension or cesarean sections could undergo the vaginal route, although the degree of dissection required could be extensive. The adhesions may be lysed more easily with LAVH. The route of hysterectomy also has been dictated by known adhesions. Just as with endometriosis and prior surgery, adhesiolysis can be accomplished with the laparoscope and the uterus addressed with LAVH.

Lack of uterine descent had been an indication for abdominal hysterectomy. The concern was that the upper pedicles may not be accessible. LAVH may overcome this problem; however, Mengert[26] showed that, until the cardinal ligaments and uterosacral ligaments are transected, descent of the uterus will not improve. LAVH does not normally improve mobility and descent of the uterus unless the uterosacral cardinal ligament complex is incised. LAVH cannot overcome limited vaginal space.

Endometrial cancer has been an indication for abdominal hysterectomy so that intra-abdominal tissue can be assessed and pelvic lymph nodes sampled for biopsy. Reports of vaginal hysterectomy for stage I endometrial cancer stimulated interest in LAVH. Using LAVH for stage I endometrial cancer is promising because of a clear advantage to sampling the lymph nodes in planning adjunctive therapy.[8, 37] The nodes can be sampled laparoscopically.

Uterine leiomyomata are not listed on the indications for LAVH because an injury to the uterus or to the uterine supporting structures may be present. Surgeons have not yet been able to convert transabdominal to vaginal hysterectomy for large uteri.[3] Vaginal morcellation techniques may be better if uterine size is less than 16 weeks. Uterine enlargement in excess of 16 weeks may directly limit visualization because of the mass effect. Leiomyoma is one of the most common indications for abdominal hysterectomy. When uterine weight is compared, LAVH is nearer to vaginal hysterectomy than to abdominal hysterectomy.

TECHNIQUE FOR LAPAROSCOPICALLY ASSISTED VAGINAL HYSTERECTOMY

The hysterectomy is started with the laparoscopic portion as described in the levels of hysterectomy (Fig. 3). Hemostasis can be obtained with extracorporal suture, the ultrasonic scalpel, computerized bipolar cautery, or traditional bipolar cautery. The Döderline hysterectomy technique, which uses an anterior colpotomy for initial entry into the peritoneal cavity, and the Heaney technique, which uses the posterior colpotomy, can be used to complete the vaginal portion of the hysterectomy.[40]

COMPARISON OF LAPAROSCOPICALLY ASSISTED VAGINAL HYSTERECTOMY, VAGINAL HYSTERECTOMY, AND ABDOMINAL HYSTERECTOMY

No studies have compared all three techniques simultaneously in a prospective manner, so assessment is dependent on reports comparing only two tech-

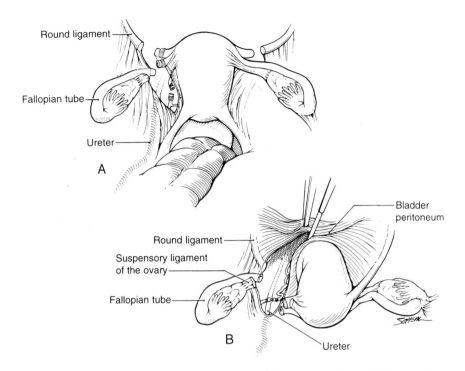

Figure 3. Laparoscopically assisted hysterectomy. *A,* The round ligament is transected. Next, the tube and suspensory ligament of the ovary are transected. *B,* The bladder peritoneum is opened.

niques and on review articles.[25] Surgical time is longer with LAVH than with abdominal hysterectomy, although the length of time necessary for the procedure is decreasing with increased surgeon experience.[3, 32, 36] Longer surgical suite time, use of disposable instruments, and the startup cost associated with purchasing highly technical equipment may make the procedure less cost-efficient than traditional surgery.[15, 32, 36] Increased cost seemed to be related to disposable staples. The shorter hospital stay may offset the higher cost associated with laparoscopy.[3] Blood loss with LAVH is no different than with abdominal hysterectomy.[7, 15] Pain scores and requirement for postoperative pain medication are less after LAVH.[7] When the overall rate of complications is compared between these two techniques, differences are not obvious; however, the incidence of ureteral injury may be higher.[50]

In retrospective reviews of LAVH and vaginal hysterectomy, less operative pain, less need for postoperative analgesia, earlier ambulation, lower instance of postoperative fever, and shorter hospital stays occur with LAVH; however, these advantages have come with longer surgical suite times and an overall more expensive procedure.[5, 33] Other purported advantages include easier adnexectomies; better ability to inspect the pelvis and abdomen; and superior adhesiolysis, especially those formed with prior surgery.[20, 27, 33] Only one randomized trial has compared these two routes of hysterectomy.[44] Surgery and anesthesia times were longer for LAVH. Estimated blood loss was greater for vaginal hysterectomy.

No significant difference was found for postoperative fever. LAVH required more pain medication, had a lower hematocrit (unexplained because less blood loss seemed to occur), and the cost was more with LAVH, probably owing to disposable staples, increased surgical suite time, and increased anesthesia time. The incidence of ureteral injury may be higher with LAVH.[50]

PELVIC ORGAN PROLAPSE AND URINARY INCONTINENCE

Pelvic organ prolapse is an encompassing term for several conditions associated with loss of support for the vagina and uterus. Clinically, the anatomic defects are described as cystocele, enterocele, rectocele, urethrocele, and uterine descensus. These support defects also are associated with hypermobility of the urethrovesical junction, which results in urinary incontinence. Before describing surgical techniques to repair these defects, a short primer is warranted to better understand the mechanism of pelvic organ support and continence.

The anatomic supports of the vagina and uterus are the levator ani muscles, endopelvic fascia, and perineal body. Support does not come from the vaginal epithelium. The levator ani are striated muscles under voluntary control and form a "trampoline" across the pelvic outlet. When neurologically intact, they provide support by contracting with the sudden increases in intra-abdominal pressure. A layer of endopelvic fascia encircles the vagina and is contiguous with the other fascia in the pelvis, both of which are composed of fibromuscular tissue. The area that supports the bladder is called the *pubocervical fascia*. The area that supports the rectum is called the *rectovaginal fascia*. These fasciae are attached to the pelvic sidewall at the arcus tendineus fasciae pelvis. Condensation of the endopelvic fascia forms the uterosacral cardinal ligament complex, which attaches to the cervix, pelvic sidewall, and sacrum. This fascia provides passive support. It is resilient, but a sudden burst of pressure, such as with childbirth, can tear the fascia or pull it away from the pelvic sidewall. Steady pressure on the fascia may cause it to become attenuated, and it can be stretched to the point of breaking. The perineal body creates a dam on which the vagina rests. Because this area is not addressed laparoscopically, it is not discussed further.

The fascia of the vagina is separated into three levels.[12] The upper third of the vagina is suspended by the uterosacral cardinal ligament complex to the sacrum and pelvic sidewall. A defect in the suspensory portion of the vagina results in prolapse of the uterus or of the vaginal cuff in women who have had a hysterectomy, which clinically is an enterocele. The middle third of the vagina is attached to the lateral pelvic sidewall at the arcus tendineus fasciae pelvis. A defect here results in prolapse of the anterior vaginal wall, clinically a cystocele, or the posterior vaginal wall, clinically a rectocele. The lower third of the vagina is fused with the pubococcygeus muscles. Detachment of the anterior fascia from the pubococcygeus portion of the levator ani muscles is uncommon but may occur after radical vulvectomy. When present, it results in hypermobility of the urethra. Detachment of the posterior rectovaginal fascia allows the posterior vaginal wall to bulge, clinically a low rectocele. For the most part, repair of prolapse must focus on repairing the fascia.

Defects in support of the upper third of the vagina may be corrected using the McCall culdoplasty, sacrospinous ligament fixation, and abdominal sacral colpopexy. Prolapse of the middle third of the vagina may be corrected using the paravaginal repair. Prolapse of the anterior lower third of the vagina may be corrected by reattachment of the superior sulcus of the vagina to the medial margin of the pubococcygeus muscle fascia. Prolapse of the posterior lower third of the vagina is associated with detachment of the rectovaginal fascia from the perineal body. The rectovaginal fascia can be reapproximated to the perineum during vaginal perineoplasty. A rectocele may be repaired by opening the rectovaginal space. Because rectocele is approached vaginally, it is not discussed further.

Three types of urinary incontinence exist: (1) stress incontinence, (2) detrusor instability, and (3) overflow. Stress urinary incontinence may improve with surgery, but the other two do not. Therefore, an accurate diagnosis is imperative. Two types of stress urinary incontinence exist: (1) one associated with hypermobility of the urethrovesical junction (bladder neck), often called *genuine stress urinary incontinence,* and (2) intrinsic sphincter deficiency. Stress incontinence is much more common than is sphincter deficiency.

The urethra lies on pubocervical fascia, which stretches between the pelvic sidewalls at the level of the arcus tendineus fasciae pelvis. The intact fascia creates a hammock, which allows the urethra to be compressed with increased abdominal pressure. If the fascia becomes detached, torn, or stretched, it may no longer provide support, and the urethra rotates inferiorly. Urethral rotation can be demonstrated by placing a cotton-tipped swab in the urethra and using the Valsalva maneuver. Movement of the swab shows the rotational changes of the urethra. Women with genuine stress urinary incontinence lose urine with coughing, laughing, or other events associated with increased intra-abdominal pressure. The function is compromised because of displacement of the urethrovesical junction and proximal urethra. With coughing or other causes of increased intra-abdominal pressure, the ratio of intra-abdominal pressure transmitted to the urethra compared with the bladder is low.

Surgery To Treat Incontinence

The goal of incontinence surgery is a reduction of the hypermobility and restoration of normal anatomy at the urethrovesical junction and proximal urethra. Surgery for urethral hypermobility has evolved. The retropubic procedures are the most popular, based on the belief that these procedures have excellent immediate results and better long-term durability than do other approaches. The Tanagho[45] modification of the Burch colposuspension is probably the most commonly used technique. In this procedure, no dissection is carried out within 2 cm of the urethra or bladder neck. The fatty tissue along the lateral aspect of the vaginal fornix is removed. This allows fibrosis to occur. Sutures are tied loosely to avoid necrosis of the fascia and to avoid compression or kinking of the urethra.

The surgical technique for the Tanagho modification of the Burch procedure is as follows:

1. A urethral catheter should be placed. Because the balloon helps to identify the urethrovesical junction, some surgeons advocate the use of a 30-mL balloon, which may be easier to palpate than a 5-c^3 balloon.
2. Indigo carmine may be placed in the bladder, and the catheter is then clamped. Leakage of dye into the surgical field alerts the surgeon to a possible bladder perforation.
3. Five trocars are placed. The primary trocar usually is placed in an intraumbilical location. A trocar is placed lateral to the epigastric arteries and approximately 1 cm or 2 cm cephalad to the inguinal ligament in

each of the lower quadrants of the abdomen. An additional trocar is placed in the midabdomen, approximately 1 cm to 2 cm inferior to the umbilical incision and at the lateral border of each rectus muscle.

4. After the cul-de-sac is obliterated, the parietal peritoneum between the lateral umbilical ligaments is incised approximately 3 cm superior to the pubic symphysis (Fig. 4). It is dissected away from the anterior abdominal wall toward the pubic bone, and the retropubic space is entered.

5. The following anatomic landmarks are identified: the pubic symphysis, Cooper's ligaments, the obturator neurovascular bundle (aberrant obturator vessels are seen), the obturator foramina, the arcus tendineus fasciae pelvis, and the arcus tendineus fascia levator ani.

6. The bladder is mobilized medially to reveal the paravesical fat, which is dissected away from the pearly white pubocervical fascia, where sutures are placed. Caution is exercised to avoid dissection within 2 cm of the urethra.

7. The optimal locus for suture placement is at the level of the midurethra and urethrovesical junction. The urethra may be identified by palpating the catheter, and the urethrovesical junction can be identified by palpating the catheter balloon. The surgeon can identify these sites by placing the index and middle fingers of the nondominant hand in the vagina. Both fingers are initially placed on the same side of the urethra, and then the fingers are pushed superiorly.

8. A suture is passed through Cooper's ligament immediately superior to the location where it will pass through the anterior vaginal wall fascia. A double loop of suture is passed through on the fascia approximately 2 cm lateral to the midurethra. Tenting the fascia helps to identify the proper loci for placing the sutures and to better view the bladder. Placing the pubocervical fascia on tension helps to drive the suture needle through the fascia. The suture is again passed through Cooper's

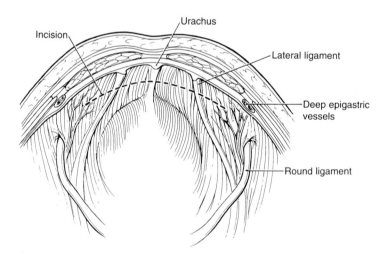

Figure 4. Peritoneal incision. The peritoneal incision is made 2 to 3 cm above the bladder and extended laterally to the deep epigastric vessels. The retropubic space is developed.

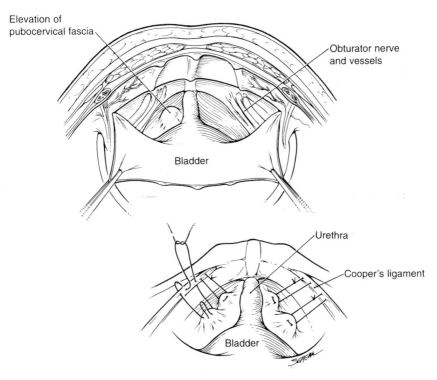

Figure 5. Burch colposuspension. After the retropubic space is opened, the pubocervical fascia is elevated so that sutures may be placed. The sutures are passed through Cooper's ligament and tied.

ligament. A similar technique is used to place a suture at the level of the urethrovesical junction but lateral to the first midurethral suture. This step is carried out bilaterally. Permanent suture material, such as nylon or dacron, is most commonly used. Protective devices for the surgeon's fingers lower the risk for needle sticks (Fig. 5).

9. The suture knots are tied extracorporeally and tightened with a knot pusher.
10. The bladder may be inspected with cystoscopy to ensure that no sutures have been passed through the detrusor muscle. Efflux of indigo carmine dye documents ureteral patency.
11. Lastly, the bladder is drained with an indwelling urethral or suprapubic catheter because normal micturition is disrupted temporarily.

Success of the Burch retropubic urethropexy is dependent on stabilizing the pubocervical fascia, which supports the urethra. Determining the correct degree of tension in these sutures and the urethrovesical angle is subjective and continues to be the art of the procedure. If the urethrovesical junction is pulled too high, the urethra may be kinked, which interferes with normal urine flow. Some quantitative measures may help with this determination. When tied properly, the supporting sutures form loops and do not approximate Cooper's ligament and fascia. When a cotton-tipped swab is placed into the urethra, it should be horizontal to the floor or point slightly upward and should have some mobility.

In 1995, Liu[21] reported long-term results of laparoscopic procedures. Sixty-five percent of patients stated that they were markedly improved. Twenty-four percent stated that they continued to have leak but were better than before surgery. Ten percent reported that they were not improved. These data are comparable with those reported for open Burch colposuspension.

CORRECTION OF PELVIC ORGAN PROLAPSE

Paravaginal Defect

Prolapse of the middle third of the vagina is associated with detachment of the pubocervical vesicle fascia and rectovaginal fascia from the pelvic sidewall at the white line. Repair includes reattachment of the paravaginal tissues as described earlier. Lateral detachment of the rectovaginal fascia accounts for some rectoceles. These fasciae should be reattached to the iliococcygeus fascia. Assessment and repair of paravaginal defects are a relatively easy extension of laparoscopic retropubic urethropexy.

In 1912, White[48] originally recognized that some cystoceles occur when the pubocervical fascia is separated from the arcus tendineus fasciae pelvis. He subsequently described reattachment of the pubocervical fascia to the arcus tendineus fasciae pelvis for correction of cystocele. In 1970, Richardson et al[39] and Shull and Baden[42] revisited the technique and the anatomic principles of repairing paravaginal defects. Richardson et al[39] emphasized that separating the pubocervical fascia from the pelvic sidewall seems to be the most likely cause of cystocele. The pubocervical fascia connects the base of the broad ligament and paracervical ring superiorly to the arcus tendineus fasciae pelvis, and laterally on both sidewalls, and to the urogenital diaphragm distally or caudad. Liu[18] described laparoscopic paravaginal repair. The patient is prepared for surgery in a fashion similar to that for the Burch procedure, and enterocele repair, vaginal vault suspension, and obliteration of the cul-de-sac are performed. Rectocele repair and perineoplasty can be completed vaginally as the last step of the procedure.

The following steps describe laparoscopic paravaginal repair[18]:

1. The retropubic space is entered in a manner identical to that for Burch colposuspension, and the retroperitoneal dissection is extended cephalad to the ischial spine.
2. The bladder should be mobilized medially to expose the paravaginal fat, and the fat should be pushed away from the underlying pearly white fascia. This is especially important in the area around the spine, where the ureter is likely to be located. The pressure generated by the carbon dioxide peritoneum accentuates the separation of superior lateral vaginal sulcus from the pelvic sidewall.
3. Placing two fingers in the vagina allows for palpation of the ischial spine and tenting the vaginal sulcus, which helps to identify the site of suture placement and helps with suture placement through the fascia. Permanent suture is used to reattach the superior lateral sulcus of the vagina to the white line. Sutures are passed through the vagina and then through the white line. The first stitch usually is placed approximately 1 cm caudad to the spine. The last stitch is placed as close to the pubic rami

as possible. Three to five interrupted sutures usually are needed to reattach the fascia to the arcus. Figure-of-eight sutures or a running continuous suture may be used to reduce the number of knots necessary for this repair. If sutures are cephalad to the spine, the pudendal artery or nerve may be injured.

4. The sutures are tied extracorporeally and tightened with a knot pusher. An assistant pushes the vaginal sulcus to the sidewall, so that the knot can be tied with less tension. The fascia and arcus are closely approximated as opposed to the loose approximation during the retropubic urethropexy (Fig. 6).

5. If the urethrovesical junction remains hypermobile, the pubocervical fascia may be stabilized with a Burch urethropexy.

6. The surgical field should be irrigated copiously, and the peritoneal defect is closed.

7. Cystoscopy is used to ascertain that no sutures have been placed into the bladder. Efflux of indigo carmine dye ensures integrity of the ureters.

8. A urethral catheter or a suprapubic catheter may be placed.

Richardson et al[39] reported that 95% of patients had a satisfactory result following paravaginal repair for cystocele and urethrocele. They noted that this technique provided an anatomic correction of cystocele and urethrocele, relief of stress urinary incontinence, preservation of normal voiding, and no persistent voiding dysfunction. They also demonstrated that the incidence of de novo detrusor instability was less than with other procedures. Subsequently, in 1989, Baden and Shull[42] found a 95% restoration of anatomy with paravaginal suspen-

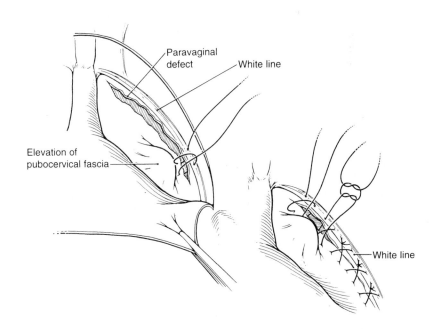

Figure 6. Paravaginal repair. The paravaginal defect is identified. The arcus tendineus is identified from the ischial spine to the pubic bone. The fascia is elevated so that sutures can be placed. The first suture is placed near the spine.

sion. They emphasized that all defects must be corrected. Liu[19] described repairing paravaginal defects and other pelvic floor defects concomitantly. He recommended a combined paravaginal and Burch procedure.

Vaginal Vault Suspension

Sacrospinous Ligament Suspension

The sacrospinous vaginal vault suspension attaches the upper and lateral margin of the rectovaginal fascia to the sacrospinous ligament. The ischial spine can be palpated through the vagina and marked with the laparoscope, which facilitates intra-abdominal identification of the ligament. Nichols[31] popularized the vaginal approach to the sacrospinous ligament.

The following steps describe a sacrospinous ligament suspension[23]:

1. A urethral catheter is placed. Indigo carmine may be placed into the bladder and diluted to an approximately 50-mL volume and the bladder catheter clamped.
2. The surgeon places two fingers into the vagina and palpates the right ischial spine and the right sacrospinous ligament. The peritoneum overlying the spine is marked with a small cautery dot or a small incision.
3. A probe is inserted into the rectum and used to deviate the rectum to the left away from the surgical field.
4. The enterocele is repaired and the cul-de-sac obliterated. The peritoneum is incised to expose the ligament and to enter the right paravaginal space.
5. A permanent suture is placed into the sacrospinous ligament approximately 2 cm or 3 cm medial to the spine toward the sacrum. Medial placement avoids proximity to the pudendal nerve and vessels. A double bite is then passed into the posterior vaginal wall, including the rectovaginal septum. A second suture is placed in a similar fashion (Fig. 7).
6. The vaginal vault is pushed to the sacrospinous ligament. Extracorporeal knots are tied and closely approximate the vagina and sacrospinous ligament.

McCall Culdoplasty

The McCall[24] procedure is designed to reattach the posterior vaginal wall (the rectovaginal fascia) to the uterosacral ligaments superior to any area where these ligaments might be broken or stretched excessively. Laparoscopic identification of uterosacral ligaments and of perirectal fascia always can be facilitated by pushing the rectum cephalad with a rectal probe.

The following steps describe a McCall culdoplasty[23]:

1. Rectosigmoid colon and small bowel are pushed out of the pelvis to expose the cul-de-sac.
2. Both ureters should be traced from the pelvic brim to the cardinal ligament.
3. A probe is placed in the vagina to help to identify the rectovaginal septum.
4. All pelvic floor defects are repaired.
5. Placing the uterosacral ligaments on tension facilitates identification. The uterosacral ligaments should be traced toward the sacrum to reveal undamaged ligaments.

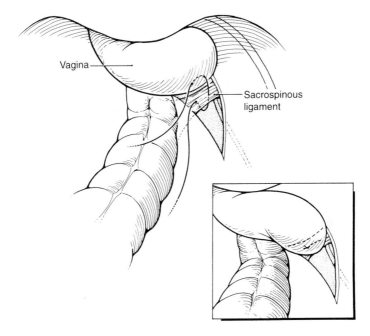

Figure 7. Sacrospinous ligament fixation. The sacrospinous ligament is identified. The vagina is elevated with a stent. A suture is placed through the ligament and then through the vagina. A second suture usually is needed.

6. The vagina is elevated with a probe toward the undamaged uterosacral ligaments.
7. A suture is placed through the undamaged ligament and the ipsilateral perirectal fascia. The suture is then passed through the posterior wall of the vagina, including the rectovaginal septum, and then placed through the opposite uterosacral ligament and perirectal fascia. When tied, the suture creates a purse-string closely approximating the vaginal to the uterosacral cardinal ligament complex (Fig. 8).
8. Second and third purse-string sutures may be placed if needed, but caution must be exercised to avoid constricting the rectum.

Sacral Colpopexy

The following steps describe sacral colpopexy[1, 29]:

1. A probe is placed in the vagina to help identify the pubocervical fascia and the rectovaginal fascia. Often, an annulus of firm tissue surrounds the large enterocele.
2. The sigmoid colon is pushed to the left, and the peritoneum is opened to expose the presacral space. The right ureter and the middle sacral vessels should be identified.
3. The mesh graft may be passed through the laparoscopic port into the pelvis.

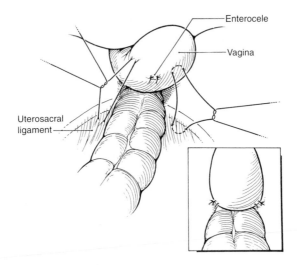

Figure 8. McCall suspension. The enterocele is ligated. A suture is placed through the uterosacral ligament and through the vagina. At least one suture is placed on each side, although multiple sutures may be needed.

4. The mesh graft is attached to the vaginal cuff with three to five permanent sutures.
5. The graft is used to pull the vagina over the levator ani plate without undue tension on the anterior wall.
6. The graft is sutured to the longitudinal ligament of the sacrum with two or three sutures. It is usually best to secure the sutures to the ligament of the sacrum with knots first and then to secure the mesh to the sutures. Injury to the middle sacral vessels results in hemorrhage that is difficult to control and, if present, may necessitate laparotomy.
7. The sigmoid colon should be positioned over the area of the graft. This rarely requires suturing the peritoneal incision.

Abdominal sacral colpopexy attaches the vagina to the hollow of the sacrum with fascia or mesh. When performed laparoscopically, this technique seems somewhat cumbersome, and potentially dangerous bleeding occurs, especially with dissection of the sacrum.

The sacral colpopexy is technically difficult to perform and perhaps is best performed with laparotomy. The mid-vagina must be attached to the pelvic sidewall because if this is not performed, the sidewalls prolapse further even though the upper vagina is well supported.

BENEFITS OF LAPAROSCOPIC SURGERY

The safety, efficacy, and cost-effectiveness of laparoscopic surgery continue to be analyzed. Shorter length of hospital stay, decreased recuperation time, and reduced postoperative morbidity have been touted as potential economic benefits of laparoscopy over laparotomy. The duration of hospital stay has decreased significantly in the past decade. With minimally invasive surgery, specifically laparoscopy, hospital stays have decreased. On a case-by-case basis, even the most extensive laparoscopic procedures require less recuperation time than when those same procedures are performed by laparotomy.[2] This may be an advantage of no abdominal incision. A 9% decrease in hospital costs has occurred with laparoscopy compared with the same procedures for pelvic organ prolapse documented in at least one study[6]; however, the startup cost for laparoscopy, which requires an additional set of complex and expensive instruments, may significantly reduce the overall cost benefit.[6]

Cosmesis is an obvious benefit. Instead of a large incision, the patient has several trocar incisions ranging from 5 mm to 12 mm, which are more esthetically pleasing than are traditional vertical or transverse incisions. Smaller incisions also reduce the risk for and severity of wound complications, such as wound infection and dehiscence.

With laparoscopy, the need for postoperative analgesia is reduced.[6] Most women are able to return to work and other routine duties more quickly than are those who had laparotomy.[43, 47] Laparoscopy may be associated with less postoperative adhesion formation because of less peritoneal trauma from packing, dehydration injury, and prolonged retraction.[13] Quality assurance also may be enhanced because endoscopic procedures can be recorded on videotape or documented with photography. Even newer technology using computer disks may allow for optimal digital recording.

Conversion from traditional abdominal hysterectomy to laparoscopically assisted surgery is perhaps the greatest benefit[30]; however, LAVH lasting 120 minutes probably is not a better procedure than a vaginal hysterectomy, which requires only 60 minutes to complete.

COMPLICATIONS

Often, a new surgical technique is associated with a new potential complications. Defining new techniques that may be performed more quickly and more efficiently by laparoscopy may be difficult. Also, the learning curve for many procedures is prolonged, and the decrease in cost may not be realized until the surgeon has significant experience, which reduces operative time.[14]

Unique to Laparoscopy

Insertion of laparoscopic trocars has unique complications that are separate from the surgical procedure. Laceration of the epigastric vessels is a common complication.[7, 28, 44] In obese patients, the epigastric vessels commonly cannot be transilluminated, nor can vessels be seen through the peritoneum. Herniation of the bowel has been reported when the trocar incisions are 12 mm in dimension.[4] Some surgeons now advocate closure of fascial defects that are more than 10 mm.

Intra-abdominal complications related to trocar placement include perforation of a viscus. Bladder perforation occurs when the trocar is not inserted sufficiently superior to the pubic symphysis or in situations when the bladder is unusually high on the abdominal wall, as is often the case after laparotomy. Bowel injuries are less common than are urinary tract injuries but are potentially more severe. Bowel perforation may occur with trocar insertion, with electrocautery spread, and directly during dissection of adhesions. These injuries may be difficult to identify. Patients may become critically ill before the injury is suspected.

Unique to the Procedures

LAVH shares complications of vaginal hysterectomy and abdominal hysterectomy. The incidence of cuff cellulitis, cuff hematoma, and atelectasis is similar among the techniques. During the vaginal portion of the procedure, hemorrhage from the cuff or the lower pedicles may occur. Cystotomy also may occur as the anterior colpotomy incision is made. This also may occur when a bladder flap is being dissected from the cervix, especially if scarring of the bladder is present.[44]

Fortunately, many cystotomies can be repaired endoscopically. The ureter also may fall in harm's way with dissection around the ovarian vessels, uterine arteries, or uterosacral cardinal ligament complex.[50] Visualization of the ureter is perhaps the best way to ensure that it is not included in a pedicle. The ureter normally is not seen or dissected because it runs through the cardinal ligament. Some surgeons advocate cystoscopy for all procedures, which probably is not warranted when hysterectomy and oophorectomy are performed without a pelvic floor procedure. Caution is warranted when a posterior colpotomy incision is made because the large bowel is at risk. The prevalence of these complications is unknown and may be much higher than commonly thought because of under-reporting.

During the performance of a Burch procedure, the urinary tract is at risk for injury. The urethra may be ligated or lacerated. The ureter may be ligated or kinked to the point of obstruction. The most common complication is cystotomy. Many, if not most, cystotomies can be repaired using laparoscopic suturing techniques. The other injuries may require laparotomy. Retropubic hematoma and abscess formation may occur. Urinary tract sepsis usually responds to antibiotic therapy. Ureteral obstruction is associated with paravaginal suspension. In one study, gross hematuria developed in one patient after placement of a suprapubic catheter.

In 1979, Cordoza et al[9] reported that 18% of women undergoing retropubic urethropexy developed detrusor instability. Other complications may include suture placement into the detrusor muscle, bladder neck obstruction, extensive dissection around the bladder neck, and hemorrhage. Detrusor instability may occur after several months. If the cul-de-sac is not addressed, enterocele may form and genital prolapse may occur. The overall rate of complications is estimated at 7.3%[18] The sacrospinous repair is associated with injury to the pudendal vessels because they course under the ligament at the spine.

TRAINING

A consensus regarding how best to teach surgeons to perform laparoscopic procedures has not been reached; however, this may be true of all technical procedures. Training is problematic for surgeons who are not in a formal training program. Fortunately, the problem is uncommon because many of these laparoscopic techniques are now commonly learned by resident physicians. Some surgeons believe that 25 to 30 cases are needed to master laparoscopic surgical technique, although designating this number of cases is arbitrary. This requirement would be lengthy and even prohibitive for most physicians. If the procedures are done in a manner similar to the open technique, surgeons have a good understanding of the procedure and have only the unique aspects of laparoscopy with which to become familiar. Because this is true for most gynecologic surgeons, other physicians advocate a three-step process for laparoscopic training.

The first step is a didactic course, in which the general techniques are outlined and strategies designed to minimize complications are discussed. A dry laboratory with a pelvic trainer may be part of this initial training. Having a trainer is an excellent way to practice and to maintain skills. Step two is in vivo training in an animal laboratory. Surgeons can gain hands-on experience with instrumentation necessary to successfully perform laparoscopic surgery. Multiple sites on the abdominal wall can be penetrated with all types and sizes of trocars. Laparoscopic suturing techniques, staplers, cautery instruments, cutting tools, and ultrasonic instrumentation are some of the tools with which surgeons might become familiar. Bladder flap dissection and cystotomy repair can be performed in animals, which effectively mimics the procedure in humans. The third step in training involves working in a surgical suite with a skilled endoscopic surgeon. In theory, the three-step approach should reduce the volume of cases needed before surgeons can work independently. The skills that a surgeon must possess and the number of supervised cases needed before performing laparoscopic procedures independently have not been defined. Attempts to establish the minimum number of cases and the minimum skills needed have proven to be elusive.[35]

SUMMARY

What is the future for laparoscopy? Any procedure thought to be impossible to perform by laparoscopy or procedures that, based on conventional wisdom, should not be done laparoscopically are being performed or developed as the reader peruses this article. Technical advances in the endoscopic equipment and development of laparoscopic instruments have allowed for performance of sophisticated procedures with laparoscopic assistance. Appropriate laparoscopic skills allow surgeons to perform these procedures in a fashion nearly identical to an open procedure; however, modifications of historically proven techniques are controversial regarding the expenses generated, equipment necessary .to perform the procedure, training necessary, and potential for complications.

Has the obituary of laparotomy been written? The benefits of laparoscopically assisted or performed procedures are continuing to be analyzed. LAVH has been touted as a way to reduce the number of abdominal hysterectomies while increasing the number of vaginal hysterectomies. Therefore, indications for LAVH would ideally more resemble indications for abdominal hysterectomy than vaginal hysterectomy; however, LAVH does not seem to have increased the total number of vaginal hysterectomies. Conversely, the number of abdominal hysterectomies seems to be roughly the same, whereas the number of vaginal hysterectomies has decreased and the number of LAVHs has increased. Therefore, surgeons seem to be substituting LAVH for vaginal hysterectomy.

Studies comparing laparoscopic Burch procedures and open Burch procedures are just now being reported. Many early reports described procedures that are not classic Burch colposuspensions. These changes make it impossible to assume that overall success and rate of complications are the same. The same can be said for techniques for correction of pelvic organ prolapse. Although laparoscopic performance and laparoscopic assistance are increasing in popularity, most cases are not handled in this way. Clearly, not every surgeon has embraced using the laparoscope to treat patients who would otherwise have undergone abdominal or vaginal surgery.

References

1. Addison WA, Livinghouse CH, Sutton GP, et al: Abdominal sacral colpopexy with Mersilene mesh in the retroperitoneal position in the management of posthysterectomy vaginal vault prolapse and enterocele. Am J Obstet Gynecol 153:140–148, 1985
2. Azziz R, Steinkampf MP, Murphy A: Postoperative recuperation: relation to the extent of endoscopic surgery. Fertil Steril 51:1061–1064, 1989
3. Boike GM, Elfstrand EP, DelPriore G, et al: Laparoscopically assisted vaginal hysterectomy in a university hospital: Report of 82 cases and comparison with abdominal and vaginal hysterectomy. Am J Obstet Gynecol 168:1690–1701, 1993
4. Boike GM, Miller CE, Spirtos NM, et al: Incisional bowel herniations following operative laparoscopy: A series of nineteen cases and review of the literature. Am J Obstet Gynecol 172:1726–1733, 1995
5. Bronitsky C, Payne RJ, Stucky S, et al: A comparison of laparoscopically assisted vaginal hysterectomy vs traditional total abdominal and vaginal hysterectomies. J Gynecol Surg 9:219–225, 1993
6. Brumsted J, Kessler C, Gibson C, et al: A comparison of laparoscopy and laparotomy for the treatment of ectopic pregnancy. Obstet Gynecol 71:889–892, 1988
7. Carter JE, Ryoo J, Katz A: Laparoscopic-assisted vaginal hysterectomy: A case control comparative study with total abdominal hysterectomy. J Am Assoc Gynecol Laparosc 1:116–121, 1994
8. Childers JM, Surwit EA: Case report: Combined laparoscopic and vaginal surgery for the management of two cases of stage I endometrial cancer. Gynecol Oncol 45:46–51, 1992
9. Cordoza LD, Stanton SL, Williams JE: Detrusor instability following surgery for genuine stress incontinence. Br J Urol 51:204–207, 1979
10. Coulam CB, Pratt JH: Vaginal hysterectomy: Is previous pelvic operation a contraindication? Am J Obstet Gynecol 116:252–260, 1973
11. Davis GD, Wolgamott G, Moon J: Laparoscopically assisted vaginal hysterectomy as definitive therapy for stage III and IV endometriosis. J Reprod Med 38:577–581, 1993
12. DeLancey JOL: Anatomic causes of vaginal prolapse after hysterectomy. Am J Obstet Gynecol 166:1717–1728, 1992
13. Filmar S, Gomel V, McComb PF: Operative laparoscopy versus open abdominal surgery: A comparative study on postoperative adhesion formation in the rat model. Fertil Steril 48:486–489, 1987
14. Gant NF: Infertility and endometriosis: comparison of pregnancy outcomes with laparotomy versus laparoscopic techniques. Am J Obstet Gynecol 166:1072–1081, 1992
15. Howard FM, Sanchez R: A comparison of laparoscopically assisted vaginal hysterectomy and abdominal hysterectomy. J Gynecol Surg 9:83–90, 1993
16. Kovac RS, Cruikshank SH, Retto HF: Laparoscopy-assisted vaginal hysterectomy. J Gynecol Surg 6:185–193, 1990
17. Kovac SR, Christie SJ, Bindbeutel GA: Abdominal versus vaginal hysterectomy: A statistical model for determining physician decision making and patient outcome. Med Decis Making 11:19–28, 1991
18. Liu CY: Laparoscopic cystocele repair: Paravaginal suspension. *In* Laparoscopic Hysterectomy and Pelvic Floor Reconstruction: Minimally invasive surgery. Cambridge, MA, Blackwell Scientific, 1995, pp 311–329
19. Liu CY: Laparoscopic cystocele repair: Paravaginal suspension. *In* Laparoscopic Hysterectomy and Pelvic Floor Reconstruction. Cambridge, MA, Blackwell Science, 1996, pp 330–340
20. Liu CY: Laparoscopic hysterectomy: A review of 72 cases. J Reprod Med 37:351–354, 1992
21. Liu CY: Laparoscopic retropubic colposuspension. *In* Laparoscopic Hysterectomy and Pelvic Floor Reconstruction: Minimally Invasive Surgery. Cambridge, MA, Blackwell Scientific, 1995, pp 311–329
22. Liu CY: Laparoscopic retropubic colposuspension: A review of 58 cases. J Reprod Med 38:526–530, 1993

23. Liu CY, Reich H: Correction of genital prolapse. *In* Hulka JF, Liu CY (eds): Textbook of Laparoscopy. Philadelphia, WB Saunders, 1998, pp 352–362
24. McCall ML: Posterior culdeplasty: Surgical correction of enterocele during vaginal hysterectomy. A preliminary report. Obstet Gynecol 10:595–602, 1957
25. Meeks GR, Harris RL: Surgical approach to hysterectomy: Abdominal, laparoscopy-assisted, or vaginal. Clin Obstet Gynecol 40:886–894, 1997
26. Mengert WF: Mechanisms of uterine support and position: I. Factors influencing uterine support (an experimental study). Am J Obstet Gynecol 31:775–781, 1936
27. Minelli L, Angiolillo M, Caione C, et al: Laparoscopically assisted vaginal hysterectomy. Endoscopy 23:64–66, 1991
27a. Munro MG, Parker WH: A classification system for laparoscopic hysterectomy. Obstet Gynecol 82:624–629, 1993
28. Nezhat C, Nezhat F, Silfen SL: Laparoscopic hysterectomy and bilateral salpingo-oophorectomy using multifire GIA surgical stapler. J Gynecol Surg 6:287–288, 1990
29. Nezhat CH, Nezhat F, Nezhat C: Laparoscopic sacral colpopexy for vaginal vault prolapse. Obstet Gynecol 142:901–904, 1994
30. Nezhat F, Nezhat C, Gordon S, et al: Laparoscopic versus abdominal hysterectomy. J Reprod Med 37:247–250, 1992
31. Nichols DH: Sacrospinous fixation for massive eversion of the vagina. Am J Obstet Gynecol 142:901–904, 1982
32. Olsson J, Ellstom M, Hahlin M: A randomized prospective trial comparing laparoscopic and abdominal hysterectomy. Br J Obstet Gynaecol 103:345–350, 1996
33. Padial JR, Sotolongo J, Casey MJ, et al: Laparoscopy-assisted vaginal hysterectomy: Report of seventy-five consecutive cases. J Gynecol Surg 8:81–85, 1992
34. Parker WH, Berek JS: Management of selected cystic adnexal masses in postmenopausal women by operative laparoscopy: A pilot study. Am J Obstet Gynecol 163:1574–1577, 1990
35. Peterson HB, Hulka JF, Phillips JM: American Association of Gynecologic Laparoscopists' 1988 membership survey on operative laparoscopy. J Reprod Med 35:587–589, 1990
36. Phipps JH, John M, Nayak S: Comparison of laparoscopically assisted vaginal hysterectomy and bilateral salpingo-oophorectomy with conventional abdominal hysterectomy and bilateral salpingo-oophorectomy. Br J Obstet Gynaecol 100:698–700, 1993
37. Photopulos GJ, Stovall TG, Summitt RL: Laparoscopic-assisted vaginal hysterectomy, bilateral salpingo-oophorectomy, and pelvic lymph node sampling for endometrial cancer. J Gynecol Surg 8:91–94, 1992
38. Reich H, DeCaprio J, McGlynn F: Laparoscopic hysterectomy. J Gynecol Surg 5:213–216, 1990
39. Richardson AC, Lyon JB, Williams NL: Treatment of stress incontinence due to paravaginal fascial defect. Obstet Gynecol 57:357–362, 1981
40. Saye WB, Espy GB, Bishop MR, et al: Laparoscopic Döderlein hysterectomy: A rational alternative to traditional abdominal hysterectomy. Surg Laparosc Endosc 3:88–94, 1993
41. Sheth SS: The place of oophorectomy at vaginal hysterectomy. Br J Obstet Gynaecol 98:662–666, 1991
42. Shull BJ, Baden WF: A six year experience with paravaginal defect repair for stress incontinence. Am J Obstet Gynecol 160:1432–1440, 1989
43. Silva PD: A laparoscopic approach can be applied to most cases of ectopic pregnancy. Obstet Gynecol 72:944–946, 1988
44. Summit RL, Stovall TG, Lipscomb GH, et al: Randomized comparison of laparoscopy-assisted vaginal hysterectomy with standard vaginal hysterectomy in an outpatient setting. Obstet Gynecol 80:895–901, 1992
45. Tanagho EA: Colpocystourethropexy: The way we do it. J Urol 116:751–753, 1976
46. Vancaille TG, Butler DJ: Laparoscopic enterocele repair—description of a new technique. Gynecol Endosc 2:211–216, 1993
47. Vermesh M, Silva PD, Rosen GF, et al: Management of unruptured ectopic gestation

by linear salpingostomy: A prospective randomized clinical trial of laparoscopy versus laparotomy. Obstet Gynecol 73:440–444, 1989

48. White GR: An anatomic operation for the cure of cystocele. Am J Obstet Dis Woman Child 56:286–290, 1912
49. Wilcox LS, Koonin LM, Pokras R, et al: Hysterectomy in the United States, 1988–1990. Obstet Gynecol 83:549–555, 1994
50. Woodland MB: Ureter injury during laparoscopy-assisted vaginal hysterectomy with the endoscopic linear stapler. Am J Obstet Gynecol 167:756–777, 1992

Address reprint requests to

G. Rodney Meeks, MD
Department of Obstetrics and Gynecology
University of Mississippi Medical Center
2500 North State Street
Jackson, MS 39216–4505

e-mail: rmeeks@ob-gyn.umsmed.edu

LAPAROSCOPY IN UROLOGY

Sean P. Hedican, MD

During the past decade, we have witnessed exponential advances and applications of laparoscopy in all fields of surgical practice. Perhaps in no other surgical subspecialty have these advances been more prevalent than in urology. Previous surgical procedures recognized as the "gold standards" of practice are being replaced by procedures that promise equivalent success rates with the added benefits of reduced postoperative pain, hospital stay, and return to full activity. As instrumentation and the skill of minimally invasive surgeons have improved, the limits of laparoscopy have continued to expand. The list of procedures that are now performed laparoscopically spans the entire realm of urology, including diagnostics, cancer staging, extirpation, and reconstruction. This article focuses on surgeries that are part of accepted treatment practice in the year 2000. Transperitoneal and extraperitoneal (or retroperitoneal) approaches have been described for all of these procedures. This article primarily discusses transperitoneal techniques but provides references, when appropriate, for alternative approaches.

PELVIC LYMPHADENECTOMY

Resurgence of interest in laparoscopy first occurred in urology with the introduction of laparoscopic pelvic lymphadenectomy for the staging of prostate cancer before definitive surgical or radiation therapy. First described in 1991 by Schuessler et al,[74] the procedure involves harvesting of the obturator node packet when evaluating prostate cancer patients but can be extended to include nodes overlying the external and common iliac vessels in patients with bladder, urethral, penile, and scrotal cancers.[33, 84] Equivalent nodal yields have been shown in comparison to open lymphadenectomy,[60] and complication rates vary from 4% to 14% depending on surgeon experience.[48] The most common complications are vascular injuries and damage to surrounding viscera, including the bladder, bowel, and ureter.[43]

From the Department of Urology, University of Iowa Health Care, Iowa City, Iowa

TECHNIQUE

A mechanical bowel preparation consisting of a bottle of magnesium citrate and an enema is administered on the day before surgery. A Foley catheter is inserted, and the scrotum is wrapped with gauze to prevent pneumoscrotum. The patient is placed in the supine position with arms tucked at the sides and all pressure points padded. The patient is secured to the surgical table with wide cloth tape or straps across the chest and upper thighs. This allows the table to be placed in deep Trendelenburg position and airplaned all of the way toward the primary surgeon to facilitate movement of the bowel out of the surgical field. The primary surgeon stands on the side opposite the dissection.

Several different trocar arrangements have been reported for performing a pelvic lymphadenectomy.[33, 84] The procedure typically is performed with four to five trocars placed in a diamond or inverted-horseshoe configuration, with a 10- to 12-mm port situated at the umbilicus for the camera (Fig. 1). The peritoneum is incised just inferior to the pulsation of the external iliac vessels, and identification, clipping, and division of the vas deferens allow for access to the obturator space (Fig. 2). Some investigators advocate a V-type peritoneotomy to improve nodal yield.[75] The node packet is clipped distal to Cloquet's node and swept proximal to the bifurcation of the iliac vessels. As much lymphatic tissue as possible is removed from posterior to the external iliac vein, with caution exercised not to injure the posteriorly located obturator nerve or the ureter as it crosses the packet proximally. Patients are usually begun on a clear liquid diet on the day of surgery and are discharged home the following day. Normal activities usually can be resumed within 1 week.

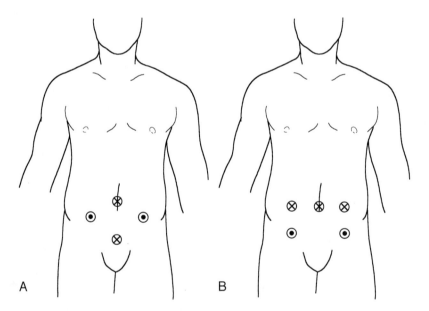

Figure 1. Trocar placement for laparoscopic pelvic lymphadenectomy. Circles containing an X represent 10- to 12-mm ports, and those containing a dot represent 5-mm ports. *A*, Diamond configuration. *B*, Inverted-horseshoe configuration.

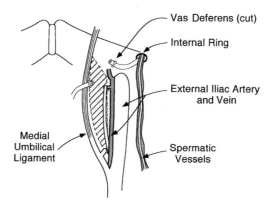

Figure 2. The area of lymph node packet removed *(hatched area)* during laparoscopic pelvic lymphadenectomy for prostate cancer staging.

DISCUSSION

The widespread use of prostate-specific antigen testing,[59] together with reproducible interpretation of biopsy findings, has improved the ability to predict which patients are at highest risk for nodal spread of their disease.[61, 63] Model systems, such as the Partin Nomogram and others, have decreased the routine application of separate nodal staging procedures in prostate cancer patients.[61] Disagreement remains over what degree of risk for spread is acceptable without performing a separate staging procedure before initiating definitive therapy.[77] Laparoscopic pelvic lymphadenectomy for staging of prostate cancer is most applicable to patients planning to undergo a radical perineal prostatectomy, external beam radiation, or prostate brachytherapy if direct access to the nodes is unavailable at the time of primary therapy.

EVALUATION AND MANAGEMENT OF CRYPTORCHIDISM

Diagnostic evaluation of the nonpalpable testicle is perhaps one of the earliest laparoscopic procedures adopted by urologists.[12] The presence of blind-ending testicular vessels seen in 16% of patients is the *sine qua non* of an absent testicle on that side.[62] If vessels are seen exiting the internal ring, then a groin exploration can be performed and the atrophic testicular tissue identified and removed. This procedure can be facilitated by laparoscopic confirmation of movement of the testicular vessels with traction on the identified testicular remnant.[18] An intra-abdominal testicle (see Color Fig. 3, p 1468) is identified in 38% of cases.[62] Previously, in this scenario, laparoscopy was merely used to guide the open approach.[12, 62] Further miniaturization of laparoscopic lenses and instrumentation has led to the development of several different techniques for laparoscopic-assisted orchiopexy.

TECHNIQUE

Patient preparation and positioning are identical to those described for laparoscopic pelvic lymphadenectomy; however, bowel preparations are usually

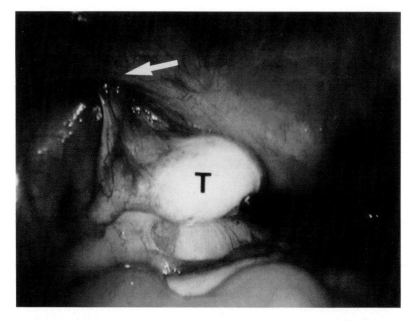

Figure 3. Laparoscopic identification of an intra-abdominal testicle (T) adjacent to the internal ring *(white arrow)*.

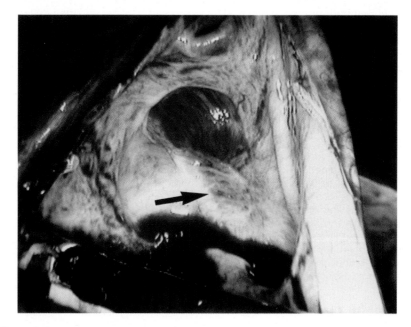

Figure 5. Laparoscopic inspection of the base of an unroofed renal cyst demonstrates the thin layer of tissue separating the cyst from the blue-tinged urine of the collecting system *(black arrow)*.

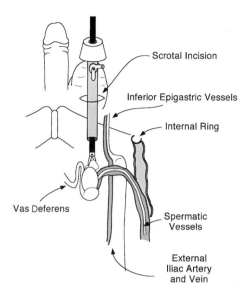

Scrotal Incision

Inferior Epigastric Vessels

Internal Ring

Vas Deferens

Spermatic Vessels

External Iliac Artery and Vein

Figure 4. An atraumatic grasper is inserted through the 5- or 10-mm port and passed medially to the epigastric vessels following complete laparoscopic mobilization of the testicular vessels. The gubernaculum is grasped and the testicle is pulled into the scrotal incision, to be secured in the dartos pouch. Release of the overlying peritoneum can be performed if the vessels are noted to be under tension.

unnecessary in small children. A 5-mm or 10-mm camera port is placed at the umbilicus, and two additional 2-mm or 5-mm ports are inserted just inferior to the umbilicus along the edge of the rectus muscle. The gubernaculum of the intra-abdominal testicle is divided and the gonadal vessels mobilized proximally until the testicle can freely reach the opposite internal ring. A scrotal incision and dartos pouch are created, and a grasper then is used to pierce the internal ring medial to the epigastric vessels from within the abdomen and is advanced out through the dartos pouch. A 5-mm or 10-mm port then is backloaded over the grasper into the peritoneal cavity. An atraumatic grasper is inserted through this new port, and the testicle is grasped, pulled out through the new defect in the abdominal wall, and secured to the dartos pouch in standard fashion (Fig. 4).[18]

DISCUSSION

Success rates for laparoscopic orchiopexy have been reported to be as high as 95%.[41] This is an impressive finding in view of the nearly 30% atrophy rate reported in one historical review[16] of all cryptorchid testicles treated with several different techniques. In that review, testicular locations included patients with intra-abdominal and inguinal testes.[16] Some investigators continue to advocate the use of laparoscopy to guide the open surgical approach. One group described their technique of performing preperitoneal dissection and passage of the testicle immediately adjacent to the pubic tubercle in all cases in which the testicle was located in an intra-abdominal position.[27] Gheiler et al[27] report a 95% success rate with this approach compared with a 70% success rate in patients explored by a standard extended inguinal incision. Similar results also have been reported by Esposito and Garipoli[21] using a laparoscopic technique to perform both stages of a two-stage Fowler-Stephens procedure for intra-abdominal testes. Their technique involves clipping the spermatic vessels by the laparoscope and, 6 to 12 months later, performing a laparoscopic orchiopexy by mobilizing a wide pedicle of peritoneal tissue surrounding the vas deferens and its vasculature.[21] In an editorial, Docimo[17] questioned the need for transection of the testicular vessels when laparoscopy is used because of the extent of vascular mobilization that can be performed laparoscopically.

LAPAROSCOPIC MANAGEMENT OF BENIGN RENAL DISEASE

Cyst Decortication

Persistent pain, infection, recurrent hematuria, and collecting system or adjacent organ compression are all indications for decortication of simple renal cystic or autosomal dominant polycystic kidney disease.[4, 49]

Technique

Preparation of all patients undergoing laparoscopic renal surgery for benign or malignant disease is the same. All patients receive an oral cathartic and an enema the day before surgery to decompress the colon. The patient is placed in a flank position with the kidney rest elevated and the table flexed to elongate the distance between the ribs and iliac crest. The surgeon stands on the side opposite the abnormality for a transperitoneal approach and on the same side for a retroperitoneal approach. Posterior and polar cysts can be reached by a direct retroperitoneal approach[56]; however, most anteriorly located cysts are often best pursued through a transperitoneal exposure. A 10-mm to 12-mm trocar is inserted by the umbilicus, and additional 5-mm trocars are inserted in the epigastrium and ipsilateral lower quadrant midway between the umbilicus and the iliac crest. The line of Toldt is taken down sharply and the colon reflected medially to reveal the underlying kidney. Gerota's fascia is incised to establish a medially or laterally based flap of well-vascularized fat to be inserted into the base of the cyst after decortication.

If a bilateral decortication is planned, a 5-mm trocar can be placed in both lower quadrants for a total of four ports in an inverted-Y configuration. An alternative is to use three ports placed in a vertical row in the midline (two 5-mm and one 10–12 mm). Patients undergoing bilateral decortications are positioned initially in a supine position, with airplaning of the table used to elevate each flank as it is undergoing surgery.

If renal cysts are in close proximity to the collecting system, an external ureteral stent can be placed by a cystoscope at the beginning of the procedure. The stent is then injected with indigo carmine or methylene blue before aspiration of the cyst. This author prefers to administer indigo carmine just before insufflating the pneumoperitoneum to allow the urine contained within the pelvis to achieve a blue discoloration (see Color Fig. 5, p 1468). When the wall of the cyst has been identified, a laparoscopic aspirating needle is used to aspirate the contents, to confirm the absence of blue staining.

When confirmed, the cyst may be unroofed using electrocautery scissors as close as possible to the renal parenchyma. If concern exists regarding the possibility of malignancy, the cyst fluid can be sent for cytology and the wall of the cyst sent for pathologic inspection. A laparoscopic argon beam coagulator probe (Pfizer Valley Lab, Boulder, CO) can be used to cauterize the edge and base of the cyst if bleeding occurs and the cyst wall is a reasonable distance from the collecting system. If a deep cyst cavity is present, the previously created strip of Gerota's fascia with attached fat pad can be placed in the base of the cavity and secured to its edges with clips, which is important for cysts that extend deep into the renal sinus and are immediately adjacent to the renal pelvis (Fig. 5).

If a leak of indigo carmine is confirmed, or if aspiration of the cyst yields blue-tinged fluid, then an internal double-pigtail stent and retroperitoneal drain should be placed. A 15 F round Jackson-Pratt drain can be brought out through the most lateral trocar site and positioned in the retroperitoneum. Patients usually are begun on clear liquids the night of surgery and are discharged home the following day if their hemoglobin level is stable and they are tolerating a regular diet.

Discussion

Surgeries performed for pain usually are preceded by a percutaneous aspiration of the cyst to document resolution of the pain on decompression,[4] which helps to predict the potential for successful resolution of pain following decortication. Extensive cyst decortications also have proven useful in managing renal pain in patients with adult polycystic kidney disease.[4, 49, 85] Some surgeons also have suggested that decompression of cysts in this patient population may prevent further progression of renal dysfunction and hypertension.[85]

PYELOPLASTY

Laparoscopic pyeloplasty was first described by Schuessler et al[73] in 1993 and was introduced as a means of replicating the high success rate of open surgery and avoiding the increased risk for hemorrhage and decreased long-term patency rates of endoscopic approaches.[24, 47, 53]

Technique

If a patient has not already had a stent placed before the procedure, one is inserted by the cystoscope at the beginning of surgery, and a Foley catheter is placed. The patient is then positioned in a semiflank position, with the kidney rest elevated and the table flexed. Three or four ports are used to perform the procedure (Fig. 6). A 10-mm to 12-mm port is inserted at the umbilicus and midway between the umbilicus and the superior iliac crest. Depending on surgeon preference, a 5-mm, 10-mm, or 12-mm port then is inserted in the epigastrium. A fourth 5-mm trocar often is required to aid in elevation of the renal pelvis during dissection and suturing of the anastomosis. This trocar is placed between the 12th rib and the iliac crest in the posterior axillary line (Fig. 6).

The line of Toldt is incised sharply, and the colon is reflected medially to expose the retroperitoneum. Gerota's fascia is incised over the lower pole of the

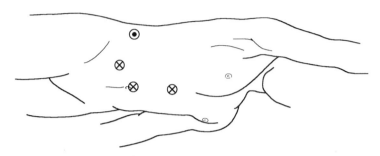

Figure 6. Typical trocar arrangement for right transperitoneal laparoscopic pyeloplasty and nephrectomy. Circles containing an X represent 10- to 12-mm ports, and the circle containing a dot represents an optional 5-mm port.

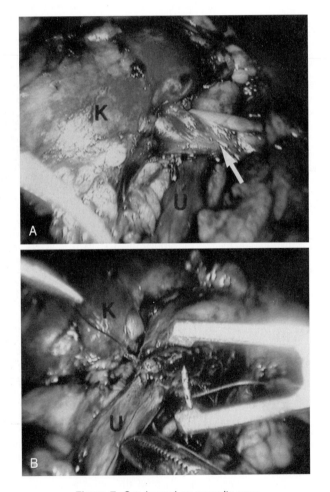

Figure 7. *See legend on opposite page*

kidney and traced medially to identify the edge of what is usually a distended renal pelvis. Caution is exercised in this region because of risk for lower pole crossing vessels, which are identified in as many as 54% of cases approached laparoscopically (Fig. 7A).[40] The region of the ureteropelvic junction then is dissected completely free of all surrounding fibrotic bands. Caution is exercised not to mobilize too much of the proximal ureter to prevent ischemia to the region of the anastomosis. If lower pole crossing vessels are identified, complete dissection is carried out around the vessels to allow for repositioning of the renal pelvis and reconstructed ureteropelvic junction anterior to the vessels (Fig. 7A–C).[34]

Several different options for laparoscopic reconstruction of the ureteropelvic junction have been described, including the dismembered pyeloplasty, Y–V plasty, and Heineke-Mikulicz repair.[40] In the presence of an anterior lower pole crossing vessel, a dismembered pyeloplasty with transposition of the anastomosis anterior to the aberrant vessels is required (Fig. 7A–C).[8, 34] The region of narrowing is identified and transected circumferentially, with caution exercised not to transect the ureteral stent. If a stenotic segment is identified, it is excised. The ureter then is spatulated laterally, and the pelvis is opened medially. A flexible nephroscope may be inserted into the renal pelvis by the closest laparoscopic port if associated upper tract stones are present. Calculi then are removed using a flexible stone basket passed by the working channel of the nephroscope.[8, 54]

The Endostitch (US Surgical, Norwalk, CT) automated, intracorporeal suturing device then is used to place corner sutures of 4-0 polyglycolic acid. If

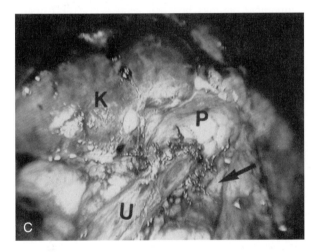

Figure 7. Right laparoscopic dismembered pyeloplasty performed for aberrant lower pole crossing vessels. *A,* Identification of crossing vessels *(arrow)* supplying the lower pole of the kidney (K). The ureter (U) courses behind the crossing vessels, causing obstruction of the ureteropelvic junction. *B,* The ureteropelvic junction has been circumferentially incised, and the ureter (U) and renal pelvis have been repositioned anterior to the crossing vessels. The posterior row of sutures is complete, the ureteral stent has been reinserted into the pelvis, and the anterior row is being placed, using the Endostitch device. The lower pole of the kidney (K) also is visible. *C,* The completed anastomosis between the ureter (U) and the renal pelvis (P) now lies anterior to the aberrant crossing vessels *(arrow)* supplying the lower pole of the kidney (K).

crossing lower pole vessels are present, the pelvis is pulled up from posterior to the vessels by placing a traction suture through its cut edge. This same suture is used to elevate the pelvis and to complete the dissection around the lower portion of the pelvis to allow for tension-free reconstruction anterior to the vessels (Fig. 7A–C). The medial corner suture is tied and then passed posterior to the ureter using a right-angle grasper. This step exposes the posterior surface of the anastomosis, and the posterior row then is completed using the Endostitch. After completion of the posterior row, the medial corner suture is passed back posterior to the ureter, and the ureteral stent is reinserted in the renal pelvis. The anterior row is then completed using the automated suturing device (Fig. 7B). A 15 F round Jackson-Pratt drain is brought out through the lateral trocar and secured to the skin.

The patient is started on a clear-liquid diet the night of surgery or the following day. The Foley catheter is left in place until the second postoperative day, when it is removed, and, if the retroperitoneal drain output does not increase appreciably, the drain then is removed. Patients usually are discharged home on the third postoperative day. The stent remains in place for 4 to 6 weeks.

Discussion

A successful radiographic patency rate of 98% was reported in the largest published series of laparoscopic pyeloplasties, with the longest mean follow-up period to date (18 mo).[40] This rate is equivalent to those reported for open pyeloplasty.[5, 72] The overall incidence of complications remains low at 12%; most are minor.[8] Comparable findings between laparoscopic and open pyeloplasty with respect to long-term pain relief using analog pain scores also have been demonstrated.[3] Also, patients undergoing laparoscopic pyeloplasty have been shown to have significant reductions in postoperative analgesia requirements, hospital stay, and mean time until return to full activity compared with their counterparts undergoing the open technique.[5]

SIMPLE NEPHRECTOMY

Since the description of the first case in 1991 by Clayman et al,[11] more than 800 cases of laparoscopic simple nephrectomy have been reported in the world literature.[44, 50, 65]

Technique

The kidney can be approached in a retroperitoneal or transperitoneal fashion. The patient is prepared and positioned as described for laparoscopic renal surgery. Gill[28] described an excellent technique for performing laparoscopic retroperitoneal nephrectomy. Because the author's preference is to perform laparoscopic nephrectomies through a transperitoneal exposure, he focuses this discussion on that technique.

Port placement for transperitoneal laparoscopic nephrectomy is similar to that for laparoscopic pyeloplasty described earlier (see Fig. 6). The line of Toldt is incised sharply and the colon reflected medially. Division of colonic attachments to the spleen and liver is recommended to allow for wide access to the retroperitoneum. Gerota's fascia is then incised over the upper or lower pole, and the kidney is "shelled out" from the surrounding fat pad. The ureter can be isolated as it crosses the psoas muscle and traced back to the hilum. The renal vessels then are identified, and all surrounding tissue and lymphatics are dissected carefully from around the vein and artery. All branching vessels, including lumbar, gonadal, and adrenal veins, are clipped separately and transected before the main renal vein is divided. The artery is secured with three clips placed proximally and one distally. A vascular Endo-GIA (US Surgical, Norwalk, CT) stapler is used to transect the vein and also can be used to transect the artery, depending on the preference of the surgeon. The ureter may be divided before or after the hilar vessels. It is often desirable to divide the ureter last because bluntly elevating it, adjacent to the renal pelvis, affords excellent exposure of the hilar vessels.

When freed, the kidney can be placed in an Endocatch (US Surgical); (10-mm) or Endocatch II (15-mm) device, depending on the size of the specimen. In noninfected and noncancerous specimens, morcellation can be performed in the Endocatch. The Endocatch is an entrapment sac mounted on a compressible ring that is opened intracorporeally. When the specimen is inside the Endocatch, the sac is disengaged from the loop by pulling the drawstring closed.

If potentially infectious material is present within the kidney, the specimen should be placed in an 8- or 10-inch impermeable LapSac (Cook Urological, Spencer, IN) or removed intact through a small extension of one of the trocar incisions to prevent dissemination of bacteria.[81] After placing the specimen superior to the liver or spleen, a grasper is closed on the sealed end of a LapSac, which is then rolled around the grasper and introduced intracorporeally by one of the port sites. The closed end of the LapSac is directed into the pelvis, and graspers are used to hold open the mouth of the sac as the kidney is inserted. When inside the sac, the drawstring is pulled out through one of the 10-mm to 12-mm trocar sites and the specimen morcellated using a large clamp or empty sponge stick under direct vision. A high-speed tissue morcellator (Cook Urological), no longer commercially available, also has been used to fragment specimens.[81] The hilum is inspected and hemostasis obtained.

Discussion

Originally reserved for benign conditions well suited for laparoscopy, the clinical scenarios in which laparoscopic nephrectomy are being performed have continued to expand together with surgical experience.[50] Even patients with giant hydronephrosis,[35] massively enlarged polycystic kidneys,[20] multiple previous abdominal procedures,[7] or significant perirenal scarring[7, 55] are considered candidates for this procedure. Bilateral nephrectomies also have been performed in patients before or after transplantation.[19, 26] Indications for bilateral surgery most commonly include repeated infections, hematuria, hypertension, calculi, or painful cystic disease.[19, 26] In the hands of experienced surgeons, complication rates for simple laparoscopic nephrectomy range from 6% to 12%, and the conversion rate to open surgery was approximately 3%.[30, 65] The added benefits of significant decreases in analgesia requirement, length of hospital stay, and time until resumption of normal activity also have been recognized compared with the open technique.[46]

DONOR NEPHRECTOMY

As experience with laparoscopic nephrectomy has continued to grow, the arena of functional organ procurement has been explored. Gill et al[29] examined the feasibility in a porcine model, and in 1995, Ratner et al[66] reported the first case of live laparoscopic kidney donation. That first case has led to perhaps one of the most significant surgical advances in kidney transplantation since its inception.

Technique

The technique for laparoscopic donor nephrectomy is similar to that for a simple nephrectomy, with several noteworthy exceptions. Patient positioning, preparation, and port placement are the same initially (see Fig. 6). The upper and lower poles are exposed, and the kidney is "shelled out" of surrounding Gerota's fat, with the exception of the lateral tissue, which is initially left intact to prevent torsion around the vessels. A generous amount of periureteric tissue also is left intact to prevent devascularization of the ureter.[23] Dissection of the renal artery is carried out to the edge of the aorta, and the artery can be sprayed lightly with papaverine if spasm occurs. The adrenal, gonadal, and any lumbar branches of the vein are clipped distal to the main renal vein and divided. The vein should be dissected proximally to at least the surface of the aorta. When the vessels have been dissected completely, the ureter is clipped distally and transected. The posterior and lateral attachments to the kidney are taken down, and mannitol and furosemide are administered before division of the hilar vessels.

A 5-cm to 8-cm incision is made in the periumbilical, or Pfannenstiel, region and carried inferiorly to the peritoneum without violating it, so that the pneumoperitoneum is maintained. The incision also can be made in a subcostal location for right-sided donations.[23, 68] An antibiotic-soaked laparotomy pad is placed in the incision. The artery is divided between clips (two placed proximally) or with a vascular Endo-GIA stapler. The vein likewise is transected using an Endo-GIA stapler. The kidney can be placed in a large Endocatch to facilitate its identification and removal after the peritoneum is incised and a hand is inserted into the abdomen. The incision then is closed using interrupted figure-of-eight sutures of #1 prolene or nylon as the kidney is being flushed and prepared for transplantation on a back table. After closure of the incision, the dissection bed and vascular stumps are inspected at low pressures and hemostasis obtained.

Discussion

In the two largest published series to date, immediate laparoscopic donor graft function was found in all 110 patients in one series[23] and was delayed in 2 patients in the other.[25] Graft survival in the postoperative period was found in 91% to 97% of patients.[23, 25] Two of the 10 patients with graft failure in one series had graft vascular thrombosis.[23] Both of these were right-sided donors, and the investigators hypothesized that the shorter right renal vein found on laparoscopic procurements (on average, 1.2 cm shorter) may have contributed to these cases of thrombosis.[68] As a result, many investigators now perform only left-sided donations or recommend open vascular control of right-sided donors after laparoscopic dissection of the kidney.[68] The overall complication rate was 10% to 14%,[23, 25] which is comparable to the 16% rate reported for open donation.[14] Mean analgesia requirements, days of hospitalization, and time until return to full activity all were shown to be significantly less than a comparable series of open donors.[25, 67, 69]

Early indications suggest that laparoscopy is expanding the potential donor pool by its promise of reduced postoperative morbidity and potential economic impact.[22, 67] At one institution, with one of the largest reported experiences, the number of live donations increased by 100% during the period in which laparoscopic donation was available compared with a similar period before it was offered.[22] At that same institution, 20% of patients indicated that they would not have donated a kidney if laparoscopic donation had been unavailable.[22] More institutions now are offering this procedure and, as patients are becoming better educated, they are seeking out facilities where this procedure is being performed.

LAPAROSCOPIC MANAGEMENT OF RENAL AND UPPER TRACT MALIGNANCY

Laparoscopic extirpation of malignancies is a topic of controversy in all fields of surgery.[13, 58] The fear of laparoscopic tumor spillage, port site or peritoneal seeding, and, ultimately, local tumor recurrences has been substantiated by experience with laparoscopic resection of colorectal, gallbladder, and ovarian malignancies.[58, 64] A review of several large series, however, demonstrates that port site recurrences occur in as few as 0.2% of laparoscopic procedures for gynecologic malignancies[9] and in 0.8% of procedures performed for the treatment of colon cancer.[64] Morcellation of organs containing malignant tumors has increased the level of concern regarding the potential for cancer spread.[57] Some investigators also suggest that features unique to laparoscopy may directly contribute to tumor cell dissemination and growth.[13] Dispersion of cancer cells by carbon dioxide convection, vasodilatory effects of carbon dioxide, and prolonged wound contact of tumor cells trapped along the outside of port sheaths all have been theorized to have a potential role in cancer cell implantation.[13]

Clayman, in Urban et al,[81] designed a laparoscopic entrapment sac (LapSac) created from a double layer of nylon and plastic. Laboratory tests demonstrated impermeability of the LapSac to bacteria and tumor cells.[81] Also, a high-speed morcellation device with recessed blades (Cook Urological) was developed to facilitate organ fragmentation within the sac.[81] These two developments allowed for intracorporeal entrapment of cancer-containing organs, which then could be removed intact or fragmented without the same risk for cancer cell spillage. Although not indestructible, to date, results of solid cancer morcellations performed within entrapment sacs have been encouraging,[6] as is discussed in the following paragraphs.

RADICAL NEPHRECTOMY

Lack of tumor cell permeability in LapSac studies eventually led to the evaluation of laparoscopy to treat renal malignancy. Original published series were limited to patients with smaller lesions (mean, 3.7 cm).[42] Since those early reports, the limitations for which laparoscopic radical nephrectomy are performed have continued to expand. Walther et al[82] have described their series of cytoreductive laparoscopic radical nephrectomies in patients before receiving adjuvant interleukin-2 therapy for metastatic renal cell carcinoma. In that series of 11 patients, the mean tumor volume was 10.8 cm.[82]

Technique

Patient preparation, positioning, and port placement are identical to those used for simple nephrectomy (see Fig. 6). Initial exposure of the kidney remains the same, except that Gerota's fascia is not violated. The kidney, contained within Gerota's fat, is mobilized to the extent required to expose the region of the hilar vessels. This step may be facilitated by identification of the ureter or gonadal vein on the left, which is traced cephalad to the hilum. The artery and vein are thoroughly dissected and transected as outlined for simple nephrectomy. It is often advantageous to leave the ureter intact until the hilar vessels are divided because this facilitates elevation and exposure by the assistant through a lateral trocar.

Removal of the ipsilateral adrenal gland at the time of nephrectomy largely depends on tumor location, size, and surgeon preference. If the lesion is small and in the midregion, or lower pole, of the kidney, it may be desirous to leave the adrenal gland behind. On the left side, this requires division of the renal vein distal to the adrenal branch or separate clipping and division of the adrenal vein. If the left adrenal gland is to be removed, the renal vein is transected proximal to the adrenal branch or the left adrenal branch is divided separately. The edge of the adrenal gland is usually easy to identify by entering Gerota's fascia in the region of the upper pole and noting the classic yellow-orange appearance of the gland. The plane between kidney and adrenal is then separated using a combination of electrocautery scissors and hemostatic clips.

On the right side, the adrenal vein usually drains directly into the inferior vena cava. If the right adrenal gland is to be left behind, the adrenal vein does not need to be identified or addressed. The adrenal gland merely is separated from the upper pole of the kidney as described earlier. If the right adrenal gland is to be included in the specimen, separate identification of the substantial right adrenal vein is necessary after division of the renal hilar vessels. This structure can be identified by gentle dissection of the lateral edge of the inferior vena cava in a cephalad direction. The vein is short and can be avulsed easily if the surgeon is not careful. Two clips should be placed on the vena cava side and one on the adrenal side of the vein before division. This is greatly facilitated by using a right-angle clip applier.

Intact specimen removal is performed by extending an incision from one of the trocars just large enough to admit the specimen. The incision is made in the upper or lower midline, subcostal, or lower quadrant, depending on surgeon preference and the patient's body habitus. The kidney can be placed in an Endocatch or LapSac to facilitate removal or simply grasped and removed by feeling for the specimen. Caution must be exercised so as not to rupture the tumor or denude Gerota's fascia on removal. If necessary, the incision should be enlarged, so it is best to entrap cancerous specimens even when an intact removal is planned.

If morcellation of the specimen is desired, the LapSac is introduced into the dissection space. Entrapment and morcellation then are performed similar to simple nephrectomy, except that caution is exercised to avoid tumor spillage. Sterile towels are used to surround the site while morcellation is performed to prevent any material from contacting the operative field. After complete morcellation of the specimen, the port incision is copiously irrigated with sterile water to facilitate lysis of any liberated tumor cells. The surrounding sterile towels are removed, and the surgeon's gloves and gown are changed. The dissection bed then is inspected and irrigated with sterile water. Wound closure then is performed, and postoperative care is identical to that for simple nephrectomy.

Discussion

The most obvious concern surrounding laparoscopic radical nephrectomy is the possibility of compromising the success of a patient's cancer surgery. In one multi-institutional report, Cadeddu et al[6] reviewed 157 laparoscopic radical nephrectomies performed for pathologically confirmed renal cell carcinomas. All lesions were clinically localized T1 or T2 cancers. A total of 142 (90%) specimens were morcellated, and the rest were removed intact. Mean follow-up was 19.2 months, and the open conversion rate was 3.8%. A total of four patients (2.5%) developed a cancer recurrence; in three patients, cancer recurred with distant metastases; and in one patient, a recurrence of renal cell cancer developed in the ureteral stump.[6] The 5-year actuarial disease-free rate of 91% + 4.8 SE is similar to reported open survival rates for similar-stage disease.[15, 52, 79] No cases of renal fossa or port site recurrences occurred.[6] Although 5-year and 10-year follow-up data will be critical in determining the relative efficacy of this cancer surgery, the initial results seem favorable.

RADICAL NEPHROURETERECTOMY

The gold standard therapy for clinically localized transitional cell carcinoma arising within the renal pelvis or upper ureter remains radical nephroureterectomy.[70] This procedure requires exposure of the upper aspect of the retroperitoneum and the deepest portion of the pelvis. The procedure can be performed by a two-incision approach or by an extended incision from the flank.[70] In 1991, Clayman et al[10] described the first laparoscopic nephroureterectomy. Since that initial description, two approaches using laparoscopy have evolved. One involves complete removal of the organ using a combination of cystoscopy and laparoscopy, and the other, a combination of laparoscopic and open surgery.

Technique

Clayman et al[10] have described the technique of endoscopically releasing the intravesical component of the ureter to enable complete laparoscopic removal of the distal ureter, including the intravesical segment.[76] In this approach, the patient first is placed in the dorsal lithotomy position, and a ureteral balloon catheter is inserted into the affected ureter. A Collins or Orandi cautery knife then is used to unroof the intravesical component of the ureter and to ablate the edges of the incised tract. The patient then is repositioned in the standard modified flank position for laparoscopic radical nephrectomy, which is performed as described earlier. Initial port placement is the same (see Fig. 6), with the exception of an additional 10-mm to 12-mm port placed in the midline suprapubic region to assist in dissection of the distal ureter.

The ureter is dissected distally, with the overlying peritoneum being incised. The vas deferens is transected between clips in male patients as is the round ligament in female patients. The ipsilateral medial umbilical ligament and any overlying vascular branches also can be transected (Fig. 8) to allow for complete dissection to, and elevation of, the ureterovesical junction. The ureter and a cuff

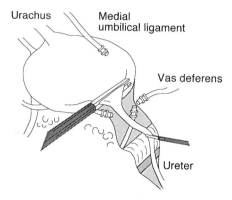

Urachus

Medial
umbilical ligament

Vas deferens

Ureter

Figure 8. Following complete dissection of the ureter, the distal bladder cuff of the nephroureterectomy specimen is obtained by firing an Endo-GIA stapler across the tented-out ureterovesical junction.

of bladder are tented outward and an Endo-GIA stapler is fired across the cuff (Fig. 8). The entire specimen then is placed in an entrapment sac, as described previously, and brought out through a port site. The ureter can be secured to the neck of the sac, delivered initially, and sent separately for pathology if a primary ureteral tumor is known to be present. Although morcellation can be performed, the propensity for tumor implantation associated with transitional cell carcinoma has encouraged most surgeons to perform intact extractions.[1, 37, 78, 80] This procedure is performed by minimally extending one of the port site incisions, as described previously for radical nephrectomy.[76] A 15 F round Jackson-Pratt drain is then inserted by a lateral port site and positioned in the pelvis.

Postoperatively, a cystogram is performed on postoperative day 3, and the Foley catheter is removed if no extravasation occurs. If drain output remains minimal, the drain also is removed. Diet advancement and hospitalization are otherwise similar to those for other laparoscopic renal procedures.

Gill et al[32] have described another innovative way of handling the distal ureter endoscopically before performing a retroperitoneal laparoscopic nephro-ureterectomy. These investigators place two 2-mm suprapubic ports directly into the bladder to grasp the edge of the ureter, assisting in dissection of its intravesi-cal component. A 2-mm endoloop then is passed through one of the trocars and is used to secure and tag the end of the ureter. In this approach, the ureter is advanced sequentially into the bladder as the dissection continues, allowing the completely dissected distal ureter to be pulled into the retroperitoneum at the time of laparoscopic retroperitoneal dissection. Because the entire procedure is performed by a retroperitoneal approach, no attempt to close the bladder is made.[32]

Cases of tumor implantation at the site of distal ureters removed by a "pluck" technique[2, 36] have led the author to support the use of open distal ureterectomy through a low-midline, or Pfannenstiel, incision. In this approach, a laparoscopic radical nephrectomy is performed, as described earlier, but the ureter is left intact and dissected distally to a point beyond the iliac vessels. The kidney and attached Gerota's fat are placed in an entrapment sac and positioned low in the iliac fossa. The patient is repositioned supine and a small midline, Pfannenstiel, or Gibson incision then is made. The ipsilateral space of Retzius is entered, and the kidney is grasped and removed from the incision. A standard open distal ureterectomy then is performed. If a transperitoneal laparoscopic approach to the kidney was used, the incised edge of the peritoneum is reapproximated to the sidewall, at the end of surgery, to prevent herniation of bowel contents into the space of Retzius.

Discussion

Several significant series of laparoscopic nephroureterectomy have been reported.[32, 45, 51] As observed initially in patients undergoing percutaneous procedures, upper tract transitional cell carcinoma has a propensity for tumor implantation at sites of intervention.[37, 80] To date, two cases of port site recurrences after laparoscopic staging procedures for transitional cell carcinoma of the bladder have been reported,[1, 78] but none following nephroureterectomy. For this reason, caution is advised when using this technique, and specimens are removed intact. The clear advantages of this approach over its open counterpart with respect to total analgesic requirements, hospital stay, and time of return to full activity warrant continued interest, provided that lengthy follow-up demonstrates no increased risk for recurrence.[51] Also, 2-year cystoscopic follow-up of patients in one series revealed no evidence of staple-related complications when bladder cuffs were obtained with an Endo-GIA stapler.[51]

SUMMARY

Mention of all of the procedures in urology that have been attempted, or are being done, laparoscopically is beyond the scope of this article. The laparoscopic procedures outlined in this article are gaining increasing support as surgeons attempt to redefine gold standard minimally invasive therapies in the new millennium. Additional procedures, such as laparoscopic retroperitoneal lymph node dissections for low-stage, nonseminomatous germ cell testicular cancers[38, 39, 83] and laparoscopic renal cryoablation of small renal cancers,[31] are soon to be added to this list. As laparoscopic instrumentation and equipment continue to improve, it will become possible to explore even more procedures laparoscopically. Advances in imaging techniques, lasers, miniaturized robotics, and other areas may further define what is meant by the term *minimal access surgery* in the decades to follow.

References

1. Andersen JR, Steven K: Implantation metastasis after laparoscopic biopsy of bladder cancer. J Urol 153:1047, 1995
2. Arango O, Bielsa O, Carles J, et al: Massive tumor implantation in the endoscopic resected area in modified nephroureterectomy. J Urol 157:1839, 1997
3. Bauer JJ, Bishoff JT, Moore RG, et al: Laparoscopic versus open pyeloplasty: Assessment of objective and subjective outcome. J Urol 162:692, 1999
4. Bennett WM, Elzinga L, Golper TA, et al: Reduction of cyst volume for symptomatic management of autosomal dominant polycystic kidney disease. J Urol 137:620, 1987

5. Brooks JD, Kavoussi LR, Preminger GM, et al: Comparison of open and endourologic approaches to the obstructed ureteropelvic junction. Urology 46:791, 1995
6. Cadeddu JA, Ono Y, Clayman RV, et al: Laparoscopic nephrectomy for renal cell cancer: Evaluation of efficacy and safety. A multicenter experience. Urology 52:773, 1998
7. Chen RN, Moore RG, Cadeddu JA, et al: Laparoscopic renal surgery in patients at high risk for intra-abdominal or retroperitoneal scarring. J Endourol 12:143, 1998
8. Chen RN, Moore RG, Kavoussi LR: Laparoscopic pyeloplasty. Urol Clin North Am 25:323, 1998
9. Childers JM, Aqua KA, Surwit EA, et al: Abdominal-wall tumor implantation after laparoscopy for malignant conditions. Obstet Gynecol 84:765, 1994
10. Clayman RV, Kavoussi LR, Figenshau RS, et al: Laparoscopic nephroureterectomy: Initial case report. J Laparoendosc Surg 1:343, 1991
11. Clayman RV, Kavoussi LR, Soper NJ, et al: Laparoscopic nephrectomy: Initial case report. J Urol 146:278, 1991
12. Cortesi N, Ferrari P, Zambarda E, et al: Diagnosis of bilateral abdominal cryptorchidism by laparoscopy. Endoscopy 8:3, 1976
13. Cuschieri A: Laparoscopic management of cancer patients. J R Coll Surg Edinb 40:1, 1995
14. D'Alessandro AM, Sollinger HW, Knechtle SJ, et al: Living related and unrelated donors for kidney transplantation: A 28-year experience. Ann Surg 222:353, 1995
15. Davis BE, Weigel JW: Management of advanced renal cell carcinoma. AUA Update Series 9: Lesson 3, 1990
16. Docimo SG: The results of surgical therapy for cryptorchidism: A literature review and analysis. J Urol 54:1148, 1995
17. Docimo SG: Editorial comment: Two-step laparoscopic Fowler-Stephens orchiopexy. J Urol 158:1954, 1997
18. Docimo SG, Jordan GH: Laparoscopic surgery in children. *In* Marshall FF (ed): Textbook of Operative Urology. Philadelphia, WB Saunders, 1996, p 207
19. Doublet JD, Peraldi MN, Monsaint H, et al: Retroperitoneal laparoscopic nephrectomy of native kidneys in renal transplant recipients. Transplantation 64:89, 1997
20. Elashry OM, Nakada SY, Wolf JS, et al: Laparoscopy for adult polycystic kidney disease: A promising alternative. Am J Kidney Dis 27:224, 1996
21. Esposito C, Garipoli V: The value of 2-step laparoscopic Fowler-Stephens orchiopexy for intra-abdominal testes. J Urol 158:1952, 1997
22. Fabrizio MD, Ratner LE, Kavoussi LR: Laparoscopic live donor nephrectomy: Pro. Urology 53:665, 1999
23. Fabrizio MD, Ratner LE, Montgomery RA, et al: Laparoscopic live donor nephrectomy. Urol Clin North Am 26:247, 1999
24. Faerber GJ, Richardson TD, Farah N, et al: Retrograde treatment of ureteropelvic junction obstruction using the ureteral cutting balloon catheter. J Urol 157:454, 1997
25. Flowers JL, Jacobs S, Cho E, et al: Comparison of open and laparoscopic live donor nephrectomy. Ann Surg 226:483, 1997
26. Fornara P, Doehn C, Fricke L, et al: Laparoscopic bilateral nephrectomy: Results in 11 renal transplant patients. J Urol 157:445, 1997
27. Gheiler EL, Barthold JS, Gonzalez R: Benefits of laparoscopy and the Jones technique for the nonpalpable testis. J Urol 158:1948, 1997
28. Gill IS: Retroperitoneal laparoscopic nephrectomy. Urol Clin North Am 25:343, 1998
29. Gill IS, Carbone JM, Clayman RV, et al: Laparoscopic live-donor nephrectomy. J Endourol 8:143, 1994
30. Gill IS, Kavoussi LR, Clayman RV, et al: Complications of laparoscopic nephrectomy in 185 patients: A multi-institutional review. J Urol 154:479, 1995
31. Gill IS, Novick AC, Soble JJ, et al: Laparoscopic renal cryoablation: Initial clinical series. Urology 52:543, 1998
32. Gill IS, Soble JJ, Miller SD, et al: A novel technique for management of the en bloc bladder cuff and distal ureter. J Urol 161:430, 1998
33. Glascock JM, Winfield HW: Laparoscopic pelvic lymph node dissection. *In* Marshall FF (ed): Textbook of Operative Urology. Philadelphia, WB Saunders, 1996, p 169

34. Hedican SP, Adams JP II: Laparoscopic surgery of the ureter. *In* Marshall FF (ed): Textbook of Operative Urology. Philadelphia, WB Saunders, 1996, p 144

35. Hemal AK, Wadwa SN, Kumar M: Transperitoneal and retroperitoneal laparoscopic nephrectomy for giant hydronephrosis. J Urol 162:35, 1999

36. Hetherington JW, Ewing R, Philip NH: Modified nephroureterectomy: A risk of tumour implantation. Br J Urol 58:368, 1986

37. Huang A, Low RK, White RD: Nephrostomy tract tumor seeding following percutaneous manipulation of a ureteral carcinoma. J Urol 153:1041, 1995

38. Janetschek G, Hobisch A, Hittmair A, et al: Laparoscopic retroperitoneal lymphadenectomy after chemotherapy for stage IIB nonseminomatous testicular carcinoma. J Urol 161:477, 1999

39. Janetschek G, Hobisch A, Holtl L, et al: Retroperitoneal lymphadenectomy for clinical stage I nonseminomatous testicular tumor: Laparoscopy versus open surgery and impact of learning curve. J Urol 156:89, 1996

40. Jarret TW, Fabrizio MD, Lamont DJ, et al: Laparoscopic pyeloplasty: Five-year experience [abstract 79]. J Urol 161:24, 1999

41. Jordan GH: Editorial: Will laparoscopic orchiopexy replace open surgery for the nonpalpable undescended testis? J Urol 158:1956, 1997

42. Kavoussi LR, Kerbl K, Capelouto CC, et al: Laparoscopic nephrectomy for renal neoplasms. Urology 42:603, 1993

43. Kavoussi LR, Sosa E, Chandhoke P, et al: Complications of laparoscopic pelvic lymph node dissection. J Urol 149:322, 1993

44. Keely FX, Tolley DA: A review of our first 100 cases of laparoscopic nephrectomy: Defining risk factors for complications. Br J Urol 82:615, 1998

45. Keely FX, Tolley DA: Laparoscopic nephroureterectomy: Making management of upper-tract transitional-cell carcinoma entirely minimally invasive. J Endourol 12:139, 1998

46. Kerbl K, Clayman RV, McDougall EM, et al: Transperitoneal nephrectomy for benign disease of the kidney: A comparison of laparoscopic and open surgical techniques. Urology 43:607, 1994

47. Kletscher BA, Segura JW, LeRoy AJ, et al: Percutaneous antegrade endoscopic pyelotomy: Review of 50 consecutive cases. J Urol 153:701, 1995

48. Lang G, Ruckle H, Hadley H, et al: One hundred consecutive laparoscopic pelvic lymph node dissections: Comparing complications of the first 50 cases to the second 50 cases. Urology 44:221, 1994

49. Lifson BJ, Teichman JM, Hulbert JC: Role and long-term results of laparoscopic decortication in solitary cystic and autosomal dominant polycystic kidney disease. J Urol 159:702, 1998

50. McDougall EM, Gill IS, Clayman RV: Laparoscopic urology. *In* Gillenwater JY, Grayhack JT, Howard SS, et al (eds): Adult and pediatric urology, ed 3. St. Louis, Mosby, 1996, p 829

51. McDougall EM, Clayman RV, Elashry O: Laparoscopic nephroureterectomy for upper tract transitional cell cancer: The Washington University experience. J Urol 154:975, 1995

52. McNichols DW, Segura JW, DeWeerd JH: Renal cell carcinoma: Long-term survival and late recurrence. J Urol 126:17, 1981

53. Meretyk I, Meretyk S, Clayman RV: Endopyelotomy: Comparison of ureteroscopic retrograde and antegrade percutaneous techniques. J Urol 148:775, 1992

54. Moore RG, Averch TD, Schulam PG, et al: Laparoscopic pyeloplasty: Experience with the initial 30 cases. J Urol 157:459, 1997

55. Moore RG, Chen RN, Hedican SP: Laparoscopic subcapsular nephrectomy. J Endourol 12:263, 1998

56. Munch LC, Gill IS, McRoberts JW: Laparoscopic retroperitoneal renal cystectomy. J Urol 151:135, 1994

57. Nakada SY, McDougall EM, Clayman RV: Laparoscopic extirpation of renal cell cancer: Feasibility, questions, and concerns. Semin Surg Oncol 12:100, 1996

58. Nduka CC, Monson JR, Menzies-Gow N, et al: Abdominal wall metastases following laparoscopy. Br J Surg 81:648, 1994
59. Pannek J, Partin AW: Prostate-specific antigen: What's new in 1997. Oncology 11:1279, 1997
60. Parra RO, Andrus C, Boullier J: Staging laparoscopic pelvic lymph node dissection: Comparison of results with open pelvic lymphadenectomy. J Urol 147:875, 1992
61. Partin AW, Kattan M, Subong E, et al: Combination of prostate-specific antigen, clinical stage, and Gleason score to predict pathological stage of localized prostate cancer: A multi-institutional update. JAMA 277:1445, 1997
62. Peters CA, Kavoussi LR: Pediatric endourology and laparoscopy. *In* Walsh PC, Retik AB, Stamey TA, et al (eds): Campbell's Urology, ed 6. Philadelphia, WB Saunders, 1992, p 1
63. Polascik TJ, Pearson JD, Partin AW: Multivariate models as predictors of pathological stage using Gleason score, clinical stage, and serum prostate specific antigen. Semin Urol Oncol 16:160, 1998
64. Ramos JM, Gupta S, Anthone GJ, et al: Laparoscopy and colon cancer: Is the port site at risk? A preliminary report. Arch Surg 129:897, 1994
65. Rassweiler J, Fornara P, Weber M, et al: Laparoscopic nephrectomy: The experience of the Laparoscopy Working Group of the German Urologic Association. J Urol 160:18, 1998
66. Ratner LE, Ciseck LJ, Moore RG, et al: Laparoscopic live donor nephrectomy. Transplantation 60:1047, 1995
67. Ratner LE, Hiller J, Sroka M, et al: Laparoscopic live donor nephrectomy removes disincentives to live donation. Transplant Proc 29:3402, 1997
68. Ratner LE, Kavoussi LR, Chavin KD, et al: Laparoscopic live donor nephrectomy: Technical considerations and allograft vascular length. Transplantation 65:1657, 1998
69. Ratner LE, Kavoussi LR, Sroka M, et al: Laparoscopic assisted live donor nephrectomy: A comparison with the open approach. Transplantation 63:229, 1997
70. Richie JP: Nephroureterectomy for carcinoma of the renal pelvis and ureter. *In* Marshall FF (ed): Textbook of Operative Urology. Philadelphia, WB Saunders, 1996, p 277
71. Roach M, Marquez C, Hae-Sook Y, et al: Predicting the risk of lymph node involvement using pre-treatment prostate specific antigen and Gleason score in men with clinically localized prostate cancer. Int J Radiat Oncol Biol Phys 28:33, 1993
72. Scardino PT, Scardino PL: Obstruction at the ureteropelvic junction. *In* Bergman H (ed): The Ureter. New York, Springer-Velag, 1981, p 697
73. Schuessler WW, Grune MT, Tecuanhuey LV, et al: Laparoscopic dismembered pyeloplasty. J Urol 150:1795, 1993
74. Schuessler WW, Vancaillie TG, Reich H, et al: Transperitoneal endosurgical lymphadenectomy in patients with localized prostate cancer. J Urol 145:899, 1991
75. See WA, Cohen MB, Winfield HW: Inverted V peritoneotomy significantly improves nodal yield in laparoscopic pelvic lymphadenectomy. J Urol 149:772, 1993
76. Shalhav AL, Elbahnasy AM, McDougall EM, et al: Laparoscopic nephroureterectomy for upper tract transitional-cell cancer: Technical aspects. J Endourol 12:345, 1998
77. Spevack L, Killion LT, West JC Jr, et al: Predicting the patient at low risk for lymph node metastasis with localized prostate cancer: An analysis of four statistical models. Int J Radiat Oncol Biol Phys 34:543, 1996
78. Stolla V, Rossi D, Bladou F, et al: Subcutaneous metastases after coelioscopic lymphadenectomy for vesical urothelial carcinoma. Eur Urol 26:342, 1994
79. Thrasher JB, Paulson DF: Prognostic factors in renal cancer. Urol Clin North Am 20:247, 1993
80. Tomera KM, Leary FJ, Zincke H: Pyeloscopy in urothelial tumors. J Urol 127:1088, 1981
81. Urban DA, Kerbl K, McDougall EM, et al: Organ entrapment and renal morcellation: Permeability studies. J Urol 150:1792, 1993
82. Walther MM, Lyne JC, Libutti SK, et al: Laparoscopic cytoreductive nephrectomy as preparation for administration of systemic interleukin-2 in the treatment of metastatic renal cell carcinoma: A pilot study. Urology 53:496, 1999

83. Winfield HW: Laparoscopic retroperitoneal lymphadenectomy for cancer of the testis. Urol Clin North Am 25:469, 1998
84. Winfield HW, Donovan JF, See WA, et al: Laparoscopic pelvic lymph node dissection for genitourinary malignancies: Indications, techniques, and results. J Endourol 6:103, 1992
85. Ye M, Chen J, Zhang L, et al: Long-term results of cyst decapitating decompression (CDD) operation for autosomal dominant polycystic disease (AD-PKD) [abstract 1114]. J Urol 157:286, 1997

Address reprint requests to

Sean P. Hedican, MD
University of Iowa Health Care
Department of Urology
200 Hawkins Drive, 3236 RCP
Iowa City, IA 52242–1089

e-mail: Sean-Hedican@uiowa.edu

LAPAROSCOPIC LUMBAR INTERBODY SPINAL FUSION

B. Todd Heniford, MD, Brent D. Matthews, MD,
and Isador H. Lieberman, BSc, MD, FRCS(C)

Anterior lumbar interbody spinal fusion (ALIF) is performed for various conditions, including spondylolisthesis, symptomatic degenerative disc disease, and as a salvage for failed posterior spinal fusion.[2] As early as 1923, surgeons were performing anterior lumbar discectomies for tuberculous spondylitis through a midline laparotomy incision.[12] Attempts to fuse the spine with tibial bone grafts were successful in many cases. In 1931, Carpener[4] described the technique of anterior, transabdominal lumbar spinal fusion for spondylolisthesis through a long oblique incision from the 12th rib posteriorly to the lower midline abdomen anteriorly.[3, 4] This approach was an extension of the flank incision general surgeons had been using for lumbar sympathectomies.[31] Freebody et al[9] popularized ALIF for degenerative spine conditions in 1963, and over the next 4 decades, several anterior transperitoneal and retroperitoneal approaches to the lumbosacral spine were described.[5, 9, 10, 14] The least invasive method is a muscle splitting, extraperitoneal approach through a vertical or oblique 4-cm to 6-cm left lower quadrant incision.[8, 20] This approach provides adequate exposure of the lumbosacral intervertebral discs but is restrictive when mobilizing deeper structures, such as the major abdominal and pelvic vessels and sympathetic plexus. Modifications in these techniques, such as the use of crossed Steinmann pins and newer retractor systems to hold and protect the great vessels and abdominal organs, have greatly enhanced the open procedure.[23]

Interest in applying minimally invasive techniques to ALIF began in 1991.[25] Over the next several years, a laparoscopic technique for ALIF was developed.[11, 19, 33] The role of the general surgeon in the surgical management of spinal disorders dramatically increased in response to the need for a skilled laparoscopist to collaborate with spine surgeons to perform laparoscopic ALIF.[29]

From Minimal Access Surgery (TBH), Carolinas Laparoscopic Advanced Surgery Program (BDM), Department of Surgery, Carolinas Medical Center, Charlotte, North Carolina; and the Department of Orthopaedic Surgery, The Cleveland Clinic Foundation, Cleveland, Ohio (IHL)

HISTORICAL PERSPECTIVE

As laparoscopic procedures were revolutionizing the field of general surgery, spine surgeons and general surgeons were also experimenting with minimally invasive approaches to the spine. In 1991, only 6 years after Muhe[24a] performed the first laparoscopic cholecystectomy in Germany, Obenchain[25] reported the first laparoscopic ALIF, performing a lumbar discectomy for a herniated disc. Within 3 years, Cloyd et al[5] reported on 21 laparoscopic anterior lumbar discectomies. Concurrent to Obenchain's series of anterior lumbar discectomies and after 2 years of instrument development and animal studies, Zucharman et al[39] performed the first laparoscopic ALIF in 1993.[39] Geis, Mack, McAfee, Regan, and Yuan were also instrumental to the development of this new technique, reporting their preliminary results over the next few years.[15, 16, 21, 30]

SURGICAL TECHNIQUE

Patient Selection, Preoperative Evaluation, and Patient Preparation

Patients with chronic mechanical lower back pain secondary to degenerative disc disease, spondylolisthesis (grade I or II), or postlaminectomy syndromes may be candidates for ALIF as part of their surgical treatment. Nonoperative treatment with aggressive physical therapy should be attempted before considering any surgical intervention. If nonoperative treatment fails, surgical options include open anterior or posterior lumbar spinal fusion and laparoscopic anterior spinal fusion. Patients who choose laparoscopic anterior lumbar spinal fusion are evaluated preoperatively by the spine and laparoscopic surgeons. The spine surgeon evaluates the disc disease, and the laparoscopic surgeon determines the feasibility of a minimally invasive approach. The authors recommend, for the first few cases, that the ideal candidate for a laparoscopic anterior spinal fusion be a tall, slim female with no previous abdominal or pelvic surgery and single level L5–S1 disc disease.

Contraindications to a laparoscopic approach include previous open anterior surgery of the lumbar spine and an active peritoneal or pelvic infection. Relative contraindications include previous lower abdominal or pelvic surgery and morbid obesity.

CT scans or magnetic resonance images of the lumbosacral spine obtained to evaluate the pathologic disc should include images of the aorta, vena cava, and iliac veins and arteries. These radiographic studies help to identify the level of the aortic bifurcation and iliac vein confluence in relation to the pathologic disc space. The location of these vessels, especially with L4–L5 disc disease, determines the accessibility and portal of entry to the disc space.

Operating Room, Patient Positioning, Equipment, and Technique

Patients can be treated with a routine mechanical bowel preparation, although the authors do not advocate this because the bowel tends to fill with fluid and air over the ensuing 24 hours. Patients are placed supine on a radiolucent surgical table in steep Trendelenburg position (Fig. 1). The steep Trendelen-

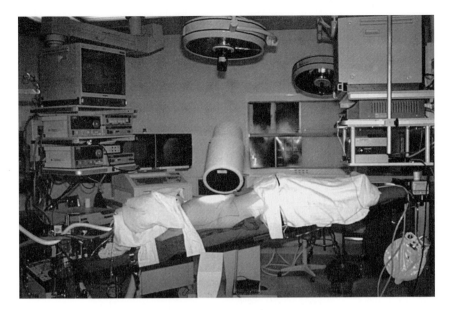

Figure 1. Operating room table with the patient in steep Trendelenburg position, a C-arm fluoroscope over the lumbar spine, a video monitor at the foot of the bed, and an image intensifier monitor over the patient's left shoulder.

burg position facilitates cephalad retraction of the small intestine, colon, and omentum. Both arms are draped at the patient's sides, providing room for the C-arm fluoroscope, two surgeons, and an assistant. The patient's arms are not in the way of the C-arm if they can be placed inferior to the level of the spine. If the arms cannot be placed posterior to the level of the spine, they are crossed over the chest on a pillow and secured with tape. The legs are secured to the surgical table, over a folded pillow with the knees flexed 20°. This position relieves tension on the psoas muscle and common iliac vessels. The shoulders are padded to prevent the patient from sliding with steep Trendelenburg position. Sequential pneumatic compression devices are applied to both legs. An orogastric tube and Foley catheter are inserted.

Pneumoperitoneum is established to 15 mm Hg with a Hasson technique or Veress needle. Port selection is at the discretion of the laparoscopic surgeon, depending on his or her surgical style. Typically, four ports are placed, with a 10-mm port at the umbilicus for a 30° videoendoscope, a 5-mm port in the right and left lower quadrants (equal distance between the umbilicus and pubic bone) for retraction and dissection, and a 5-mm suprapubic port (Fig. 2). The suprapubic port is initially used for retraction but subsequently enlarged to perform the anterior spinal fusion. The video monitor is positioned at the foot of the surgical table and the image intensifier monitor at the head of the bed opposite the spine surgeon.

Anterior L5–S1 Disc Exposure

With the patient positioned in 30° of Trendelenburg, the small intestine and omentum are retracted cephalad, and the sigmoid colon is retracted laterally.

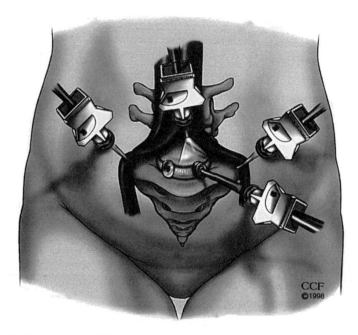

Figure 2. Anterior view of the trocar placement for laparoscopic anterior L5–S1 spinal fusion. (Courtesy of Isador H. Lieberman, MD, Cleveland Clinic Foundation, Cleveland, OH.)

The location of the aortic bifurcation, iliac vein confluence, and right and left ureters are identified. The midline posterior peritoneum over the sacral promontory is lifted anteriorly and incised longitudinally. The retroperitoneal space is entered, and the fine, gossamer tissue planes are bluntly separated. This space contains the presacral plexus of nerves, which are difficult to identify as discrete structures. These are bluntly dissected laterally to expose the middle sacral vessels. The middle sacral vessels are ligated and divided between hemoclips, which exposes the L5–S1 annulus (Fig. 3). The left common iliac vein not only overlies the left lateral third of the annulus but also may be adherent to it and must be carefully dissected laterally (Fig. 4).

A laparoscopic extraperitoneal approach to the L5–S1 disc space is an alternative to the previously described transabdominal technique.[27] The initial approach is similar to a totally extraperitoneal laparoscopic inguinal herniorrhaphy. After making an infraumbilical skin incision, the anterior rectus sheath is incised and the rectus muscle is retracted laterally, exposing the posterior rectus sheath. A balloon-tipped trocar is placed superior to the posterior rectus sheath and directed toward the pubic symphysis. A laparoscope is inserted into the trocar, and the balloon is inflated under direct vision. The balloon trocar is replaced with a 10-mm trocar. Under direct vision, 5-mm trocars are placed in the left and right lower quadrants similar to the transperitoneal L5–S1 approach. A space is developed between the peritoneum, abdominal wall, and pelvis. The dissection of the preperitoneal space posteriorly exposes the L5–S1 disc space, aortic bifurcation, iliac vessels, and ureters. The remainder of the procedure proceeds similar to the transabdominal approach. In the authors' experience

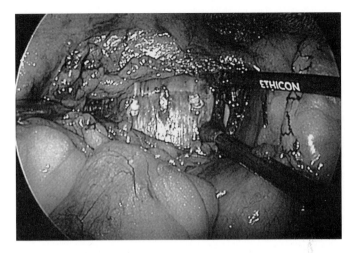

Figure 3. Anterior view of the L5–S1 disc space.

with an extraperitoneal approach, it is difficult to maintain pneumoperitoneum and keep the iliac vessels out of the surgical field.

Anterior L4–L5 Disc Exposure

Trocar placement and patient positioning are identical to L5–S1 disc exposure, except that the authors tend to place the trocars 2 cm to 3 cm higher and use the upper portion of the umbilicus as opposed to the lower portion. The sigmoid colon is retracted laterally as described earlier. Additional retraction of the sigmoid colon may be provided by a suture or endoloop placed around an

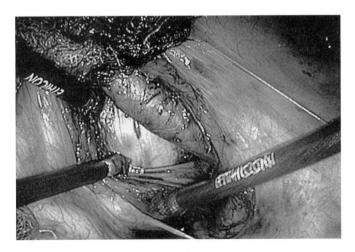

Figure 4. Anterior view of the left iliac vein crossing the L4–L5 disc space.

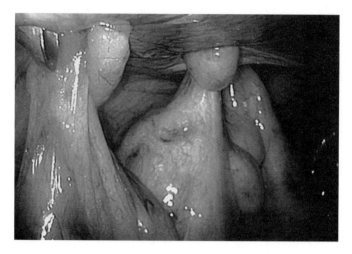

Figure 5. The sigmoid colon is retracted with the aid of three transabdominal sutures (endoloops) secured to appendiceal epiplocae.

epiploic appendage and passed through the anterior abdominal wall of the left lower quadrant (Fig. 5). The midline posterior peritoneum is incised longitudinally approximately 3 cm more cephalad than for the L5–S1 disc exposure. The aortic bifurcation is identified with gentle blunt dissection. The L4–L5 disc space is inferior to this area. The left iliac artery and vein must be retracted to the right. Retraction of these vessels is facilitated by dissecting lateral to the iliac artery and vein and ligating ascending segmental vessels and lumbar or iliolumbar venous branches. The iliac vessels are retracted with Kitner forceps. If the aortic bifurcation and iliac vein confluence lie cephalad to the L4–L5 disc space, exposure is similar to that for the L5–S1 disc space. Laparoscopic anterior lumbar spinal fusion at L4–L5 should be attempted only after successful experience with L5–S1 fusion. A greater degree of difficulty exists with exposing the L4–L5 disc space, and the risk for injury to the iliac vessels and lumbar branches is increased. Frequently, the left iliac vein tethers the inferior vena cava, so one must work in a mobile window over the L4–L5 annulus, displacing the vessels from one side to the other as necessary.

Anterior L2–L4 Disc Exposure

The L2–L4 disc space can be approached similarly to the exposure described for the L4–L5 disc space. Patient positioning is identical to L5–S1 and L4–L5 disc exposures, but the trocars are placed slightly superior. The small intestine and omentum are retracted cephalad, and the sigmoid colon is retracted laterally. The posterior peritoneum is incised lateral (left) to the aorta and medial to the left ureter and mesenteric vessels. A crossing lumbar vein and artery are located in the area of the L3–L4 disc spaces. These vessels can be ligated and divided between hemoclips but are best avoided if they do not interfere with access to the disc space. Because the iliac vessels are caudal to the surgical field with this approach, L2–L4 anterior disc space exposure is more straightforward than is L4–L5 disc space exposure.

Interbody Fusion Material

Laparoscopic anterior interbody fusion requires some form of structural bone graft or implant that can be delivered through a 18-mm or 21-mm working trocar and can restore the native height of the disc space. Fusion devices include autogenous iliac bone, allograft femoral bone, and titanium cages. Autogenous iliac crest bone dowels, harvested at the time of open or laparoscopic anterior spinal fusion, have the best potential to achieve interbody fusion[32]; however, unlike cervical spine fusion with autogenous bone graft, the structural stability of autogenous bone between the load-bearing vertebral bodies of the lumbar spine is a concern. Threaded allograft femoral bone dowels are available in sizes (16-mm, 18-mm, and 20-mm diameters) amenable to laparoscopic placement. Advantages of using allograft bone dowels include decreased bone graft site morbidity, the potential to become incorporated into the spinal fusion, and minimal radiographic artifact on postoperative imaging of the lumbar spine.[38] Disadvantages of allograft bone dowels include a potentially higher pseudoarthrosis rate (because of resorption and fragmentation of the graft) compared with autogenous bone graft and an increased risk for disease transmission.[34] The newest fusion devices are cylindrical, fenestrated, titanium-threaded cages. These interbody fusion cages, available in eight sizes, are placed in a manner similar to threaded allograft bone dowels. Before placement, the titanium cages are packed with morselized autogenous bone graft. The interbody fusion cages provide structural stability to the spine during bony ingrowth and fusion without becoming incorporated into the spinal fusion[36]; however, the titanium cages, unlike autogenous bone grafts, may produce significant radiographic artifacts on postoperative imaging. Regardless of the implant device used, exact placement with respect to the midline is critical to achieve a successful fusion and minimize implant-related complications.

Discectomy and Interbody Fusion

After the appropriate disc space is exposed, a spinal needle is passed percutaneously from the midline suprapubic position and into the diseased disc (Fig. 6). A cross-table lateral radiograph using the C-arm is performed to confirm that the diseased disc space has been identified properly and to determine the angle of trajectory for placement of the suprapubic operating trocar (18 mm to 21 mm). The operating trocar should be parallel to the endplates of the disc in the sagittal plane. When the proper angle of trajectory has been determined, an incision is made for the operating trocar.

The annulus over the disc space is divided, and the disc is evacuated with rongeurs and curettes until bleeding cancellous bone is exposed. A dilator and distraction plug are driven into the interspace to restore the native disc space height, distract the vertebral bodies, and apply tension to the annulus before vertebral reaming and graft or cage placement (Fig. 7). Lastly, the interbody grafts or cages are implanted according to their respective techniques under laparoscopic and fluoroscopic guidance. After confirming hemostasis, the posterior peritoneum is reapproximated with interrupted, absorbable sutures.

Throughout the entire procedure, C-arm fluoroscopy is used to evaluate placement of the cages. Virtually all cage failures result from improper positioning too far lateral, too deep, or not deep enough. It is easy to lose sight of the midline if one is not paying appropriate attention to the video image by angling the 30° scope to get a parallax view or not paying attention to the C-arm

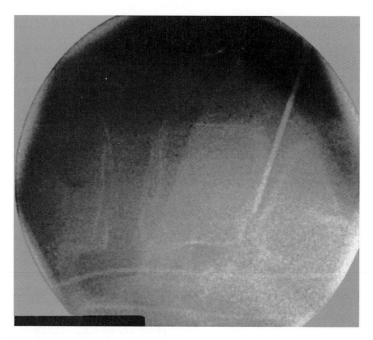

Figure 6. Lateral fluoroscopic view of a spinal needle placed into the L5–S1 disc space to identify the diseased disc and to determine the proper trajectory for placing the working (20-mm) trocar.

radiographs, which may be oblique. To prevent this, one should consistently use the C-arm from a midline trajectory and cross-table lateral position to guide placement of the cages (Fig. 8).

Lateral L2–L5 Disc Exposure and Interbody Fusion

This retroperitoneal approach requires the patient to be placed into a lateral decubitus position with the right side down. Three trocars are used, one in the midaxillary line below the 12th rib, one in the anterior axillary line at the level of the L2 vertebral body, and one in the anterior axillary line caudal to the anterior superior iliac spine. A potential space is developed in the retroperitoneum between the peritoneum and the psoas muscle with balloon insufflation through the midaxillary line trocar. The other two trocars are placed under direct vision after the potential space is enlarged. To expose the lumbar disc spaces and vertebral bodies, the transversalis fascia, peritoneum, perinephric fascia, ureter, and aorta are retracted anteriorly, and the psoas muscle is retracted posteriorly. The diseased disc space is confirmed fluoroscopically. Access to the disc space may require ligation of the segmental vessels at the equator of the vertebral body. The lumbar disc is evacuated with rongeurs and curettes, and interbody fusion follows with titanium-threaded cages, allograft bone dowels, or autogenous bone graft. Instead of placing interbody fusion cages on the left and right sides of the anterior disc space as described for anterior lumbar spinal fusion, one is placed anteriorly and one posteriorly from the lateral aspect of the disc space. An alternative is to use one long cage placed obliquely across the disc space.

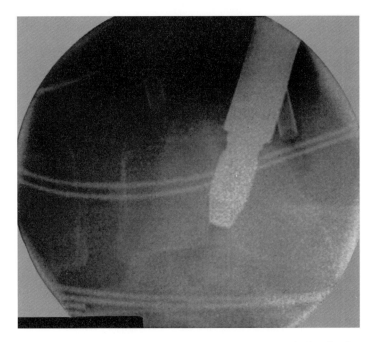

Figure 7. Lateral fluoroscopic view of distraction plug placed into the L5–S1 disc space.

RESULTS

The authors have performed 140 laparoscopic ALIFs involving three spine surgeons and five laparoscopic surgeons. Most were single-level or two-level cases, although the authors have done a few three-level ALIFs. All cases were completed using the BAK interbody fusion system (Sulzer Spine Tech, Minneapolis, MN) with titanium cages. The operative time varied from 80 to 360 minutes. Operative time was longer for multilevel fusions and during each surgeon's learning curve. The average hospital stay for a single-level case was 2 days in the absence of complications and 4 days for two-level cases. One surgical team (one spine and one laparoscopic surgeon) performed the first 50 cases of this series, and the exposure-related complication rate was less than 5%. The overall (three spine and five laparoscopic surgeons) exposure-related complication rate was 10%, including four vessel injuries, one bowel injury, and one postoperative bowel obstruction. In four (2.9%) patients, surgery was converted to open ALIF, two for vessel injuries, one because of obesity, and one because of iliac vein immobility after an open posterior spinal fusion. One patient with an iliac vein injury developed a postoperative deep venous thrombosis (DVT). Postoperative exposure-related complications included a permanent retrograde ejaculation rate of 2% and a transient retrograde ejaculation rate of 5% in men and a 10% prevalence of transient left leg sympathetic effect in the entire group. The cage complication rate was 15% caused by pseudoarthrosis, misplacement, traction radiculopathy, and retropulsed disc material. The clinical outcomes were graded as improved in 70%, no change in 20%, and worsening of symptoms or complications in 10%.

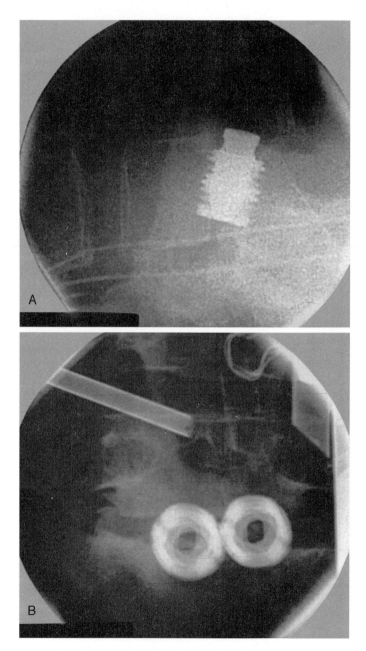

Figure 8. Lateral fluoroscopic view (*A*) and anterior view (*B*) of a L5–S1 titanium-threaded cage interbody fusion.

Only a few series have reported on more than 30 patients. In the largest reported series, a prospective multicenter study by Regan et al[30] evaluating laparoscopic transperitoneal (n = 240) and open retroperitoneal (n = 305) ALIF using interbody BAK fusion cages, hospital stay (mean, 3.3 days versus 4.0 days, P = 0.005) and blood loss (mean, 141.7 mL versus 207.2 mL, P = 0.005) were less and operative time was longer (mean, 201.2 min versus 144.9 min; P < 0.001) in the laparoscopic group.[30] The mean operative time decreased from 215.0 minutes to 164.7 minutes from the first five to the last five cases. A 10% conversion rate to open technique occurred in the laparoscopic group. Reasons for conversion in these 24 patients were an iliac vein injury or bleeding (n = 6), obstructed access to the lumbar spine by bowel or one of the major vessels (n = 5), adhesions (n = 8), and technical reasons (n = 6). Two great vessel injuries occurred in the open ALIF group. No significant difference was found in the postoperative complication rate (19.1% versus 14.1%) or the device-related reoperative rate (4.7% versus 2.3%) among the laparoscopic and open ALIF groups, respectively. Other than the reoperative rate, no long-term follow-up was provided.

In another study by Olsen et al,[26] laparoscopic ALIF was attempted in 75 patients using a carbon fiber fusion cage packed with cancellous bone harvested from the iliac crest. The mean operative time was 192 minutes. All but two (97.3%) procedures were completed laparoscopically. Reasons for conversion to open technique were pelvic adhesions and presacral scarring. Four (5.3%) perioperative complications occurred: two bladder lacerations repaired without the need for a laparotomy, one retrograde ejaculation, and one displaced posterior fragment requiring reoperation. The mean time to discharge was 36 hours. Twenty-three patients have been followed up for more than 2 years. All of these patients reported some level of improvement. Eighteen patients considered their symptoms to be significantly improved, and five patients considered their symptoms to be moderately improved. Mean pain scores on a modified pain scale of 1 to 10 showed a mean preoperative score of 8.7 and a mean postoperative score of 2.3.

Long-term follow-up, documenting fusion rates after laparoscopic ALIF, has been reported by only a few investigators. Mahvi and Zdeblick[17] reported on 16 patients with at least 6 months' follow-up. None of the 16 patients had motion on flexion–extension radiographs, and all were considered stable. Katkhouda[13] reported that 85% of patients with single-level fusions and only 40% of patients with multilevel fusions were asymptomatic without motion on flexion–extension radiographs with 8 months' follow-up. McAfee et al[21] reported on 18 patients who underwent laparoscopic lateral retroperitoneal spinal fusion at L1–L5. No cases of implant migration or pseudoarthroses were found at a mean follow-up examination of 24.3 months (range, 12–40 mo).

COMPLICATIONS

Hemorrhage

As previously described, Regan et al[30] converted six (2.4%) laparoscopic cases because of bleeding in a large prospective, multicenter study evaluating open (n = 305) and laparoscopic (n = 250) ALIFs. Four patients had iliac vein injuries, and two patients had excessive bleeding from the disc space. Only two (0.7%) great vessel injuries occurred in the open ALIF group. Zdeblick[36] converted 3.0% of cases because of vascular injuries during laparoscopic ALIF. Two of three conversions in this series occurred in the first three cases. Olsen et al[26] reported no vascular injuries in 75 consecutive laparoscopic anterior discectomies with interbody fusion. The rate of iliolumbar vein, iliac vein, or vena cava injury in open ALIF is 3.0%.[34] Rates as high as 15.6% have been reported in multilevel open ALIF by an anterolateral or paramedian retroperitoneal approach.[1] The mechanism of injury for most vascular complications in open spinal fusion is traction on the vein during exposure.[28] Excessive traction can tear the iliac vein or avulse any of the segmental, branching veins. A similar injury can occur during laparoscopic anterior lumbar spinal fusion.[37] A problem unique to laparoscopic anterior lumbar spinal fusion is that 15 mm Hg pneumoperitoneum may compress or even collapse the iliac vein, making it difficult to identify during the dissection and susceptible to injury. Consequently, caution is warranted when dissecting in the area of the iliac veins. If an injury to one of the vessels occurs, the surgeon should attempt to control it by tamponade with Kitner forceps or a gauze sponge placed through one of the large trocars. If this is unsuccessful, rather than attempting to repair it laparoscopically, the surgeon should convert to a laparotomy, repair the injury, and complete the procedure using the open technique.

Retrograde Ejaculation

If the superior hypogastric plexus of the autonomic nervous system is injured while dissecting near the pelvic brim, the seminal vesicles fail to contract and the bladder neck does not close during ejaculation. This results in retrograde ejaculation. The prevalence of retrograde ejaculation in open anterior lumbar surgery is 1.7%.[34] The prevalence after laparoscopic ALIF is slightly higher, ranging from 2.7% to 5.1%.[17, 30] Dissecting inferior to the pelvic brim and the use of electrocautery while dissecting in this area are discouraged. The dissection should be restricted to the lumbar spine superior to the pelvic brim.

Injuries to the pelvic splanchnic nerves or the pudendal nerves can cause impotence. This is an extremely uncommon complication of open anterior lumbar surgery and laparoscopic ALIF and is probably an operator-dependent issue. If the dissection is focused with minimal use of electrocautery, the risk is small. Nevertheless, all male patients must be made aware of this risk regardless of a laparoscopic or open anterior approach to the lumbar spine.

Deep Venous Thrombosis and Pulmonary Embolism

The prevalance of DVT in open anterior lumbar surgery is 0.3% to 4.5%.[18, 22, 35] Pulmonary embolism occurs in 1.0% to 2.2% of cases.[7] Postoperative DVT and pulmonary embolism have been reported less frequently after laparoscopic ALIF. Reasons for a decreased rate of DVT and pulmonary embolism after laparoscopic anterior lumbar spinal fusion are not completely understood. Nevertheless, perioperative sequential pneumatic compression devices are recommended in all patients. Anticoagulant agents, such as low-molecular-weight heparin, may be appropriate, but at the discretion of the surgeons.

SUMMARY

Laparoscopic ALIF is an evolving technique requiring the participation of a laparoscopic surgeon experienced in advanced laparoscopic techniques and knowledgeable in anterior lumbar spinal exposures. Initial enthusiasm for this technique was fostered by the development of interbody fusion devices and a method of exposing the anterior lumbar spine, which takes advantage of the ability of minimally invasive surgeries to improve exposure and visualization while minimizing collateral tissue damage and injury to healthy tissue. Preliminary studies have demonstrated laparoscopic ALIF feasibility. These same studies have been able to prove only minor advantages with the laparoscopic versus open technique using the current implants and bone grafting techniques for single-level disc disease. General acceptance of laparoscopic ALIF awaits further investigation. Reasons for a lack of general acceptance include the expense of the interbody fusion devices and laparoscopic equipment, the unfamiliarity of this advanced laparoscopic technique to spine and general surgeons, and the steep learning curve of the procedure. Intraoperative complications that arise are often severe, such as vascular injuries. Many skeptics appropriately believe that initial enthusiasm and zealousness must be tempered with scientific effort that provides data from long-term follow-up.[24] For laparoscopic ALIF to gain general acceptance, randomized comparisons of laparoscopic ALIF to open ALIF and posterior lumbar spinal fusion and controlled studies with long-term follow-up documenting symptomatic outcome variables and spinal fusion rates must be completed.

As new modalities are developed, minimally invasive techniques may facilitate their utility. The indications, procedures, and surgical principles of ALIF are unchanged, and physicians must not invent indications to justify the technique; however, eventually we may be able to redefine the indications to take full advantage of the endoscopic techniques and biological advances.

References

1. Baker JK, Reardon PR, Reardon MJ, et al: Vascular injury in anterior lumbar surgery. Spine 18:2227, 1993
2. Blumenthal SL, Baker J, Dossett A, et al: The role of anterior lumbar fusion for internal disc disease. Spine 13:566, 1988
3. Burns BH: An operation for spondylolisthesis. Lancet 224:1233, 1933
4. Carpener N: Spondylolisthesis. Br J Surg 19:374, 1931
5. Cloyd DW, Obenchain TG, Savin M: Transperitoneal laparoscopic approach to lumbar discectomy. Surg Laparosc Endosc 5:85, 1995
6. Crofts KM, Wong DA, Murr PC: Anterior paramedian retroperitoneal surgical approach to the lumbar spine. Orthopedics 17:699, 1994
7. Ferree BA, Stern PJ, Jolson RS, et al: Deep venous thrombosis after spinal surgery. Spine 1:315, 1993
8. Fraser RD, Gogan WJ: A modified muscle-splitting approach to the lumbosacral spine. Spine 17:943, 1992
9. Freebody D, Bendall R, Taylor RD: Anterior transperitoneal lumbar fusion. J Bone Joint Surg 53:617, 1971
10. Hacker RJ: Comparison of interbody fusion approaches for disabling low back pain. Spine 22:660, 1997
11. Hildebrandt U, Pistorius G, Olinger A, et al: First experience with laparoscopic spine fusion in an experimental model in the pig. Surg Endosc 10:143, 1996
12. Ito H, Tsuchia J, Asami G: A new radical operation for Pott's disease. J Bone Joint Surg 16:498, 1934
13. Katkhouda N: Laparoscopic Anterior Spinal Fusion. Presented at the 51st Annual Meeting of the Southwestern Surgical Congress. San Diego, CA, April 18, 1999
14. Lane LD, Moore SE: Transperitoneal approach to the intravertebral disc in the lumbar area. Ann Surg 127:537, 1948

15. Mack MJ, Regan JJ, Bobechko WP, et al: Application of thoracoscopy for diseases of the spine. Ann Thorac Surg 56:736, 1993
16. Mack MJ, Regan JJ, McAfee PC, et al: Video-assisted thoracic spine surgery for the anterior approach to the thoracic spine. Ann Thorac Surg 56:736, 1993
17. Mahvi DM, Zdeblick TA: A prospective study of laparoscopic spinal fusion: Technique and operative complications. Ann Surg 224:85, 1996
18. Marsicano J, Mirovsky Y, Remer S, et al: Thrombotic occlusion of the left common iliac artery after an anterior retroperitoneal approach to the lumbar spine. Spine 19:357, 1994
19. Matthews HH, Evans MT, Molligan HJ, et al: Laparoscopic discectomy with anterior lumbar interbody fusion. Spine 20:1797, 1995
20. Mayer HM: A new microsurgical technique for minimally invasive anterior lumbar interbody fusion. Spine 22:691, 1997
21. McAfee PC, Regan JJ, Geis WP, et al: Minimally invasive anterior retroperitoneal approach to the lumbar spine: Emphasis on the Lateral BAK. Spine 23:1476, 1998
22. McAfee PC, Regan JR, Zdeblick TA, et al: The incidence of complications in endoscopic anterior thoracolumbar spinal reconstructive surgery: A prospective multicenter study comprising the first 100 consecutive cases. Spine 15:1624, 1995
23. McComis GP, Holt RT: Anterior approaches to the lumbosacral joint. Spine 11:155, 1997
24. McCulloch JA: Point of view. Spine 20:2034, 1995
24a. Muhe E: Die erste cholecystektomie durch das laparoskop. Langenbeck's Arch Surg 369:804, 1986
25. Obenchain TG: Laparoscopic lumbar discectomy: Case report. J Laparoendosc Surg 1:145, 1991
26. Olsen D, McCord D, Law M: Laparoscopic discectomy with anterior interbody fusion of L5–S1. Surg Endosc 10:1158, 1996
27. Onimus M, Papin P, Gangloff S: Extraperitoneal approach to the lumbar spine with video assistance. Spine 21:2491, 1996
28. Rajaraman V, Vingan R, Roth P, et al: Visceral and vascular complications resulting from anterior lumbar spinal interbody fusion. J Neurosurg 91:60, 1999
29. Regan JJ, Guyer RD: Endoscopic techniques in spinal surgery. Clin Orthop 335:122, 1997
30. Regan JJ, Yuan H, McAfee PC: Laparoscopic fusion of the lumbar spine: A prospective multicenter study evaluating open and laparoscopic lumbar fusion. Spine 24:402, 1999
31. Royle ND: The treatment of spastic paralysis by sympathetic rami-section. Surg Gynecol Obstet 39:701, 1924
32. Silcox DH: Laparoscopic bone dowel fusions of the lumbar spine. Orthop Clin North Am 29:655, 1998
33. Southerland SR, Remedios AM, McKerrell JG, et al: Laparoscopic approaches to the lumbar vertebrae: An anatomic study using a porcine model. Spine 20:1620, 1995
34. Weis JC, Betz RR, Clements DH, et al: Prevalence of perioperative complications after anterior spinal fusion for patients with idiopathic scoliosis. J Spinal Disord 10:371, 1997
35. West JL, Anderson LD: Incidence of deep venous thrombosis in major adult spinal surgery. Spine 17:254, 1992
36. Zdeblick TA: Laparoscopic spinal fusion. Orthop Clin North Am 29:635, 1998
37. Zelko JR, Misko J, Swanstrom L, et al: Laparoscopic lumbar discectomy. Am J Surg 169:496, 1995
38. Zucharman J, Hsu K, Picetti G, et al: Clinical efficacy of spinal instrumentation in lumbar degenerative disc disease. Spine 17:834, 1992
39. Zucharman JF, Zdeblick TA, Bailey SA, et al: Instrumented laparoscopic spinal fusion: Preliminary results. Spine 20:2029, 1995

Address reprint requests to
B. Todd Heniford, MD
Chief of Minimal Access Surgery
Department of Surgery
Carolinas Medical Center
1000 Blythe Boulevard, Medical Education Building 601
Charlotte, NC 28203

0039–6109/00 $15.00 + .00

THORACOSCOPIC ESOPHAGOMYOTOMY FOR ACHALASIA

James W. Maher, MD

PATHOPHYSIOLOGY

Achalasia is the most common of the primary motor disorders of the esophagus. The term *achalasia* is of Greek origin and translates as "failure to relax." This allusion refers to the lower esophageal sphincter (LES), which exhibits a lack of receptive relaxation in response to swallowing with achalasia. Although wonderfully descriptive, this term ignores that a generalized failure of progressive peristaltic activity also is present in the esophagus. Thus, achalasia is characterized by an LES that does not relax and an aperistaltic esophagus. Examination of the dorsal motor nucleus and the vagus nerve may reveal mild degenerative changes and reduced numbers of ganglion cells in the myenteric plexus. The esophageal smooth muscle exhibits hypertrophy. Nevertheless, the cause of this disease is unclear.

A picture similar to achalasia is presented by Chagas' disease, which produces a syndrome of cardiomegaly, megaesophagus, and megacolon. Examination of pathologic material from Chagas' disease shows a loss of ganglion cells within the myenteric plexus secondary to infestation with the protozoan *Trypanosoma cruzi*. No satisfactory experimental model exists for achalasia, but a high bilateral cervical vagotomy produces an achalasia-like picture in dogs.

CLINICAL SYMPTOMS AND SIGNS

Achalasia has no predilection for gender and may occur at any time in life. The onset of dysphagia may be subtle, and patients commonly have symptoms for years before seeking medical care. The degree of dysphagia may vary from

From the Department of Surgery, University of Iowa Health Care, Iowa City, Iowa day to day; however, these patients commonly have dysphagia for solids and liquids from an early stage. Because they have aperistalsis and a tonically closed LES, these patients empty their esophagus only when the hydrostatic pressure of the column of food and liquid within the esophagus exceeds that of the LES. This process can be helped somewhat by the contraction of the striated muscular portion of the esophagus in the upper third of the esophagus, which still functions. Increasing intrathoracic pressure with the Valsalva maneuver also may aid in achieving emptying of the esophagus. Many patients empirically learn maneuvers that can help them to empty the esophagus, such as grunting or straining. The increased hydrostatic pressure in the esophageal lumen leads to gradual esophageal dilation with food retention.

Chest pain caused by esophageal spasm is a common symptom and may precede the development of dysphagia. Regurgitation of undigested food is a common complaint and may lead to nocturnal aspiration or even aspiration pneumonia. Weight loss occurs in many patients, but it is insidious and must be carefully sought or it will be missed.

Some patients complain of burning epigastric pain that may be mistaken for gastroesophageal reflux (GER). This fact is paradoxic because these patients have a high pressure sphincter that does not relax. Fermentation of rotting food may occur within the esophagus, which may produce an acidic pH and hence the resultant burning sensation.

DIAGNOSIS

Physical examination is unhelpful. Diagnosis relies on manometric and radiographic criteria.

Radiology

Barium swallow can be valuable. It should be carried out with the patient in the supine position so that the esophagus does not empty by gravity. The esophagus typically shows varying degrees of dilation caused by the constantly increased hydrostatic pressure within the esophageal lumen, although this sign may be absent early in the disease. In late stages, the esophagus may exhibit a "sigmoid" appearance. The typical finding is a smooth, symmetric "bird's beak" at the gastroesophageal junction (Fig. 1). This contrasts with the "apple-core" type of irregular narrowing seen in patients with esophageal cancer. When the patient is placed in the upright position, the esophagus may begin to empty. As the disease progresses, retained food commonly is present within the esophageal lumen. Occasionally, patients demonstrate an epiphrenic diverticulum.

Manometry

The diagnosis of achalasia is best made by manometry. Typically, these patients demonstrate an increased or normal LES pressure that does not relax in response to deglutition (Fig. 2), although some patients demonstrate incomplete relaxation of the sphincter. Occasionally, the sphincter may seem to relax. This finding usually represents movement of the measuring aperture away from the sphincter during the longitudinal shortening of the esophagus that may occur

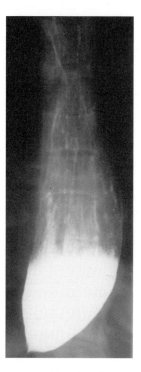

Figure 1. Barium swallow in a patient with achalasia showing bird beak narrowing of the esophagogastric junction and esophageal dilation.

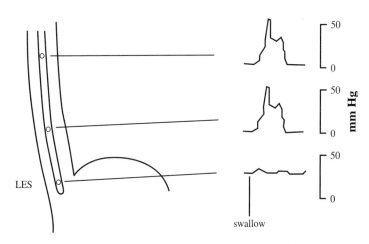

Figure 2. Classic manometric findings of achalasia: high pressure lower esophageal sphincter that fails to relax when swallowing. Peristalsis is absent. Esophageal body waves are simultaneous and identical. This is known as a *common cavity* phenomenon and indicates a dilated lumen.

with swallowing. Physicians should differentiate this finding from true receptive relaxation of the sphincter because the true relaxation of the sphincter is incompatible with the diagnosis of achalasia. The two can be distinguished by placing a "sleeve-type sensor" that measures LES pressure over several centimeters.

The other characteristic finding is aperistalsis in the distal two thirds of the esophagus. Some patients demonstrate increases in pressure with swallowing, but these increases are simultaneous rather than peristaltic and are all identical images of each other. They are referred to as a *common-cavity phenomenon* and indicate the presence of esophageal dilation. Some patients demonstrate high-pressure simultaneous contractions in addition to the usual findings of achalasia. These high-pressure waves often are associated with chest pain, and the condition is termed *vigorous achalasia*.

Twenty-Four–Hour pH Monitoring

Some patients with achalasia complain of a burning sensation in the esophagus. These patients may exhibit three patterns on 24-hour pH monitoring. Most patients have no significant reflux and have normal 24-hour pH studies as one would expect in an individual with a tonically contracted sphincter. Some patients also inexplicably exhibit GER. The pH tracing in these patients exhibits the usual sharp decreases in pH, representing GER episodes that are followed by a slow return toward a normal pH as saliva neutralizes remaining acid. A few patients, however, exhibit slow decreases in pH, followed by rapid return of the pH toward normal. These incidents are believed to represent fermentation of retained food with production of acid by-products. The rapid return of pH toward normal is believed to be secondary to swallowed saliva. The computer that reads pH studies interprets this fermentation pattern incorrectly as GER episodes. Thus, clinicians should examine the tracing. Following pneumatic dilation or surgical myotomy, patients may complain of symptoms that represent pathologic reflux caused by disruption of the sphincter, so it is helpful to have a baseline pH study before therapy so that post-treatment symptoms, if they occur, may be better interpreted in light of the preoperative pattern.

Endoscopy

Endoscopic examination should be carried out in all patients for two main reasons. The first is to establish the diagnosis. An infiltrating cancer of the cardia may produce a picture that is indistinguishable from achalasia except by endoscopy with biopsy (this is known as *pseudoachalasia*). Strictures also may be ruled out. A typical endoscopic examination demonstrates a dilated esophagus with retained food. The distal esophagus may be somewhat tortuous and difficult to navigate. The gastroesophageal junction is closed, but the endoscope passes with gentle pressure. No mucosal lesions are present. The endoscope should be retroflexed in the cardia to rule out an occult submucosal cardiac cancer.

Endoscopic evaluation is also helpful immediately preoperatively to document that the esophagus is clean and empty of food before surgery. This helps to prevent aspiration at the time of induction of anesthesia. If the esophagus is not empty, it should be emptied with a large-bore lavage tube. The author also has occasionally observed esophageal candidiasis preoperatively. If present, this should be treated before surgery because the increased friability of the mucosa may make perforation more likely at esophagomyotomy.

MEDICAL THERAPY

Commonly used medical therapies for achalasia include smooth muscle relaxants, such as long-acting nitrates and calcium channel blockers. These medications do tend to reduce LES pressure, but the amount of symptomatic relief obtained is inconsistent and typically not long lasting. Use of a standard rigid dilator may produce relief for 2 or 3 days, but because the standard 50F to 60F circumference dilators do not disrupt esophageal muscle, no long-term relief should be expected.

HYDROSTATIC OR PNEUMATIC BALLOON DILATION

Dilation of the distal esophagus beyond its normal diameter is effective in eliminating dysphagia if it ruptures the LES. These dilators were formerly made from fluid-filled bags, the inflation diameter of which was limited by a layer of cloth (Brown-McHardy bag or Mosher bag). They now take the form of a flexible, nonstretch balloon that is inserted over a guidewire placed at the time of endoscopy. These balloons are 30 mm to 40 mm in diameter. Inflation of the balloon typically produces severe chest pain as the sphincter is torn. Many endoscopists believe that if a patient does not experience this pain, the procedure is unsuccessful. Although blood often is seen on the balloon, the esophageal perforation rate is only 5%. Patients should be observed overnight to rule out perforation of the esophagus, which is ordinarily signalled by continuing chest pain and tachycardia, or undergo postdilation contrast studies if they are to be discharged. Most perforations are localized, and many can be managed by placement of a nasoesophageal tube for suction, parenteral antibiotics, and parenteral nutrition; however, if symptoms do not abate rapidly, the patient should undergo immediate thoracotomy for closure of the perforation.

Appreciable symptomatic improvement is seen in 60% to 77% of patients, but pathologic GER occurs in approximately 25% to 30% of patients.[13] Reflux is a difficult problem in patients with achalasia because the mechanism that prevents GER (the sphincter) and the mechanism that clears GER (peristalsis) are deficient. This complication may be ameliorated somewhat by the availability of the potent proton pump inhibitor medicines. In the past, most patients with achalasia were treated initially with hydrostatic dilation to avoid the morbidity of surgical therapy. This approach is reasonable; however, more than two dilations does not seem to improve results, and a somewhat higher risk for perforation exists. Repeated dilations may produce fibrosis in the esophageal submucosa and thus make surgical myotomy more difficult.

BOTULINUM TOXIN INJECTION

Intrasphincteric injection of botulinum toxin has been used[7a] as treatment for achalasia. This toxin probably works by reducing the cholinergic tone of the LES. Subjective and objective improvement have been reported[7a] in many patients, with few reported adverse reactions. Clinical improvement typically lasts 2 to 6 months; however, patients often require repeat treatment. The fibrosis induced by the injections may render myotomy difficult if it is later required. Although studies directly comparing botulinum toxin injection with pneumatic dilation and surgical myotomy are needed, botulinum toxin injection rapidly has become another therapeutic option in the treatment of patients with achalasia.

SURGICAL THERAPY

Controversy exists as to the best method for achieving surgical relief of the dysphagia associated with achalasia. Many surgeons believe that a properly performed esophagomyotomy, which extends less than 1 cm past the squamoco-lumnar junction, relieves dysphagia without producing pathologic GER. In a remarkable study, Ellis[4] demonstrated that, at 10 to 20 years after transthoracic esophagomyotomy as described earlier, 88% of patients remain improved over their preoperative status and that symptomatic reflux developed in only 5% of patients. The lack of clinically significant GER with this approach probably is related to the fact that the limited myotomy does not traverse the gastric sling fibers, which have an important role in the prevention of GER. A limited transthoracic esophagomyotomy does not disturb the phrenoesophageal membrane, which also may contribute to GER control. Other investigators believe that a complete myotomy cannot be ensured unless the myotomy is extended well down onto the stomach. This maneuver invariably produces GER, which they believe may be managed with one of several antireflux procedures.[2, 3, 6, 9] Early results with this type of approach are promising; however, relieving one physiological obstruction with myotomy and then adding another obstruction in the form of an antireflux procedure seems counterintuitive. Surgeons cannot restore patients' peristalsis; the esophagus must empty passively. In fact, Topart et al[12] reported that, although early results were promising with esophagocardio-myotomy plus fundoplication, long-term results included return of dysphagia in 14 of 17 patients. Distal esophageal diameter increased from 3.9 cm preoperatively to 6.0 cm at 10 years of follow-up, which suggests that significant esophageal obstruction was produced by the 360° wrap. A 29% reoperation rate occurred. Others have suggested that esophagocardiomyotomy be combined with a partial fundoplication to prevent GER.[9] Long-term results of this strategy are unavailable; however, partial laparoscopic fundoplication does not seem to be as effective in preventing GER in healthy patients as does a 360° fundoplication. Jobe et al[5] reported on a series of 100 patients undergoing laparoscopic Toupet fundoplication. Twenty percent (15/74) complained of recurrent GER at a mean of 22 months postoperatively. Twenty-four–hour pH studies were abnormal in 90% of these patients (9/10). Twenty-four–hour pH studies also were performed in 31 asymptomatic patients at follow-up. Thirty-nine percent of these patients (12/31) had pathological GER. If results are this bad in patients with normal peristalsis and acid clearance, it is hard to imagine that an aperistaltic esophagus would fare better.

Andreolla and Earlam[1] reviewed the world literature on esophagomyotomy for achalasia and concluded that, when surgery was done through an abdominal incision, GER was almost twice as common as when it was done through a thoracic incision, regardless of whether an antireflux procedure was performed.

Thoracoscopic and laparoscopic techniques have been adapted to the performance of esophagomyotomy. The controversies regarding the extent of myotomy and the addition of an antireflux procedure are the same.[7, 8, 10, 11] The early results with these procedures mimic the results of open procedures. The morbidity rate is much lower. If long-term results confirm the early results, balloon dilation one day may be supplanted by thoracoscopic or laparoscopic esophagomyotomy.

Transthoracic Esophagomyotomy

Transthoracic myotomy is described first because it is the gold standard of therapy for patients with achalasia with known long-term results. It is also helpful in patients who suffer mucosal injury at the time of thoracoscopic myotomy. In this situation, the myotomy may be closed, achieving two-layered closure, and the esophagus may be rotated counterclockwise to allow a new myotomy to be performed approximately 90° medial to the old myotomy.

Preparation

The esophagus must be empty preoperatively. Endoscopy on the day before surgery allows retained food to be emptied from the stomach. After the esophagus is clean, the patient should remain on a clear-liquid diet until surgery. If esophageal candidiasis is present, surgery should be delayed until this condition has cleared with medical therapy. A nasoesophageal tube should be inserted just before induction of anesthesia, and the esophagus should be emptied of saliva. If weight loss is severe, the patient should have preoperative measurement of nutritional parameters. If these indicate malnutrition, the patient should receive appropriate nutritional supplements.

Technique

A double-lumen endotracheal tube is useful to improve exposure. It is also helpful to insert a flexible endoscope into the esophagus before turning the patient into the right lateral decubitus position. The endoscope helps the surgeon to determine the proper extent of myotomy. The procedure is performed through a left 6th rib thoracotomy. The esophagus is dissected and encircled with a Penrose drain, which is placed on traction. The myotomy is begun approximately 10 cm superior to the hiatus. It is extended through the longitudinal and circular layers. The submucosa is recognized easily because it protrudes through the myotomy. The thickened muscularis is elevated with a right-angle clamp and divided with the cautery, with caution not to cauterize the submucosa. The myotomy is extended less than 1 cm past the squamocolumnar junction. A vein retractor may be used to retract the hiatus to improve exposure of the distal esophagus. The transition to stomach may be recognized in several ways:

- The muscularis begins to assume a normal thickness.
- Transverse submucosal veins that are characteristic of the cardiac submucosa begin to appear.
- Finally, many times, Belsey's fat pad is seen.

Nevertheless, endoscopy is the most reliable way to judge completeness of the myotomy. The squamocolumnar junction is easily recognized with the endoscope, allowing for the extent of myotomy to be accurately determined. When the myotomy has relieved the obstruction, the gastroesophageal junction, which was previously closed, opens with only gentle insufflation through the endoscope. The muscularis then may be dissected for approximately half of the esophageal circumference. The Penrose drain is removed, and the esophagus retracts back into the mediastinum. A single chest tube is used to drain the chest. It may be removed in the recovery area if the chest radiograph shows complete lung expansion. These patients may resume a regular diet the next morning. They are instructed to chew their food well and to drink plenty of liquids with their meals. They still have an aperistaltic esophagus. Solid food empties primarily by peristalsis, whereas liquids empty primarily by gravity. Adding liquids to food, therefore, aids passive esophageal emptying. Patients are discharged when they are comfortable on oral analgesic therapy.

Complications

Most investigators[1-12] have reported no deaths following esophagomyotomy. Mucosal perforations occur but are rare and may be repaired with fine sutures when they occur. If a perforation occurs near the distal end of the myotomy, the author prefers to close the myotomy, rotate the esophagus, and perform the myotomy on the opposite side of the esophagus.

Residual dysphagia is a problem in less than 5% of patients. If a patient still has dysphagia and a manometric high-pressure zone is present, the patient may benefit from another myotomy. If the previous surgery was performed through the chest, the reoperation should be performed through the abdomen, and vice versa.

GER occurs in less than 5% of patients. In most cases, it can be treated with standard medical therapy. If GER is severe, an antireflux procedure with a partial fundoplication or even resection may be appropriate.

Transthoracic Esophagocardiomyotomy with Modified Belsey Procedure

This surgery is performed in a fashion similar to esophagomyotomy described earlier, except that the myotomy is extended 2 cm or 3 cm onto the stomach. A Belsey 270° partial fundoplication is performed, with the exception that only two sutures are used to construct each layer of the fundoplication.

Thoracoscopic Myotomy

Technique

Thoracoscopic myotomy should be performed in a fashion nearly identical to the open technique, with a few exceptions. A double-lumen endotracheal tube is mandatory to allow for collapse of the left lung. The upper gastrointestinal endoscope is used as described for the open technique. The tip of the esophagoscope may be deflected intraoperatively by the endoscopist to lift the esophagus out of the mediastinum into a more visible location. Four ports are placed on the chest in a diamond pattern at the sixth interspace midaxillary and posterior axillary lines, the 9th interspace midaxillary line, and the third interspace anterior axillary line. The midaxillary sixth interspace port is used for the camera, whereas the other sixth interspace port and the ninth interspace ports are used for the surgeon's instruments. A fifth incision may be placed inferiorly to accommodate a vein retractor for hiatal retraction and suction, if necessary. After division of the pulmonary ligament, the pleura is incised over the esophagus inferiorly to the level of the hiatus. The esophagus is then retracted anteriorly, and the posterior plane is developed bluntly until the right pleura is visualized. Next, the esophagus is retracted posteriorly, and the anterior plane is developed in an identical fashion until the esophagus can be encircled with a Penrose drain. The two ends of the drain are secured outside of the chest with clamps. The drains should be brought through the trocar incision but outside of the trocars so that they do not interfere with passage of instruments. The traction exerted aids in exposure of the distal portion of the myotomy. The myotomy is begun with the hook cautery as the thickened muscularis is elevated over an angled clamp, much as described for the open technique (Fig. 3). Bleeding should be controlled with thrombin-soaked gelatinous foam because cautery might produce potential delayed mucosal injury. A vein retractor aids in exposure of the distal esophagus by retracting the hiatus. The myotomy is extended in a fashion identical to that described for open transthoracic myotomy. The endoscope is used to determine completeness of myotomy. The remainder of the procedure is identical to that for the open technique.

These patients are commonly discharged the next day. The author prefers to obtain a contrast radiograph to document the lack of leak and relief of obstruction on the morning after surgery. A regular diet then is begun.

Results

The results of thoracoscopic myotomy parallel those achieved with open transthoracic myotomy. In the author's experience, excellent or good relief of dysphagia was achieved in 88% of 21 patients. This series has been extended to 37 patients, with similar findings. Nevertheless, long-term follow-up, such as that described previously by Ellis,[4] provides the "proof of the pudding."

Resection for End-Stage Disease

The results of myotomy when esophageal dilation has progressed to the megaesophagus or sigmoid esophagus stage are not as good as the results with

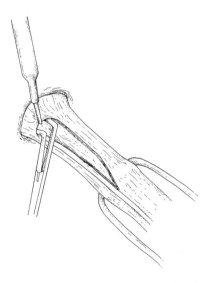

Figure 3. Completed thoracoscopic myotomy. Note that the distal end of the myotomy retracts below the hiatus when hiatal retraction has been released.

lesser degrees of esophageal dilation. Some patients still suffer with severe dysphagia because the sigmoid curling of the esophagus leaves the esophagogastric junction in a position in which the esophagus does not empty dependently. In some of these patients, and in patients with severe postmyotomy GER, esophageal resection may relieve their obstruction. Resection may be performed through a transhiatal approach with cervical esophagogastrostomy or visceral interposition. This approach relieves dysphagia but is associated with the morbidity and mortality of esophagectomy. Treatment at an early stage with esophagomyotomy prevents the need for this radical approach in most patients.

SUMMARY

The adaptation of minimally invasive approaches to the therapy of achalasia has yielded immense benefits for patients because it allows the best treatment to be provided with minimal morbidity.

References

1. Andreolla NA, Earlam RJ: Heller's myotomy for achalasia: Is an added anti-reflux procedure necessary? Br J Surg 74:765–769, 1987
2. Bonavina L, Nosadini A, Bardini R, et al: Primary treatment of esophageal achalasia: Long-term results of myotomy and Dor fundoplication. Arch Surg 127:222–227, 1992
3. Donahue PE, Schlesinger PK, Sluss KF, et al: Esophagocardiomyotomy: Floppy Nissen fundoplication effectively treats achalasia without causing esophageal obstruction. Surgery 116:719–725, 1994
4. Ellis FH: Oesophagomyotomy for achalasia: A 22-year experience. Br J Surg 80:882–885, 1993
5. Jobe BA, Wallace J, Hansen PD, et al: Evaluation of laparoscopic Toupet fundoplication as a primary repair for all patients with medically resistant gastroesophageal reflux. Surg Endosc 11:1080–1083, 1997
6. Little AG, Soriano A, Ferguson MK, et al: Surgical treatment of achalasia: Results with esophagomyotomy and Belsey repair. Ann Thorac Surg 45:489–494, 1988
7. Maher JW: Thoracoscopic esophagomyotomy for achalasia: Maximum gain, minimal pain. Surgery 122:836–841, 1997
7a. Pasricha PJ, Ravich WJ, Hendrix TR, et al: Botulinum toxin for the treatment of achalasia. N Engl J Med 322:774, 1995
8. Pelligrini C, Witter LA, Patti M, et al: Thoracoscopic esophagomyotomy: Initial experience with a new approach for the treatment of achalasia. Ann Surg 216:291–299, 1992
9. Rosato EF, Acker M, Curcillo PG, et al: Transabdominal esophagomyotomy and partial fundoplication for treatment of achalasia. Surg Gynecol Obstet 173:137–141, 1991
10. Shimi S, Nathanson LK, Cuschieri A: Laparoscopic cardiomyotomy for achalasia. J R Coll Surg Edinb 36:152–154, 1991
11. Swanstrom LL, Pennings J: Laparoscopic esophagomyotomy for achalasia. Surg Endosc 9:286–292, 1995
12. Topart P, Deschamps C, Taillefer R, et al: Long-term effect of total fundoplication on the myotomized esophagus. Ann Thorac Surg 54:1046–1051, 1992
13. Vantrapen G, Hellemans J: Treatment of achalasia and related motor disorders. Gastroenterology 79:144–154, 1980

Address reprint requests to
James W. Maher, MD
Department of Surgery
4601 JCP
University of Iowa Hospitals and Clinics
200 Hawkins Drive
Iowa City, IA 52242–1086

0039–6109/00 $15.00 + .00

VIDEO-ASSISTED THORACIC SURGERY FOR DISEASES WITHIN THE MEDIASTINUM

Jeffrey C. Lin, MD, Stephen R. Hazelrigg, MD, and Rodney J. Landreneau, MD

The development of advanced video-assisted thoracic surgery (VATS) instrumentation and refinement of endoscopic surgical techniques have allowed for increasing VATS applications to disease processes of the mediastinum for diagnostic evaluation and definitive surgical treatment. VATS techniques have yielded decreased patient pain and morbidity while increasing patient and referring physician acceptance.[27, 33, 44, 70] Thoracic surgeons have recognized VATS techniques as effective approaches for the diagnosis and treatment of many common mediastinal diseases, including:

Accepted mediastinal indications for VATS
  Biopsy of mediastinal lymph nodes
  Biopsy of mediastinal masses
  Resection of benign germ cell tumors
  Resection of ectopic parathyroid
  Resection of thymus for thymic cyst, myasthenia gravis, stage I thymoma
  Resection of bronchogenic or pericardial cysts
  Esophageal cystectomy
  Enucleation of esophageal leiomyomata
  Esophagomyotomy for achalasia
  Resection of posterior mediastinal (neurogenic) tumors
  Thoracic dorsal sympathectomy for palmar or axillary hyperhidrosis
  Thoracic splanchnicectomy for chronic intractable abdominal pain

From the Division of General Thoracic Surgery, Allegheny General Hospital, Pittsburgh, Pennsylvania (JCL, RJL); and the Division of Cardiothoracic Surgery, Southern Illinois University School of Medicine, Springfield, Illinois (SRH)

Relative mediastinal indications for VATS
  Antireflux operation for gastroesophageal reflux disease
  Pericardiectomy and drainage of pericardial effusion
  VATS facilitated anterior approach to the thoracic spine
  Drainage of suppurative or descending necrotizing mediastinitis
  Sympathectomy for conditions other than upper-extremity hyperhidrosis
  Adjunctive dissection of intrathoracic goiter
  Preoperative lymph node biopsy and staging for esophageal cancer
  Esophagectomy

In this article, the role of VATS in the diagnosis and therapy of mediastinal diseases is reviewed, together with the indications and results of VATS procedures for the mediastinum.

MANAGEMENT OF PATIENTS WITH MEDIASTINAL LYMPHADENOPATHY

Despite refinements in modern diagnostic radiographic modalities, thoracic surgeons continue to maintain an important role in the diagnostic process for indeterminate mediastinal masses and lymphadenopathy. Magnetic resonance (MR) imaging and helical CT have allowed for more accurate clinical (radiologic) evaluation of the mediastinum. Transbronchial and CT-guided percutaneous needle biopsy can be effective in selected cases to confirm malignant cytology within the abnormal mediastinal lymph nodes; however, a surgical biopsy is still required in many instances to establish a histologic diagnosis. Patients with indeterminate mediastinal lymphadenopathy without evidence of disease elsewhere require surgical biopsy to establish the histologic diagnosis in 40% of cases.[59]

Cervical mediastinoscopy is the preferred minimally invasive surgical diagnostic approach to most paratracheal and subcarinal mediastinal lymphadenopathy identified by preoperative CT scanning of the chest. Cervical mediastinoscopy, as described by Harken et al[25] and popularized by Carlens,[7] is simple, safe, and effective for the diagnostic evaluation of paratracheal lymph node stations. For the evaluation of simple paratracheal lymphadenopathy, the diagnostic yield of cervical mediastinoscopy has been found to be comparable with that of VATS but can be accomplished with single-lumen ventilation and simple instruments.[20]

Limitations of cervical mediastinoscopy for accessing the lymph nodes in the anterior mediastinum and aortopulmonary window stations led to parasternal or anterior mediastinotomy approaches as described by Stemmer et al[71] and popularized by McNeill and Chamberlain.[51] Familiar to most thoracic surgeons, anterior mediastinotomy has been an effective adjunct to cervical mediastinoscopy in the evaluation of mediastinal lymphadenopathy. Other investigators developed alternative techniques of "extended" cervical mediastinoscopy to avoid the anterior mediastinotomy for access to the anterior mediastinal and aortopulmonary window lymph nodes.[10, 18, 36] Although the extended cervical mediastinoscopy techniques are effective, the increased technical complexity and the inability to assess low-lying nodes have limited their widespread clinical application.

Because of the access and visual limitations of cervical mediastinoscopy and anterior mediastinotomy, VATS techniques have been explored as an adjunctive modality to evaluate mediastinal lymphadenopathy.[43] VATS provides a comprehensive evaluation of the mediastinum when lymphadenopathy beyond the paratracheal or subcarinal lymph node stations is present. VATS conveys the ability to assess the entire ipsilateral mediastinum in greater scope. VATS can directly access the lower subcarinal and periazygos nodal stations and the anterior and posterior mediastinal regions that are inaccessible to cervical mediastinoscopy. VATS is useful when multiple sites within the mediastinum require biopsy.[43, 58]

When the lymphadenopathy is found to be benign, mediastinal lymph node sampling by VATS allows for immediate progression to pulmonary resection by VATS or thoracotomy, avoiding the need to reposition the patient. VATS-directed mediastinal lymph node sampling is a comprehensive method to evaluate mediastinal lymph node status for patients with known lung cancer, and its routine use has been advocated by some investigators, particularly for patients with known adenocarcinoma of the lung.[50] VATS also can identify potential intrapleural metastases not recognized on preoperative radiology studies, thus sparing patients the unnecessary morbidity of a nontherapeutic thoracotomy for advanced-stage disease.[68]

Although the focus of many of the reported experiences with VATS evaluation of mediastinal lymphadenopathy has been in the extended staging of potentially resectable lung cancer, VATS also is useful in the evaluation of "primary" mediastinal lymphadenopathy and lymphoid malignancy. VATS can easily provide acquisition of sufficient tissue to establish the histologic diagnosis from benign causes, such as sarcoidosis or lymphoid hyperplasia.[35] Large amounts of tissue necessary to properly evaluate for lymphoma and for other malignancies, such as germ cell tumors or thymoma, can be obtained easily while the more extensive and cosmetically unappealing anterior mediastinotomy incision is avoided. Because the surgical incision is located on the lateral chest wall, the VATS approach allows for the immediate use of radiotherapy through standard anteroposterior portals, without the fear of detrimental wound healing.[43] In female patients, the anterior mediastinotomy incision through the breast is avoided with the use of the laterally oriented VATS intercostal access sites. In general, the VATS approach is superior to anterior mediastinotomy for biopsy of mediastinal lymphadenopathy inaccessible to standard cervical mediastinoscopy; however, a few selected indications for the anterior mediastinotomy remain.[20, 43, 58] Anterior mediastinotomy is better suited for the biopsy of large or bulky anterior mediastinal mass lesions abutting the anterior chest wall (Fig. 1). A simple anterior incision with standard endotracheal tube ventilation is technically simpler than is double-lumen endotracheal intubation, especially when the trachea is distorted by the mediastinal mass, or when addressing mediastinal lymphadenopathy in elderly, frail individuals.

Technical Considerations

Double-lumen endotracheal intubation and patient positioning are performed. For VATS of the anterior mediastinum, the surgical table is rotated posteriorly to expose more of the anterior chest. The thoracoscope is introduced at the fifth intercostal space (ICS) along the midaxillary line, and additional intercostal access sites are strategically positioned at the second or third ICS midaxillary line and fifth or sixth ICS midaxillary line for the additional instruments in the manner previously described. Posterior rotation of the patient also allows the lung to fall posteriorly, enhancing visibility of the anterior mediastinal structures. A separate lung retractor may be used if visualization must be enhanced. The intercostal approach to the right mediastinum is similar to the

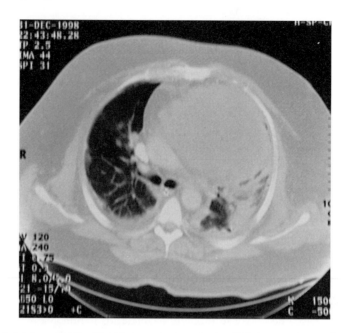

Figure 1. Large mediastinal lymphoma mass, a case in which the anterior mediastinotomy would be preferred over video-assisted thoracic surgery.

left, but for detailed evaluation of the aortopulmonary window (Figs. 2 and 3), the ICS access sites may be altered slightly (Table 1). Sharp dissection with the endoscopic Metzenbaum scissors (US Surgical, Norwalk, CT; Snowden Pencer, Atlanta, GA) is used, with judicious applications of electrocautery. Endoscopic clip ligature of vascular and lymphatic pedicles of the mediastinal lymph nodes is performed as needed. The locations of the phrenic, vagus, and recurrent laryngeal nerves are identified carefully, and dissection is directed to prevent injury to these structures.

MANAGEMENT OF ANTERIOR MEDIASTINAL MASSES AND CYSTS

VATS is well suited for resection of small benign tumors of the anterior mediastinum.[40, 62, 63, 78] Successful VATS resection of benign mediastinal teratoma has been reported. Similarly, patients with ectopic mediastinal parathyroid glands or adenomas may be considered for VATS resection.[16, 24, 57, 69] The reported worldwide experience with VATS resection of mediastinal ectopic parathyroid adenomas is small, but results with this alternative approach to sternotomy seem promising. Precise preoperative localization of the ectopic glands must be obtained, following a diligent cervical exploration for parathyroid glands in their normal position at the thoracic outlet. Sestamibi, CT, and MR scans are useful in the preoperative localization of intrathoracic parathyroid glands. VATS parathyroidectomy is planned as a directed resection following preoperative localization and not as a general exploration (Fig. 4). Additional details regarding parathyroidectomy are discussed in the article by Howe (see pp 1399–1426).

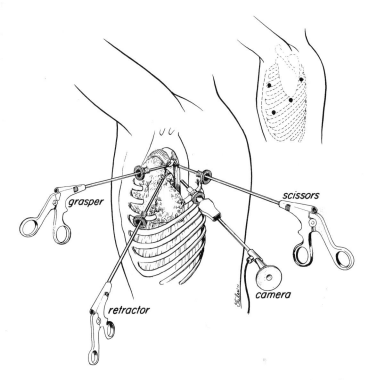

Figure 2. VATS approach for anteroposterior (AP) window and mid esophageal level pathology.

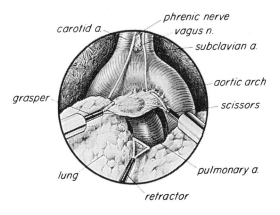

Figure 3. VATS visualization of AP window lymph nodes.

Table 1. STRATEGIC INTERCOSTAL ACCESS LOCATIONS FOR MEDIASTINAL VIDEO-ASSISTED THORACIC SURGERY

Area of Interest	Thoracoscope	Retractor or Grasper	Dissector or Stapler	Additional Instruments
Apices (dorsal sympathectomy)	6 mid	4 ant	4/5 post	—
Anterior mediastinum	5 mid/post	2/3 mid	5/6 post	7 mid
Posterior mediastinum	5 mid	4/6 ant	2 ant	3/4 ant
Midesophagus or aortopulmonary window	5/6 post	5 asc triangle	4 ant	7 mid
Distal esophagus (thoracic splanchnicectomy)	7 mid	4 ant	6/8 post	7 ant
Pericardium (left)	7 post	9 mid	5 post	—

Ant, mid, post = anterior, middle, and posterior axillary lines, respectively; 5 = fifth intercostal space, 6 = sixth intercostal space, and so forth; asc triangle = auscultatory triangle.

Although VATS has been accepted as a reasonable approach to thymic cysts, the use of VATS to accomplish thymectomy remains controversial,[8] which has been reflected in the commentaries of Pairolero[53] following the 1992 report by Landreneau et al[40] of a VATS subtotal thymectomy for a stage I thymoma (Fig. 5). A total thymectomy is the appropriate and proper surgical treatment of thymoma and myasthenia gravis, and operative experience acquired since the authors' initial report[40] has demonstrated that a "total" anatomic thymectomy can be performed with VATS.[47, 48, 78] Clinical data have substantiated the utility of VATS for carefully selected patients with thymic disorders referred for surgical intervention, including thymic cysts, myasthenia gravis, and early-stage thymoma.[47, 48, 62, 78, 81] Careful patient selection for VATS thymectomy is vitally important and must be combined with considerable experience in elementary VATS

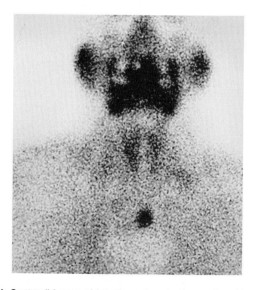

Figure 4. Sestamibi scan of intrathoracic ectopic parathyroid adenoma.

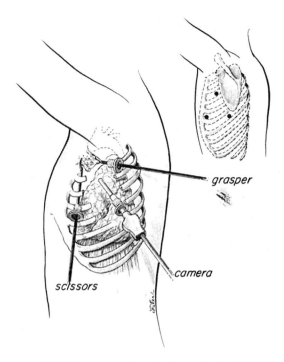

Figure 5. VATS approach for anterior mediastinal pathology.

procedures before thymic resection is attempted. Known malignant tumors and thymomas with preoperative evidence of local invasion should be resected with thoracotomy or sternotomy as deemed appropriate for the specific lesion. Conversion to an open resection is performed when unexpected findings are appreciated during VATS to minimize the risk for incomplete tumor resection.

Criticism of the VATS thymectomy has been based on potential incomplete resection, but the clinical data available demonstrate no appreciable patient response in short-term and intermediate-term evaluation for myasthenia gravis. The 1996 report by Mack et al[47] on a series of 33 patients after VATS thymectomy for myasthenia gravis, with a mean follow-up of 23 months, showed that 88% of patients were improved, which compares favorably with the 1998 report from Bril et al,[6] who reported palliation in 83% and complete remission in 44% of 52 patients after cervical thymectomy, with a mean follow-up of 8.4 years postoperatively. The report by Yim et al[81] on 107 patients after VATS thymectomy for myasthenia gravis showed that 11% of patients were in complete remission and that 78% of patients were improved at a mean postoperative follow-up of 25 months. The 1998 review by Mack and Scruggs[48] maintained that the intermediate-term data following VATS thymectomy compare well with historical series with trans-sternal thymectomy and even "maximal" thymectomy, as advocated by Jaretzki and Wolff.[34]

Technical Considerations

The general VATS surgical routine and intercostal access are the same as outlined for other anterior mediastinal pathology. The authors now routinely approach VATS thymectomy from the right chest unless the thymic mass is predominantly on the left. Although the right-sided approach makes evaluation of the aortopulmonary window difficult for ectopic thymic tissue, excellent visualization of the innominate vein–superior vena cava junction is available during the course of the dissection as described by Yim.[80] This exposure facilitates the dissection while avoiding troublesome bleeding from venous tributaries at this region. Tension on the thymus is avoided when dissection proceeds to the superior aspect of the thymus to avoid avulsion of the thymic veins (of Keynes) or injury to the innominate vein. The thymic veins are identified and doubly clipped on the side of the innominate vein before their transection. The phrenic nerve is carefully identified to avoid its potential injury, and the mediastinal pleura is incised well anterior to the nerve. The surgeon and the patient should be prepared for conversion to thoracotomy or sternotomy to ensure sufficient wide excision when intraoperative evidence of local invasion or other signs of malignant disease are present.[27]

NEUROGENIC TUMORS IN THE POSTERIOR MEDIASTINUM

Posterior mediastinal and paravertebral tumors are predominantly of neurogenic origin. Malignancy is unusual in adults; 90% are of benign nerve sheath origin (i.e., schwannomas or gangliomas). Appropriate management is by surgical excision, and recurrence is unusual. Malignant lesions also may be approached with surgical excision, but prognosis is typically dismal. Preoperative spinal MR or CT scans routinely are indicated to evaluate the intraspinal extension of tumor (i.e., "the dumbbell tumor"), which occurs in 10% of patients.[1] Small posterior neurogenic tumors, without evidence of neural canal invasion (Figs. 6 and 7), can be approached readily for resection using VATS[5, 41] (Fig. 8). Hazelrigg et al[29] have reported an 86% success rate in a series of 21 patients who underwent VATS resection for posterior mediastinal neurogenic tumors. Abnormalities included ganglioneuroma, neurofibroma, malignant schwannoma, and ganglioneuroblastoma, with tumor sizes ranging from 7 cm to 13 cm. The mean operating time was 65 minutes. Postoperative morbidity was minimal and the average length of hospital stay was 2 days.

More complex "dumbbell" tumors with an intraspinal component usually require a staged neurosurgical and thoracic surgical approach incorporating laminectomy followed by thoracotomy to resect the tumor.[23] Nonetheless, reports of combined minimally invasive surgical techniques have been described to manage such complex pathology. Successful use of VATS to resect a dumbbell tumor has been described following staged and combined posterior approaches to laminectomy.[75] The VATS approach to small discrete posterior neurogenic tumors is safe and effective.

Technical Considerations

The patient is prepared and intubated with a double-lumen endotracheal tube in standard fashion. For better exposure of the posterior mediastinum, the patient is rotated anteriorly to facilitate exposure of the posterior mediastinum during the VATS intervention (Fig. 8). This anterior rotation allows gravity to improve exposure by allowing the lung to fall away from the paraspinous region. A lung retractor may be used, if necessary, to enhance exposure. The thoracoscope is placed in the fifth ICS along the midaxillary line, and the other

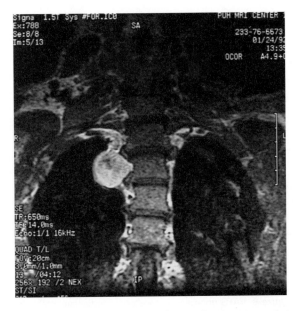

Figure 6. Coronal MR imaging view of paraspinous neurogenic tumor.

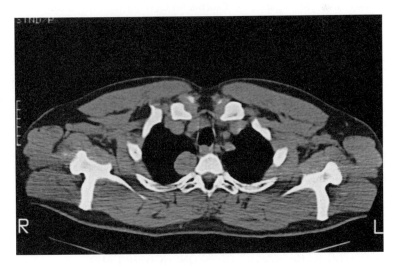

Figure 7. Computerized axial tomography view of paraspinous neurogenic tumor.

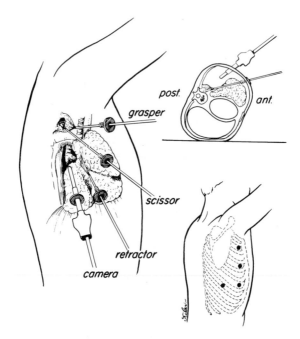

Figure 8. VATS approach for posterior mediastinal pathology.

instruments are placed in the second, forth, and sixth ICSs along the anterior to midaxillary line. This arrangement forms an L shape with the thoracoscope on the left, which is a slight departure from the triangular intercostal access site arrangement usually used for VATS. As Mack et al[46] reported, this intercostal access arrangement is similarly useful for VATS-directed anterior approaches to the spine (i.e., discectomy, corpectomy, and spinal ligamentous release). In addition to experience in advanced VATS techniques, several considerations must be followed when performing surgery in the paraspinous region. The pleura is incised circumferentially around the lesion, then the lesion is mobilized with the use of sharp dissection. The sympathetic nerve trunks and larger (> 2 mm) blood vessels are clipped as they are encountered. Smaller vessels may be managed by electrocautery. Monopolar diathermy should be avoided around the spinal foramen. Bipolar diathermy is used for coagulation in this region to prevent injury to the spinal cord or nerve roots. Strict hemostasis should be achieved to avoid complications of epidural hematoma. Similarly, the use of gelatin foam or oxidized cellulose to pack the neuroforamen should be avoided because it may expand within the spinal canal and cause compression of cord structures.

THERAPEUTIC MANAGEMENT OF BRONCHOGENIC AND PERICARDIAL CYSTS AND PERICARDIAL EFFUSION

Bronchogenic and pericardial cysts in adults are typically asymptomatic and present as an incidental finding on routine chest radiography. Diagnosis usually is confirmed with chest CT demonstrating a simple cyst with low attenuation. Expectant management in young, asymptomatic patients with classic features of a bronchogenic or pericardial cyst on CT scan is suggested, with appropriate follow-up by interval CT scanning; however, if the diagnosis of a simple cyst is uncertain because the attenuation of the cyst contents is high or if the cyst is multiloculated, then surgical resection is indicated. Likewise, if the cyst becomes clinically symptomatic or infected, then cyst excision is warranted (Fig. 9). The cystic structures typically are dissected or marsupialized easily after they are decompressed by intraoperative fine-needle aspiration.[17, 49, 67] The phrenic nerve must be identified clearly and protected during the dissection. Complete resection is ideal, but when the wall of the cyst is firmly adherent to vital mediastinal structures, it may be safer to leave the posterior wall of the cyst in situ after cauterizing the endothelial lining of the cyst.[28]

The role of VATS in the management of malignant and idiopathic benign pericardial effusions has been examined. Malignancy is the most common source of pericardial effusions, accounting for 30% to 50% of the cases of pericardial effusions referred for surgical drainage.[22] The development of a malignant pericardial effusion is often a terminal manifestation of their systemic malignant disease,[79] with a mean survival time of 2.8 months in patients with bronchogenic cancer who present with a pericardial effusion.[26] Patients with advanced malignancies or poor functional status should be temporized with a simpler and less physiologically taxing procedure, such as percutaneous pericardiocentesis. If the effusion is refractory to repeated pericardiocentesis, then a subxyphoid pericardial window can be performed; however, for patients with malignant effusions resulting from diseases with reasonable hope for treatment (e.g., breast cancer or lymphoma) and with good physiologic reserve, VATS is a good alternative to thoracotomy when a more extensive pericardial resection is indicated.[45]

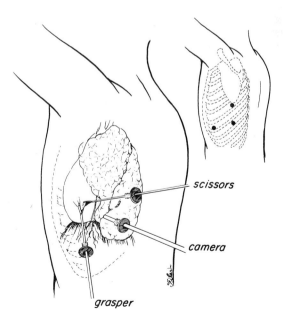

scissors

camera

grasper

Figure 9. Intercostal access used to approach left-sided pericardial cyst.

Technical Considerations

When VATS is chosen to manage such patients, it is preferable to approach the patient after an initial percutaneous drainage procedure to partially decompress the pericardium, which allows for a safer induction of general anesthesia and easier manipulation of the pericardium during VATS.[45] A left chest approach can be used to perform VATS pericardiectomy (Fig. 10); however, a right-sided approach is preferred for greater instrument access[13] (Fig. 11). In general, a left-sided approach is used only when an associated pleural effusion exists on the left side. On entry into the chest and visualization of the pericardium, the phrenic nerve is identified. Pericardiectomy is performed with endoscopic scissors anterior, and posterior if necessary, to the phrenic nerve pedicle. Minor bleeding from the pericardial edge can be managed by judicious use of diathermy. Caution should be exercised to avoid injuring the atrial appendage when the pericardial incision is carried superiorly. External defibrillation pads should be placed preoperatively on these patients routinely because of the potential risk for ventricular dysrhythmias precipitated by the use of electrocautery during the procedure.

ESOPHAGUS

Minimal access surgical techniques for the treatment of gastroesophageal reflux disease, achalasia, and paraesophageal hernias are managed better laparoscopically rather than by VATS. Specific details of minimal access surgery for these esophageal conditions and the role of minimal access surgery in esophageal malignancy are not elaborated here (see article by Maher, pp 1501–1510); however, surgical treatment of benign esophageal cysts and leiomyomata is accomplished through the chest, and VATS has been used with great success.

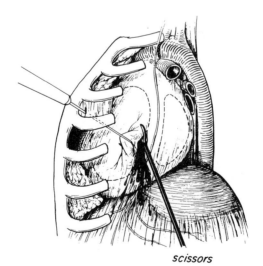

scissors

Figure 10. Left-sided VATS approach for pericardial effusion. A similar approach from the right can be used for pericardiectomy or resection of pericardial cysts.

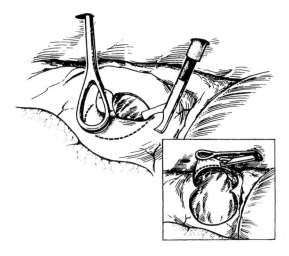

Figure 11. Right-sided VATS pericardiectomy anterior to the pulmonary hilum and phrenic nerve. Creating the window is simplified by the use of the D-loop forceps to grasp the pericardium.

ESOPHAGEAL CYSTS OR LEIOMYOMATA

Historically, surgical management of patients with benign esophageal leiomyomata or cysts has been achieved with enucleation (Fig. 12). These have been regarded as a technically simple open procedure, associated with excellent clinical results and low surgical mortality rate.[4] The recognized morbidity of traditional thoracotomy to remove benign tumor in patients with minimal or no symptoms has led some physicians[61] to recommend expectant management with interval follow-up studies by endoscopic sonography, with resection limited to patients with indeterminate diagnosis or growth of the lesion (Figs. 13 and 14). The introduction of VATS and reports of success with VATS enucleation of esophageal leiomyomata have eased the apprehension among patients and their physicians toward earlier elective resection of these lesions.[3, 12, 19]

The diagnosis of esophageal leiomyomata or duplication cysts may be suspected in patients with obstructive symptoms and evidence of smooth extrinsic compression of the esophageal lumen by an asymmetric convex process (see Fig. 12). Often, the diagnosis is made when the barium upper gastrointestinal series was ordered for other reasons in asymptomatic patients. CT, MR, or endoscopic sonography scans then should be obtained to confirm the diagnosis. A benign esophageal leiomyoma usually is demarcated sharply, smooth, and homogenous to radiographic and sonographic inspection. It is located in the submucosal plane of the esophagus, and no evidence of mediastinal lymphadenopathy is present. Esophagoscopy should reveal a smooth, normal mucosa with some luminal encroachment from external compression. If an esophageal leiomyoma is strongly suspected after radiologic studies, endoscopic biopsy should be avoided to minimize the risk for mucosal perforation at resection caused by inflammatory adhesion development at the endoscopic biopsy site.[4]

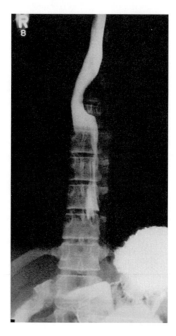

Figure 12. Anteroposterior view of extremic mass effect on midesophagus from one esophageal duplicative cyst.

Technical Considerations

VATS usually is approached from the right (Fig. 15), unless the intended surgical site is in the distal esophagus, where a left-sided approach is more appropriate (Fig. 16). Intraoperative fiberoptic esophagoscopy is an important component of VATS. Esophagoscopy allows for expedient localization of the lesion. The patient is rotated anteriorly to expose the posterior mediastinum and to allow gravity to help to retract the deflated lung. Specific intercostal access sites are selected depending on the level of the lesion (Table 1). Usually, the leiomyoma is in the middle third of the intrathoracic esophagus, and division of the azygos vein with the endoscopic stapler may facilitate exposure of the esophagus at this level. A limited longitudinal esophagomyotomy is created overlying the lesion with the endoscissors, electrocautery, or Harmonic Scalpel (Ethicon Endo-Surgery, Cincinnati, OH), with caution to avoid injury to the esophageal mucosa. Transillumination with the esophagoscope, coupled with selective insufflation, also may facilitate the dissection and detect any penetration of the mucosa. Intraoperative endoscopic sonography has been a useful adjunct in locating smaller lesions that may be difficult to localize by VATS alone (Figs. 13 and 14). When the lesion has been separated from the esophagus, retrieval is accomplished using a plastic Endobag (US Surgical, Norwalk, CT). Maneuvers with the esophagoscope to confirm mucosal integrity include direct and endoscopic examination, together with insufflation of the esophagus, while saline irrigation is introduced into the chest. The myotomized wall of the esophagus should be reapproximated to avoid late complications of dysphagia from mucosal pseudodiverticuli.[3, 4, 64] Mucosal integrity also should be routinely

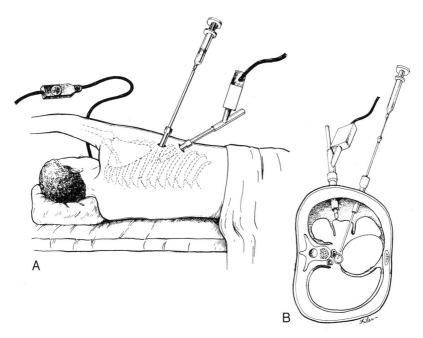

Figure 13. *A,* Esophageal ultrasonography probe, thoracoscope, and aspirating needle introduced through intercostal access for esophageal cyst localization. *B,* Aspirating needle placed through intercostal access under thoracoscopic vision.

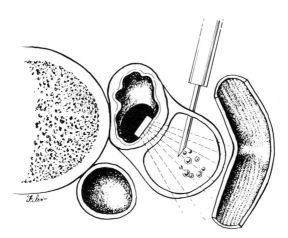

Figure 14. Microbubbles from saline injection into esophageal mass delineate cystic nature of lesion by esophageal ultrasonography.

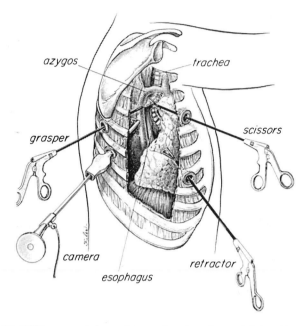

Figure 15. VATS approach for periazygos lymph nodes and right mid esophagus.

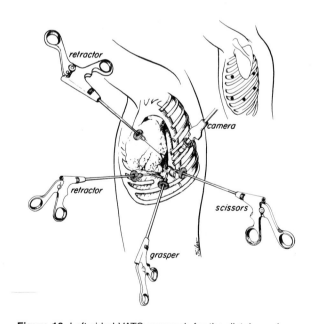

Figure 16. Left-sided VATS approach for the distal esophagus.

confirmed postoperatively with a diatrizoate meglumine solution (Gastrografini; Squibb, Princeton, NJ) esophagram.

DRAINAGE FOR MEDIASTINITIS

Descending necrotizing mediastinitis occurs when a pharyngeal, periodontal, or cervical abscess dissects along anatomic fascial planes down the neck into the mediastinum through the thoracic inlet. This catastrophic condition has been associated with a mortality rate exceeding 50%.[54] Appropriate treatment of this condition includes broad-spectrum antibiotic therapy and aggressive wide surgical débridement and drainage of the mediastinum and posterior pharyngeal space. Cervical drainage alone typically is insufficient treatment, and mediastinal drainage usually requires thoracotomy, particularly if the abscess extends to the level of the T4 vertebra or inferior.[11, 31, 76] Several reports of successful VATS drainage of the mediastinum in the setting of descending necrotizing or acute purulent mediastinitis have been published[39, 60]; however, VATS cannot be recommended for this severe condition until more clinical data can substantiate its use.

THORACODORSAL SYMPATHECTOMY AND SPLANCHNICECTOMY

Surgical nerve ablation procedures, including thoracic sympathectomy and splanchnicectomy, are effective treatment options that have been overlooked by physicians largely because of the additional morbidity of thoracotomy necessary to perform the ablation, together with the tainted history of imprecise indications for the procedure, including:

Established indications
    Hyperhidrosis
Relative indications
    Sympathetic reflex dystrophy
    Raynaud's phenomenon
    Peripheral arterial occlusive disease
    Upper extremity posttraumatic causalgia
Uncertain indications
    Bronchial asthma
    Angina pectoris

Thoracodorsal Sympathectomy

The efficacy of thoracodorsal sympathectomy for idiopathic palmar or axillary hyperhidrosis has been well documented since the initial report by Kotzareff in 1920. Dorsal sympathectomy has been performed through cervical, transaxillary, and thoracic incisions and by the thoracoscopic approach in 1942. By 1954, Kux[37] had accumulated more than 1400 thoracoscopic sympathectomies for vasospastic conditions of the upper extremities. His colleague, Wittmoser (1954), developed the first thoracoscope with multiple working channels that allowed for successful sympathectomy through a single intercostal access technique in 1950. The relatively simple technical nature of these nerve-ablative procedures and the reduction in pain-related morbidity relative to thoracotomy made these conditions ideally suited for thoracoscopic intervention. Interest in non–video thoracoscopic sympathectomy was maintained by a few selected clinicians.[38] The introduction of VATS has revived interest in performing thoracic sympathectomy. In general, sympathectomy can achieve a 85% to 95% success rate in relieving palmar hyperhidrosis and 60% to 80% for axillary hyperhidrosis.[32, 52, 74] VATS approaches to thoracodorsal sympathectomy also have been successfully used to treat patients with severe vasospastic conditions (e.g., Raynaud's syndrome) and reflex sympathetic dystrophy after upper extremity trauma. Although the results with VATS sympathectomy for these latter conditions typically are favorable (60–80% success rate), they do not uniformly approach that of sympathectomy for hyperhidrosis. A common side effect, however, is the development of compensatory or truncal gustatory sweating, which may be experienced in as many as 50% of patients.[21, 82] Also, injury to the stellate ganglion may result in temporary Horner's syndrome in 2% to 5% of patients and permanent Horner's syndrome in 1% to 2% of patients.[82]

Thoracic Splanchnicectomy

Severe, chronic, intractable pain from pancreatic or hepatobiliary cancer, chronic pancreatitis, and other advanced intra-abdominal cancers is mediated through the celiac plexus, the celiac ganglia, and the greater and lesser splanchnic nerves. Interruption of the pathway with alcohol or phenol injection of the celiac plexus can be temporarily effective in controlling this visceral pain, but diminishing results occur with repeated injections. Complications related to the injury of vascular structures in proximity to the neural structures may occur. Surgical interruption of the splanchnic nerves with or without vagotomy through left thoracotomy can be performed to interrupt the afferent visceral pain pathway.[72] Concurrent bilateral thoracic truncal vagotomy has been advocated by some investigators[72] for chronic pancreatitis to interrupt the pain-sensory pathways and to reduce gastric and pancreatic stimulation. These investigators were able to demonstrate short-term relief of pain in all patients after a left thoracic splanchnicectomy and bilateral vagotomy. Long-term relief was sustained in 67% of patients. The performance of a subsequent right thoracic sympathectomy among patients with persistent pain improved the long-term pain control to 80%. Others[73] have advocated limiting the vagotomy to the posterior trunk to interrupt the pain fibers to the pancreas, to avoid delayed gastric emptying that results from dividing the vagal innervation to the pylorus. VATS left thoracic splanchnicectomy also has resulted in excellent short-term palliation of pain in these patients similar to that achieved through thoracotomy[77] and may be a reasonable approach for chronic pain control for these selected patients without incurring the morbidity of a formal thoracotomy.

Technical Considerations

The patient is positioned to enhance exposure of the posterior mediastinum by anterior rotation (see Fig. 8). Alternatively, the patient may be kept in a supine position with the chest elevated with rolls behind the back to better expose the lateral chest wall to avoid having to reposition the patient. The table is alternatively rotated to enhance exposure to the left and right chest, with the ports placed in an anterolateral location. The lung is retracted, if necessary, with a separate retractor. The classic method of sympathectomy involves division of the interganglionic sympathetic chain from the inferior aspect of the stellate ganglion for a variable distance. The authors commonly resect the T2–T3 ganglia for the management of palmar hyperhidrosis. The interganglionic resection is effective, but some critics maintain that this "nonselective" method may result in a higher risk for Horner's syndrome and reflex truncal or facial perspiration afterward. "Selective" techniques of interrupting the preganglionic or postganglionic rami communicantes have been described.[14, 15] Based on the pioneering work of Wittmoser, Freidel et al[14, 15] advocate the postganglionic technique as the most effective while minimizing the undesired complications of Horner's syndrome or compensatory sweating. Monopolar electrocautery near the stellate ganglion should be avoided to minimize the risk for Horner's syndrome.

For VATS left splanchnicectomy, the patient is placed in right lateral decubitus position, with the surgical table rotated anteriorly to expose the posterior mediastinum (Fig. 17). The splanchnic nerves should be visible posterior to the pleura, arising from and coursing medial to the sympathetic ganglia and chain. The greater splanchnic nerve may arise from as high as the fifth thoracic sympathetic ganglion and as low as the tenth. The lesser splanchnic nerve usually arises from the 9th to 11th thoracic ganglia. Once identified, the nerves are clipped and divided at the origin and then traced down to the diaphragm, where they are clipped and divided again (Fig. 18).

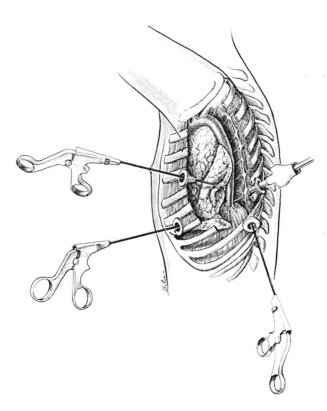

Figure 17. VATS approach for thoracic splanchnicectomy.

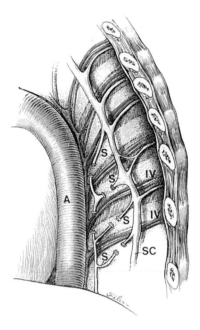

Figure 18. Left view of thoracic splanchnicectomy. SC = sympathetic chain; S = splanchnic nerve; IV = intercostal vessels; A = aorta.

SUMMARY

VATS and concepts of minimal access thoracic surgery have revitalized many aspects of general thoracic surgery, including the surgical approach to diseases and conditions of the mediastinum. Proven surgical options that have been shunned by patients and referring physicians because of the perceived morbidity of thoracotomy have been reconsidered with the emergence of these minimal access surgical options. Continued critical review of the accumulating experience in VATS techniques will refine the surgical indications for VATS and open thoracotomy.

References

1. Akwari OE, Payne WS, Onofrio BM, et al: Dumbell neurogenic tumors of the mediastinum: Diagnosis and management. Mayo Clin Proc 53:353–358, 1978
2. Bardini R, Segalin A, Ruol A, et al: Video-thoracoscopic enucleation of esophageal leiomyoma. Ann Thorac Surg 54:576–577, 1992
3. Bardini R, Asolati M: Thoracoscopic resection of benign tumours of the esophagus. Int Surg 82:5–6, 1997
4. Bonavina L, Segalin A, Rosati R, et al: Surgical therapy of esophageal leiomyoma. J Am Coll Surg 181:257–262, 1995
5. Bousamra M, Haagler GB, Patterson GA, et al: A comparative study of thoracoscopic vs. open removal of benign neurogenic mediastinal tumors. Chest 109:1461–1465, 1996
6. Bril V, Kojic J, Ilse WK, et al: Long-term clinical outcome after transcervical thymectomy for myasthenia gravis. Ann Thorac Surg 65:1520–1522, 1998

7. Carlens E: Mediastinoscopy: A method for inspection and tissue biopsy in the superior mediastinum. Dis Chest 36:343–346, 1959
8. Cooper JD: Video-assisted thoracic surgery thymectomy for myasthenia gravis: Commentary. Chest Surg Clin North Am 8:827–834, 1998
9. DePaula AL, Hashiba A, Ferraira EA, et al: Laparoscopic transhiatal esophagectomy with esophagogastroplasty. Surg Laparosc Endosc 5:1–5, 1995
10. Deslauriers J, Beaulieu M, Dufour C, et al: Mediastinoscopy: A new approach to the diagnosis of intrathoracic disease. Ann Thorac Surg 22:265, 1976
11. Estrera AS, Londory MJ, Grisham JM, et al: Descending necrotizing mediastinitis. Surg Gynecol Obstet 157:545–552, 1983
12. Everitt N, Glinatsis M, McMahon M: Thoracoscopic enucleation of leiomyoma of the oesophagus. Br J Surg 79:643, 1992
13. Flores RM, Jaklitsch MT, DeCamp MM, et al: Video-assisted thoracic surgery pericardial resection for effusive disease. Chest Surg Clin North Am 8:835–851, 1998
14. Friedel G, Linder A, Toomes H: Selective video-assisted thoracoscopic sympathectomy. Thorac Cardiovasc Surg 41:245–248, 1993
15. Friedel G, Linder A, Toomes H: Sympathectomy and vagotomy. *In* Manncke K, Rosin RD (eds): Minimal Access Thoracic Surgery. London, Chapman & Hall, 1998, pp 67–84
16. Furrer M, Leutenegger AF, Ruedi T: Thoracoscopic resection of an ectopic giant parathyroid adenoma: Indication, technique, and three years follow-up. Thorac Cardiovasc Surg 44:208–209, 1996
17. Furukawa K, Takahata S, Ichimiya H, et al: Video-assisted thoracoscopic resection of a mediastinal cyst: Report of a case. Surg Today 24:923–925, 1994
18. Ginsberg RJ, Rice TW, Goldberg M, et al: Extended cervical mediastinoscopy: A single staging procedure for bronchogenic carcinoma of the left upper lobe. J Thorac Cardiovasc Surg 94:673, 1987
19. Gossot D, Fourquier P, El Meteini M, et al: Technical aspects of endoscopic removal of benign tumors of the esophagus. Surg Endosc 7:102–103, 1993
20. Gossot D, Toledo L, Fritsch S, et al: Mediastinoscopy vs thoracoscopy for mediastinal biopsy. Chest 110:1328–1331, 1996
21. Gossot D, Toledo L, Fritsch S, et al: Thoracoscopic sympathectomy for upper limb hyperhidrosis: Looking for the right operation. Ann Thorac Surg 64:975–978, 1997
22. Gregory JR, McMurtrey MJ, Mountain CF: A surgical approach to the treatment of pericardial effusion in cancer patients. Am J Clin Oncol 8:319–323, 1985
23. Grillo HC, Mathisen D: Combined approach to "dumbbell" intrathoracic and intraspinal neurogenic tumors. Ann Thorac Surg 36:902–907, 1983
24. Gullstrand P, Olsson G, Olsson M, et al: Thoracoscopic parathyroidectomy of an ectopic mediastinal adenoma. Br J Surg 83:1757, 1996
25. Harken DE, Black H, Clauss R, et al: A single cervical mediastinal exploration for tissue diagnosis of intrathoracic disease. N Engl J Med 251:1041, 1954
26. Hazelrigg SR, Mack MJ, Landreneau RJ, et al: Thoracoscopic pericardiectomy for effusive pericardial disease. Ann Thorac Surg 56:792–795, 1993
27. Hazelrigg SR, Mack MJ, Landreneau RJ: Video-assisted thoracic surgery for mediastinal disease. Chest Surg Clin North Am 3:283–297, 1993
28. Hazelrigg SR, Landreneau RJ, Mack MJ, et al: Thoracoscopic resection of mediastinal cysts. Ann Thorac Surg 56:656–660, 1993
29. Hazelrigg SR, Boley TM, Krasna MJ, et al: Thoracoscopic resection of posterior neurogenic tumors. Am Surg (in press)
30. Heltzer JM, Krasna MJ, Aldrich F, et al: Thoracoscopic excision of a posterior mediastinal "dumbbell" tumor using a combined approach. Ann Thorac Surg 60:431–433, 1995
31. Howell HS, Prinz RA, Pickleman JR: Anaerobic mediastinitis. Surg Gynecol Obstet 143:353–359, 1976
32. Hsu C, Chen C, Lin C, et al: Video-assisted thoracoscopic T2 sympathectomy for hyperhidrosis palmaris. J Am Coll Surg 179:59, 1994
33. Hurley JP, McCarthy J, Wood AE: Retrospective analysis of the utility of video-assisted thoracic surgery in 100 consecutive procedures. Eur J Cardiothorac Surg 8:589–592, 1994

34. Jaretzki A, Wolff M: Maximal thymectomy for myasthenia gravis. J Thorac Cardiovasc Surg 96:711–716, 1988
35. Kern JA, Daniel TM, Tribble CG, et al: Thoracoscopic diagnosis and treatment of mediastinal masses. Ann Thorac Surg 56:92–96, 1993
36. Kirschner PA: Extended mediastinoscopy. *In* Jensen O, Sorensen HR (eds): Mediastinoscopy. Oderise, Denmark, Odense University Press, 1971, p 131
37. Kux E: Thorakoskopishe Eingriffe am Nervensystem. Stuttgart, Thieme Verlag, 1954
38. Kux M: Thoracic endoscopic sympathectomy in palmar and axillary hyperhidrosis. Arch Surg 113:264–266, 1978
39. Laisaar T: Video-assisted thoracoscopic surgery in the management of acute purulent mediastinitis and pleural empyema. Thorac Cardiovasc Surg 46:51–54, 1998
40. Landreneau RJ, Dowling RD, Castillo W, et al: Thoracoscopic resection of an anterior mediastinal mass. Ann Thorac Surg 54:142–144, 1992
41. Landreneau RJ, Dowling RD, Ferson PF: Thoracoscopic resection of a posterior mediastinal mass. Chest 102:1288–1290, 1992
42. Landreneau RJ, Mack MJ, Hazelrigg SR, et al: Video-assisted thoracic surgery: Basic technical concepts and intercostal approach strategies. Ann Thorac Surg 54:800–807, 1992
43. Landreneau RJ, Hazelrigg SR, Mack MJ, et al: Thoracoscopic mediastinal lymph node sampling: A useful approach to mediastinal lymph node stations inaccessible to cervical mediastinoscopy. J Thorac Cardiovasc Surg 106:554–558, 1993
44. Landreneau RJ, Mack MJ, Keenan RJ, et al: Strategic planning for video-assisted thoracic surgery. Ann Thorac Surg 56:615–619, 1993
45. Mack MJ, Landreneau RJ, Hazelrigg SR, et al: Video thoracoscopic management of benign and malignant pericardial effusions. Chest 103(suppl 4):390–393, 1993
46. Mack MJ, Regan JJ, Bobechko WP, et al: Application of thoracoscopy for diseases of the spine. Ann Thorac Surg 56:736–738, 1993
47. Mack MJ, Landreneau RJ, Yim AP, et al: Results of video-assisted thymectomy in patients with myasthenia gravis. J Thorac Cardiovasc Surg 112:1352–1360, 1996
48. Mack MJ, Scruggs G: Video-assisted thoracic surgery thymectomy for myasthenia gravis. Chest Surg Clin North Am 8:809–826, 1998
49. Mouroux J, Padovani B, Maalouf J, et al: Pleuropericardial cysts: Treatment by videothoracoscopy. Surg Laparosc Endosc 6:403–404, 1996
50. Nakanishi R, Yasumoto K: Combined thoracoscopy and mediastinoscopy for mediastinal lymph node staging of lung cancer. Int Surg 81:359–361, 1996
51. McNeill TM, Chamberlain JM: Diagnostic anterior mediastinotomy. Ann Thorac Surg 2:532, 1966
52. Nicholson ML, Hopkinson DR, Dennis MJ: Endoscopic transthoracic sympathectomy: Successful in hyperhidrosis but can the indications be extended? Ann R Coll Surg Engl 76:311, 1994
53. Pairolero PC: Commentary of Landreneau RJ, Dowling RD, Castillo W, Ferson PF: Thoracoscopic resection of an anterior mediastinal mass. Ann Thorac Surg 54:142–144, 1992
54. Pearse HE: Mediastinitis following cervical suppuration. Ann Surg 108:588–611, 1938
55. Pearson FG: An evaluation of mediastinoscopy in the management of presumably operable bronchial carcinoma. J Thorac Cardiovasc Surg 55:617, 1968
56. Pearson FG: Use of mediastinoscopy in selection of patients for lung cancer operations. Ann Thorac Surg 30:205, 1980
57. Prinz RA, Lonchyna V, Carnaille B, et al: Thoracoscopic excision of enlarged mediastinal parathyroid glands. Surgery 116:999–1005, 1994
58. Rendina EA, Venuto F, DeGiacorno T, et al: Comparative merits of thoracoscopy, mediastinoscopy, and mediastinotomy for mediastinal biopsy. Ann Thorac Surg 57:992–995, 1994
59. Ribet M, Cardot G: Approach to anterior mediastinal tumours. Ann Chir 47:161–166, 1993
60. Roberts JR: Thoracoscopic management of descending necrotizing mediastinitis. Chest 112:850–854, 1997

61. Rosch T, Lorenz R, Dancygier H, et al: Endosonographic diagnosis of submucosal upper gastrointestinal tract tumor. Scand J Gastroenterol 27:1–8, 1992
62. Roviaro G, Rebuffat C, Varoli F, et al: Videoscopic excision of mediastinal masses: Indications and technique. Ann Thorac Surg 58:1679–1684, 1994
63. Roviaro GC, Rebuffat C, Varoli F, et al: Major thoracoscopic operations: Pulmonary resection and mediastinal mass excision. Int Surg 81:354–358, 1996
64. Roviaro GC, Maciocco M, Varoli F, et al: Videothoracoscopic treatment of oesophageal leiomyoma. Thorax 53:190–192, 1998
65. Satur CM, Hsin MK, Dussek JE: Giant pericardial cysts. Ann Thorac Surg 61:208–210, 1996
66. Schmid RA, Schob OM, Klotz HP, et al: VATS resection of an oesophageal leiomyoma in a patient with neurofibromatosis recklinhausen. Eur J Cardiothorac Surg 12:659–662, 1997
67. Schwarz CD, Puschmann R, Eckmayr J, et al: Video-endoscopic removal of a mediastinal cyst. Chest 105:1254–1256, 1994
68. Shields T: The significance of ipsilateral mediastinal lymph node metastasis (N2 disease) in non-small cell carcinoma of the lung. J Thorac Cardiovasc Surg 99:48–53, 1990
69. Smythe WR, Bavaria JE, Hall RA, et al: Thoracoscopic removal of mediastinal parathyroid adenoma. Ann Thorac Surg 59:236–238, 1995
70. Soliani L, Bagioni P, Campanini A, et al: Diagnostic role of videothoracoscopy in mediastinal diseases. Eur J Cardiothorac Surg 13:491–493, 1998
71. Stemmer EA, Calvin JW, Chandor SB, et al: Mediastinal biopsy for indeterminate pulmonary and mediastinal lesions. J Thorac Cardiovasc Surg 49:405–411, 1965
72. Stone JJ, Chauvin EJ: Pancreatic denervation for pain relief in chronic alcohol associated pancreatitis. Br J Surg 77:303–305, 1990
73. Testart J: Commentary of Worsey J, Landreneau RJ: Thoracoscopic pancreatic denervation for pain control in irresectable pancreatic cancer. Br J Surg 81:149, 1994
74. Urschel HC: Video-assisted sympathectomy and thoracic outlet syndrome. Chest Surg Clin North Am 3:299–306, 1993
75. Vallieres E, Findlay JM, Fraser RE: Combined microneurosurgical and thoracoscopic removal of neurogenic dumbbell tumors. Ann Thorac Surg 59:469–472, 1995
76. Wheatley JH, et al: Descending necrotizing mediastinitis: Trans-cervical drainage is not enough. Ann Thorac Surg 111:485–486, 1996
77. Worsey J, Ferson PF, Keenan RJ, et al: Thoracoscopic pancreatic denervation for pain control in irresectable pancreatic cancer. Br J Surg 80:1051–1052, 1993
78. Yim AP: Video-assisted thoracoscopic resection of anterior mediastinal masses. Int Surg 81:350–353, 1996
79. Yim AP, Chung SS, Lee TW, et al: Thoracoscopic management of malignant pleural effusions. Chest 109:1234–1238, 1996
80. Yim AP: Thoracoscopic thymectomy: Which side to approach? Ann Thorac Surg 64:584–585, 1997
81. Yim AP, Mack MJ, Lerut T, et al: VATS thymectomy for myasthenia gravis: Results of intermediate follow up in 107 patients. Ann Thorac Surg (in press)
82. Zacherl J, Juber ER, Imhof M, et al: Long term results of 630 thoracoscopic sympathectomies for primary hyperhidrosis: The Vienna experience. Eur J Surg 580:43–46, 1998

Address reprint requests to
Rodney J. Landreneau, MD
Division Director, General Thoracic Surgery
02 Level South Tower
320 East North Avenue
Pittsburgh, PA 15212

e-mail: Rlandren@aherf.edu

MINIMAL ACCESS SURGERY, PART II   0039–6109/00 $15.00 + .00

THORACOSCOPIC EVALUATION AND TREATMENT OF THORACIC TRAUMA

Gregory A. Lowdermilk, MD,† and Keith S. Naunheim, MD

HISTORY

The history of thoracoscopy dates back to 1910, when Jacobaeus,[10] from Sweden, first reported the use of a cystoscope to examine the pleural and pericardial cavities in patients with tuberculosis. Edwards[4] reviewed the use of thoracoscopic surgery in 1924, but its use in trauma care was not reported. It was not until 1946 that Branco[2] in Brazil first used thoracoscopy in five patients with penetrating trauma to evaluate the need for thoracotomy. Thoracoscopy for thoracic trauma evaluation was again reported in 1974, when Senno et al,[24] in the United States, used a rigid bronchoscope for thoracoscopy to visualize bleeding from a stab wound. Again in 1981, 36 cases of penetrating trauma were evaluated using rigid thoracoscopy.[11]

Video-assisted thoracoscopic surgery (VATS) became a reality in the early 1990s with the evolution of endoscopic instrumentation, lighting, and video imaging. These technologic advances have allowed for more thorough and precise visualization of the thoracic cavity and its contents. VATS was introduced into trauma care in a series evaluating diaphragmatic injury in 1993.[22] Today, VATS is being used in various pulmonary, chest wall, mediastinal, neurologic, and cardiac surgical procedures. The application to trauma patients is reviewed.

EPIDEMIOLOGY

Thoracic trauma is responsible for 25% of the approximately 150,000 trauma deaths in the United States each year.[18] An estimated one third of these deaths occur immediately and the remaining two thirds occur as a result of thoracic

†Deceased.

From the Division of Cardiothoracic Surgery, Saint Louis University Health Sciences Center, St Louis, Missouri injury or a thoracic complication. Many of these latter deaths occur because of sepsis or respiratory failure secondary to pneumonia or inflammatory response syndrome. This response frequently is manifested and diagnosed in the lung as acute respiratory distress syndrome. The thoracotomy incision has been recognized as the most morbid of surgical incisions, making it even more undesirable in a patient already physiologically compromised by the effects of trauma. Landreneau et al[12] reported on 138 consecutive, nonrandomized patients with equivalent demographic and preoperative physiological parameters who underwent a VATS approach ($n = 81$) or a limited lateral thoracotomy approach to accomplish pulmonary resection for peripheral lung lesions. Pain was quantitated by postoperative narcotic requirements, the need for intercostal or epidural analgesia, and patient perception of pain using index scoring. Patients undergoing VATS experienced statistically significant less pain ($P = 0.001$). Shoulder girdle strength was equally impaired at day 3, but function was more improved in VATS patients at 3 weeks ($P = 0.01$). Patients undergoing wedge resection alone by limited lateral thoracotomy had greater impairment in early (day 3) pulmonary function (FEV_1; $P = 0.002$). The capability of evaluating and managing thoracic trauma without the need for thoracotomy could prove valuable and perhaps decrease the incidence of pulmonary complications. Thoracoscopy can provide just such an option.

INDICATIONS

The gold standard for diagnosis and management of thoracic trauma has been physical examination, chest radiography, chest CT, and aortography. These modalities are reliable in the diagnosis of great vessel, lung parenchyma, and bony injuries. The pitfalls have been recognizing diaphragmatic injuries and the specific source of a hemothorax. Before the use of video thoracoscopy, recognition of these injuries often required a thoracotomy. Currently, the role of thoracoscopy in trauma includes evaluation and control of continued chest tube bleeding, early evacuation of a retained hemothorax, evacuation and decortication of posttraumatic empyemas, evaluation and limited treatment of suspected diaphragmatic injuries, evaluation and treatment of persistent air leaks, and evaluation of mediastinal injuries.

The major contraindication to VATS for trauma is the presence of hemodynamic instability. VATS procedures require single lung anesthesia and can be somewhat time consuming, two attributes that are unacceptable in trauma patients who are hypotensive for an unknown reason. These patients are best managed with an immediate thoracotomy, an approach that allows for rapid evaluation, packing, and control of active bleeding. Other contraindications to VATS include:

Hemodynamic instability
Suspected injuries to the heart or great vessels
Major injuries to the heart or great vessels
Inability to tolerate single lung ventilation
Inability to tolerate lateral decubitus position
Obliterated pleural space
Prior thoracotomy
Indication for emergent thoracotomy or sternotomy
Bleeding diathesis

Thoracoscopy should be performed only in the surgical suite under controlled conditions by a surgeon and anesthesiologist experienced in endoscopic techniques. The surgeon should have no hesitation in converting immediately to a thoracotomy if bleeding becomes uncontrollable, the patient is hemodynamically unstable, or both.

ANESTHETIC MANAGEMENT

Expert anesthetic management of these patients is essential if good results are to be obtained. A VATS procedure should be performed only in the surgical suite with the patient under general anesthesia with single-lung ventilation. A right-sided or left-sided double-lumen endotracheal tube may be used, but many surgeons prefer a left-sided tube because of its ease of placement and stability. If the patient is small or if a double-lumen tube is unavailable, a single-lumen endotracheal tube with a bronchial blocker is preferred. Proper placement must be confirmed by bronchoscopy and auscultation after the patient is positioned in the lateral decubitus position—an essential part of the procedure, to be performed before the patient is prepped and draped. It takes only one episode of finding the tube incorrectly positioned after draping the patient to understand its importance. Continuous monitoring of oxygen saturation and arterial pressure is essential in seriously ill trauma patients managed using single-lung ventilation techniques. When only thoracoscopy is performed, postoperative pain usually can be managed without an intercostal nerve block or epidural analgesics.

TECHNIQUE

VATS procedures may require an experienced assistant, depending on the complexity of the procedure. One port may be used in rare cases when visualization alone is necessary. Normally, two or more ports are needed for manipulation of the lung and therapeutic interventions. The lung on the operative side is decompressed, and a thoracoport is introduced through an incision in the midaxillary line because this provides the most satisfactory perspective to visualize the lung, diaphragm, and mediastinum. The intercostal space chosen may depend on the suspected region most likely injured. Caution must be exercised to prevent iatrogenic bleeding from the intercostal bundle in the space entered. A 0° thoracoscope with video camera is placed through the port. Thirty and forty-five degree viewing thoracoscopes can prove useful to look "over" or "around" structures and down into crevices, such as the costophrenic angle. Although 10-mm thoracoscopes are most often used for their superior lighting, definition, and field of view, in some instances, 5-mm thoracoscopes can be used.

The pleural cavity and lung are inspected thoroughly. Evaluation of the need for additional ports in the anterior axillary and posterior axillary lines is made. Usually, at least one additional port is necessary for manipulation of the lung. One caveat is to ensure that the ports are sufficiently distal to prevent "dueling" instruments during surgery. At the termination of surgery, a single chest tube is placed posteriorly, and an additional anterior tube is recommended if a significant postoperative air leak is expected or if raw oozing surfaces are present in the anterior aspect of the pleural cavity.

DIAPHRAGMATIC INJURY

The diagnosis of a traumatic diaphragmatic injury can be a perplexing problem. Approximately 30% of all diaphragmatic injuries are missed, even after chest radiography, CT, and diagnostic peritoneal lavage are used.[6] Villavicencio et al[27] performed an analysis of thoracoscopy in trauma, which best illustrates the current progress. Literature between 1975 and 1997 was reviewed and contained 15 reports with a total of 199 patients in whom VATS or nonvideo thoracoscopy was used to evaluate suspected diaphragmatic injury. Eight of these studies were retrospective, seven were prospective, and none were randomized. The injuries consisted of 23 blunt wounds, 22 nonspecific penetrating wounds, 21 gunshot wounds, and 134 stab wounds. Of 199 suspected diaphragmatic injuries, 84 were proven by a laparotomy or thoracotomy. The correct diagnosis was made by thoracoscopy in 82 of 84 injuries. Nine of these injuries were repaired with thoracoscopy. Three procedure-related complications occurred among the 199 patients. Thoracoscopy in these 15 studies had a specificity of 97%, a sensitivity of 100%, and an accuracy of 98%.

Ochsner et al[23] reported a series in which they performed thoracoscopy with subsequent laparotomy in 14 patients with penetrating wounds to the thoracoabdominal region. Laparotomy was negative in all five patients without evidence of diaphragmatic injury on thoracoscopy. Nine patients had diaphragmatic injuries on thoracoscopic examination, which were confirmed by laparotomy. These data support the use of thoracoscopy when one suspects the presence of diaphragmatic injury. Accurate diagnosis of this injury can be safely accomplished thoracoscopically in patients who might otherwise require a thoracotomy or laparotomy to make the diagnosis.

Experienced surgeons may be able to repair penetrating wounds of the diaphragm with the thoracoscope, but no long-term results are available. Large diaphragmatic disruptions from blunt trauma require a thoracotomy or laparotomy not only to repair the diaphragm but also to evaluate the presence of significant visceral injury. Penetrating injuries around the zone of the diaphragm require thoracic and abdominal exploration to rule out a colon, liver, or gastric injury. It is possible to undertake exploration using minimally invasive surgical techniques.

HEMOTHORAX

Continued bleeding from chest trauma is an indication for surgical exploration. Criteria used as indications include drainage of more than 1500 mL in 24 hours or 200 mL/h or more for several hours. The most common sites for such blood loss are from intercostal vessels or lung lacerations. These can often be controlled thoracoscopically by using electrocautery, endoclips, staples, or suture. For difficult-to-control intercostal vessel bleeding, pericostal sutures can be placed from outside the skin after the bleeding site is localized. Lung lacerations often can be controlled with endoscopic staplers. Conversion to a thoracotomy is common for cases of intercostal vessels retracted beneath the pleura or for injured lung parenchyma vessels near the hilum. Communication with the anesthesiologist is essential to maintain a safe margin between blood loss and hemodynamic instability. Thoracoscopy for control of bleeding should be avoided in unstable patients but has been proven to be a successful therapeutic modality in stable patients meeting these criteria, with only 18% requiring a thoracotomy.[11]

Posttraumatic retained hemothorax can lead to an entrapped lung and empyema. In the past, this problem was managed by thoracotomy when chest tube drainage failed to evacuate the pleural cavity. Coselli et al[3] reported a study that strongly supports early drainage in such cases. They reviewed 4000 patients requiring a chest tube for hemothorax. A thoracotomy was necessary in 3.8% of cases because of a clotted hemothorax or empyema. The mortality rate for early evacuation (< 5 d) was 0% compared with mortality rates of 1.6% and 9.4% for patients who progressed to decortication or empyema, respectively.

The use of VATS in the early evacuation of posttraumatic retained hemothorax has been well documented. Twelve studies* have reported on a total of 99 patients. These cases report a low rate of postoperative complications, but none were performed in a prospective, randomized fashion. VATS should be performed in patients with inadequately drained hemothorax within 5 days if the patient is hemodynamically stable and has no surgical contraindications.

POSTTRAUMATIC EMPYEMA

Posttraumatic empyema has been reported in 2% to 10% of all patients sustaining thoracic trauma.[5, 9] The therapeutic application of VATS for the evacuation of posttraumatic empyemas has been widely reported.[5, 7, 9, 14, 16, 21] These studies should be reviewed with caution because they do not always describe the precise stage of empyema or the extent of decortication necessary. VATS is most effective in the early exudative or purulent phase. The empyema consists of infected clot or fibrinous deposits without significant organized fibrin deposits on the visceral pleural surface. When the second or fibrinopurulent stage has begun (at 7 to 10 d), the fibrinous peel on the lung surface tends to impair complete lung expansion and increase the risk for a persistent pleural space. Patients in the third, or fibrotic, stage of empyema have a thick peel visualized on CT scanning with major volume loss, a problem best treated with immediate thoracotomy and formal decortication.

VATS has been reported to be successful in 54% of chronic empyemas of all causes.[20] Striffeler et al[26] published their VATS experience of 67 patients with stage II empyemas from all causes. Nineteen (28%) required conversion to an open procedure because advanced disease was found. Trauma was the cause of empyema in 7% of patients, and all were successfully managed with VATS. They found no preoperative investigation, including CT scanning, to be useful in differentiating patients in whom VATS likely would be successful. Empyema recurred in two (4%) patients who required thoracotomy.

PERSISTENT AIR LEAKS

Evaluation and treatment of persistent air leaks in trauma can be approached technically in the same manner as in nontraumatic patients, such as patients with spontaneous pneumothorax and refractory air leak. Small leaks can be controlled with an endoscopic stapler. Although the use of buttress material (polytetrafluoroethylene or bovine pericardium) is helpful in controlling air leaks in patients with end-stage emphysema, it has little or no role in thoracic trauma patients. Most such patients are young with fairly normal lung

---

*References 1, 7, 9, 13–17, 19, 24, 27, and 28.

parenchyma that requires no buttress or reinforcement. The use of foreign material is contraindicated in light of the potential for infection.

Lang-Lazdunski et al[14] have reported their series of 42 trauma patients with persistent leaks, of whom five were treated with VATS. VATS was effective in treating direct lung injuries and confirming proper chest tube placement. The mean period of persistent air leak was 11 days. Four patients required stapling, and one had a extrapleural chest tube. No complications from the procedures were noted.

MEDIASTINAL INJURIES

Several investigators have proposed using VATS for exploring the heart, great vessels, and pericardium when a negative exploration is expected. The procedure has been reported to be used in patients with blunt and penetrating injuries.[8, 19] The risk for life-threatening hemorrhage is real with this approach, and it must be used with caution, if at all. It is mentioned here only for completeness.

COST

No study has analyzed the cost of using thoracoscopy for trauma versus conventional care. One study compared length of stay among patients treated with thoracoscopy and those undergoing thoracotomy for continued chest tube bleeding, diaphragmatic injury, or related hemothorax and showed no significant difference.[28]

SUMMARY

VATS has a diagnostic and therapeutic role in the treatment of patients with chest trauma, but the basic rule of safety over technology must be applied. It is

Table 1. CONVERSION TO THORACOTOMY

Study	Thoracotomy Conversion Rate
Heniford[7]	2/19
Landrenau[13]	0/7
Lang-Lazdunski[14]	1/12
Liu[16]	0/18
Mancini[17]	1/3
McManus[19]	1/2
Sosa[25]	0/3
Abolhoda[1]	4/13
Ilic[9]	0/3
Waller[28]	0/2
Lesser[15]	0/3
Wong[29]	1/14
Total	**10/99 (10%)**

an effective means for managing diaphragmatic injuries, hemothorax, empyemas, and persistent air leaks in selected hemodynamically stable patients. An overview of reported series (Table 1) demonstrates that VATS can be used successfully in the evaluation of patients with blunt and penetrating trauma. In appropriately selected cases, thoracoscopy can prove to be useful, with conversion to thoracotomy in only 10% of patients. Additional studies must be performed to determine any cost benefit compared with conventional therapy.

References

1. Abolhoda A, Livingston DH, Donahoo JS, et al: Diagnostic and therapeutic video assisted thoracic surgery (VATS) following chest trauma. Eur J Cardiothorac Surg 12:356–360, 1997
2. Branco JMC: Thoracoscopy as a method of exploration in penetrating injuries of the chest. Diseases of the Chest 12:330–335, 1946
3. Coselli JS, Mattox KL, Beall: Reevaluation of early evacuation of clotted hemothorax. Am J Surg 148:786, 1984
4. Edwards AT: Thoracoscopy in surgery of the chest. Br J Surg 12:69–75, 1924
5. Fallon WF Jr: Post traumatic empyema. J Am Coll Surg 179:483–492, 1994
6. Feliciano DV, Cruse PA, Mattox KL, et al: Delayed diagnosis of injuries to the diaphragm after penetrating wounds. J Trauma 28:1135–1144, 1989
7. Heniford BT, Carrillo EH, Spain DA, et al: The role of thoracoscopy in the management of retained thoracic collections after trauma. Ann Thorac Surg 63:940–943, 1997
8. Hermansson U, Konstantinov I, Traffs S: Lung injury with pleuripericardial rupture successfully treated by video-assisted thoracoscopy: Case report. J Trauma 40:1024–1025, 1996
9. Ilic N: Functional effects of decortication after penetrating war injuries to the chest. J Thorac Cardiovasc Surg 111:967–970, 1996
10. Jacobaeus HC: Possibility of the use of the cystoscope for investigation of serous cavities. Munch Med Wochenschr 57:2090–2092, 1910
11. Jones JW, Kitahama A, Webb WR, et al: Emergency thoracoscopy: A logical approach to chest trauma management. J Trauma 21:280–284, 1981
12. Landreneau RJ, Hazelrigg, SR, Mack MJ, et al: Postoperative pain-related morbidity: Video-assisted thoracic surgery versus thoracotomy. Ann Thorac Surg 56:1285–1289, 1993
13. Landreneau RJ, Keenan RJ, Hazelrigg SR, et al: Thoracoscopy for empyema and hemothorax. Chest 109:18–24, 1996
14. Lang-Lazdunski L, Mouroux J, Pons F, et al: Role of videothoracoscopy in chest trauma. Ann Thorac Surg 63:327–333, 1997
15. Lesser T, Bartel M: Stellenwert der thorakskopic beim thorax-trauma: Erste erfahrungen. Zentralbl Chir 122:661–665, 1997
16. Liu DW, Liu HP, Lin PJ, et al: Video-assisted thoracic surgery in the treatment of chest trauma. J Trauma 36:536–553, 1997
17. Mancini M, Smith LM, Nein A, et al: Early evacuation of clotted blood in hemothorax using thoracoscopy: Case reports. J Trauma 34:144–147, 1993
18. Mattox KL, Wall MJ: Newer diagnostic measures and emergency management. Chest Surg Clin North Am 7:213–226, 1997
19. McManus K, McGuigan J: Minimally invasive therapy in thoracic injury. Injury 25:609–614, 1994
20. Morales CH, Salinas CM, Henaco CA, et al: Thoracoscopic pericardial window and penetrating cardiac trauma. J Trauma 42:273–275, 1997
21. Nel JM, Warren BL: Thoracoscopic evaluation of the diaphragm in patients with knife wounds of the left lower chest. Br J Surg 81:713–714, 1994
22. O'Brien J, Cohen M, Solit R, et al: Thoracoscopic drainage and decortication as defined treatment for empyema thoracis following penetrating chest injury. J Trauma 36:536–553, 1994

23. Ochsner MG, Rozycki GS, Lucente F, et al: Prospective evaluation of thoracoscopy for diagnosing diaphragmatic injury and thoraco-abdominal trauma: A preliminary report. J Trauma 34:704–710, 1993
24. Senno A, Moallem S, Quijano ER, et al: Thoracoscopy with fiberoptic bronchoscopy. J Thorac Cardiovasc Surg 67:606–611, 1974
25. Sosa JL, Puente I, Lemasters L, et al: Videothoracoscopy in trauma: Early experience. J Laparoendosc Surg 4:295–300, 1994
26. Striffeler H, Gugger M, Hof VM, et al: Video-assisted thoracoscopic surgery for fibrinopurulent empyema in 67 patients. Ann Thorac Surg 65:319–323, 1998
27. Villavicencio RT, Aucar JA, Wall MJ Jr: Analysis of thoracoscopy in trauma. Surg Endosc 13:3–9, 1999
28. Waller DA, Bouboulis N, Forty J, et al: Videoassisted thoracoscopy in the evaluation of penetrating thoracic trauma. Ann R Coll Surg Eng 78:463–465, 1996
29. Wong MS, Tsoi EK, Henderson VJ, et al: Videothoracoscopy: an effective method for evaluating and managing thoracic trauma patients. Surg Endosc 10:118–121, 1996

Address reprint requests to

Keith S. Naunheim, MD
Department of Surgery
Saint Louis University Health Sciences Center
3635 Vista Avenue at Grand
St Louis, MO 63110–0250

e-mail: naunheks@wpogate.slu.edu

THORACOSCOPIC EVALUATION AND TREATMENT OF PULMONARY DISEASE

Robert J. McKenna, Jr, MD

The expectation for video-assisted thoracoscopic surgery (VATS) is that it decreases morbidity, mortality, length of hospital stay (LOS), and time to return to regular activities for patients after procedures that formerly required major incisions. Although the data have not conclusively proven these benefits, VATS has been incorporated into thoracic surgery. Thoracoscopic evaluation and treatment of pulmonary disease are evolving, but this article presents techniques for lung resection (i.e., wedge resection, lobectomy, and pneumonectomy) with VATS.

INTERSTITIAL LUNG DISEASE

Many diagnoses for interstitial lung diseases exist, and a biopsy is often required to make a diagnosis. Transbronchial lung biopsy has a lower diagnostic yield than does open lung biopsy (59% versus 94%).[2] A VATS lung biopsy has a diagnostic yield comparable with that of open lung biopsy but has a lower complication rate, shorter duration of chest tube necessity, and shorter LOS.[1]

Technique

VATS lung biopsies usually are done with one-lung ventilation but can be performed with a single-lumen tube. In the latter case, the lung is gently ventilated to allow for visualization. The thoracoscope is placed in the eighth intercostal space (ICS) in the midaxillary line; the stapler, in the sixth ICS in the midclavicular line; and a ring forceps, in the fourth ICS in the midaxillary line

---

From the Section of Thoracic Surgery, Cedars Sinai Medical Center, Los Angeles, California

---

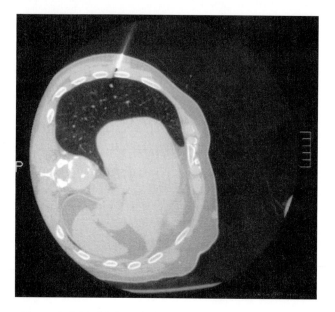

Figure 1. Axial CT view of wire being placed to localize lesion.

to manipulate the lung. All areas of the lung are accessible with this approach. The specimen is placed in a bag if cancer is suspected.

RESECTION OF LUNG NODULES

Lung nodules are more commonly resected with VATS than with thoracotomy. Compared with the open procedure, VATS has a shorter LOS, although the cost savings from a shorter LOS is equal to the additional cost of the extra equipment for VATS, so no overall cost savings is incurred.[6] A centrally located mass may be difficult to resect with VATS, and a small mass (≤ 5 mm) may be difficult to locate with VATS, so VATS wedge resection usually is undertaken for a peripherally located mass 1 cm to 5 cm in diameter.

Technique

With the patient under one-lung general anesthesia, the patient is placed in a full lateral decubitus position, as for a posterolateral thoracotomy. A trocar and a thoracoscope are placed through the eighth ICS to obtain the optimal panoramic view of the thoracic cavity. Additional incisions are needed for an instrument to hold the lung and for the endoscopic stapler. The exact location of the incisions depends on the location of the lung nodule and the best location for incisions that might be required if an additional lung resection is performed. In general, a 1-cm to 2-cm incision is placed in the midaxillary line for palpation of the lung with a finger and a 1-cm to 2-cm incision in the midclavicular line in the sixth ICS for a stapler.

Localization of Lung Nodules

Because the small incisions used for VATS limit surgeons' ability to palpate the lung, a key to successful performance of resection of a lung mass by VATS is the ability to find the lesion. Surgeons must correlate the location of a mass on CT scan with the patient's anatomy. Incisions are placed carefully to allow the surgeon's finger to reach the area of the lung where the mass is located. An experienced thoracic surgeon can almost always find a lung mass in this fashion.

Rarely, preoperative wire localization of a lung nodule is helpful when a lung mass is small (usually ≤ 5 mm) or deeper (3 cm inferior to the pleura). With CT guidance, the radiologist places a hooked wire in the nodule (Figs. 1 and 2). The wire should be cut off at skin level because there is no problem if the wire retracts into the chest. On the other hand, if the wire has been fixed to the chest wall with tape, the wire may not remain in the proper location if a pneumothorax develops and the lung retracts from the chest wall. When the wire has been positioned, the patient is transferred to the surgical suite for resection of the area of the lung with the wire. The mass usually can be palpated in the specimen without the need for a specimen radiograph to confirm that the mass has been resected. This technique is associated with minimal complications (i.e., rarely dislocation of the wire or pneumothorax).[13]

Wire localization was used more often in the early days of VATS, before surgeons realized that it was rarely necessary. Surgeons again are using wire localization because lung cancer screening with chest CT scanning identifies small lung nodules that require localization.

Wedge Resection

Endoscopic staples usually are used for wedge resections of lung nodules. Ring forceps through two incisions position the mass for the stapler. Often, the stapler is fired through both incisions to complete the resection (Fig. 3).

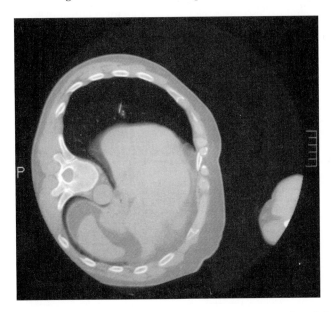

Figure 2. Wire in place in lesion. Note that lung has collapsed partially.

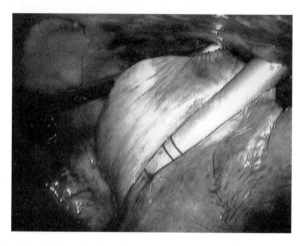

Figure 3. Stapler being fired across lung parenchyma. A second firing will be made to complete the wedge resection.

Alternatively, electrocautery can resect the mass and the lung parenchyma sutured. Optimal function of the electrocautery requires good traction and countertraction on the lung, so a fourth incision often is made. Smoke from the electrocautery device can be problematic. Suction in the thoracic cavity causes the lung to re-expand unless air can flow into the thoracic cavity through at least one of the incisions. Many thoracic surgeons find endoscopic suturing difficult, so this approach is less common than is wedge resection with staples.

Cancer has recurred in thoracoscopy incisions after biopsy.[3] If the lung mass might be a malignancy, it should be placed in a bag for removal to protect the incision. Several endoscopic bags are available for removal of the usual wedge resection.

VIDEO-ASSISTED THORACOSCOPIC SURGICAL VERSUS COMPUTED TOMOGRAPHY–GUIDED BIOPSY

The trend in recent years has been to omit a needle biopsy and proceed with resection of a suspicious lung mass because the result of the biopsy does not change the decision to perform surgery. Surgery is performed for needle biopsy that diagnoses cancer and nondiagnostic biopsy of suspicious masses.

CT-guided needle biopsy, however, seems to be cost-effective. Table 1 shows the cost comparison of outpatient needle biopsy versus VATS wedge resection. Surgical suite and anesthesiologist's times are charged in 15-minute increments. The cost of VATS includes only the time to obtain the biopsy, all the associated

Table 1. COST COMPARISON OF AN OUTPATIENT CT-GUIDED NEEDLE BIOPSY VERSUS VATS

CT-Guided Biopsy	VATS ≤ 30 Min	VATS ≥ 30 Min
$2003.80	$2011.31	$2898.31

costs, and the time for the frozen section result. This averages more than 30 minutes, so the CT-guided biopsy reduces surgical time for the patient and seems to be cost-effective.

LOBECTOMY WITH VIDEO-ASSISTED THORACOSCOPIC SURGERY

VATS lobectomy is same as for open surgery, including a lymph node dissection or sampling after the individual ligation of vessels and bronchus for the lobectomy.[15] Indications for and contraindications to the procedure include:

Indications
  Clinical stage I lung cancer
  Tumor size of less than 5 cm
  Benign disease (e.g., giant bulla or bronchiectasis)
  Physiological operability
Contraindications
  Nodal disease (benign or malignant)
  Chest wall or mediastinal invasion (T3-level or T4-level tumor)
  Endobronchial tumor seen at bronchoscopy
  Neoadjuvant chemotherapy
  Neoadjuvant radiation therapy
  Positive mediastinoscopy

Centrally located tumors require a thoracotomy to determine whether sleeve resection or a pneumonectomy is appropriate. The dissection around the vessels and in the mediastinum is more difficult after chemotherapy or radiation, so a thoracotomy is usually necessary. This section first describes the techniques that are common to all VATS lobectomies and then some features that are unique to resection of specific lobes.

One-Lung Ventilation

After induction of general anesthesia with one-lung ventilation, the patient is placed in a full lateral decubitus position. To allow the maximal time possible for the lung to collapse, one-lung ventilation is instituted while the patient is positioned and the surgeon scrubs his hands. If the lung has not sufficiently collapsed when surgery begins, the bronchoscope is passed into the ipsilateral main stem bronchus for suctioning to encourage further atelectasis.

Incisions

Proper placement of incisions is critical because suboptimal placement of the incisions may cause difficulty. The trocar and thoracoscope are placed in the eighth ICS in the midaxillary line on the right or the posterior axillary line on the left to avoid obstruction of vision by the pericardial fat pad. This step provides the best panoramic view of the thoracic cavity. The 30° lens allows the surgeon to see around structures in the hilum better than does the 0° lens. This incision usually is placed anterior to a rib and angled superiorly toward the ICS to reduce irritation of the intercostal nerve. All other incisions are made directly anterior to an ICS.

Through a 1-cm to 2-cm incision in the ascultatory triangle, a curved ring forceps manipulates the lung to allow for inspection of the pleura and exposure of the hilum to determine the proper position for the other incisions. Inferior placement of this posterior incision improves the angle of the stapler for the superior pulmonary vein and assistance with a lower lobectomy. Slightly higher placement of the incision helps with paratracheal node dissection but makes the angle for the stapler on the pulmonary vein more difficult.

The utility thoracotomy incision is a 4-cm to 6-cm incision from the anterior edge of the latissimus dorsi muscle to the anterior axillary line. It is directly lateral to the superior pulmonary vein for an upper lobectomy or one ICS inferior for a middle or lower lobectomy. The ribs are not spread, but a Weit-lander retractor may be used to hold the soft tissues of the chest wall open for easier passage of instruments and to prevent the lung from expanding when intrathoracic suctioning causes a negative pressure in the chest. The hilar structures are easily accessible for dissection through this incision. Hilar vessels can be tied just as with an open procedure because a finger usually can reach through this incision to the vessels.

A 2-cm incision is made in the midclavicular line in the largest ICS proximal to the costal margin. A ring forceps through this incision can depress the diaphragm for visualization of the inferior pulmonary ligament or retracts the middle lobe out of the visual field after the minor fissure has been completed during an upper lobectomy.

Position of the Surgeon

The surgeon usually stands on the anterior side of the patient and the dissection begins in the hilum. This approach is used for lung resection through an anterolateral, muscle-sparing thoracotomy, which makes the procedure easier than with the approach for a posterolateral thoracotomy (see section on technique for right upper lobectomy).

Hilar Dissection

Vessels in the hilum are dissected sharply through the utility thoracotomy incision with standard thoracotomy instruments, such as Metzenbaum scissors and DeBakey pickups. Hilar lymph nodes are removed as separate specimens to facilitate pathologic staging and passage of the nonarticulating endoscopic stapler (EZ 35, Ethicon, Cincinnati, OH; Endo-GIA, US Surgical, New Brunswick, NJ) across the pulmonary vessels, which requires more dissection for VATS than is customary for thoracotomy.

Staplers

The fissure, bronchus, and pulmonary vessels larger than 5 mm are transected with surgical (usually endoscopic) staples. The vascular (20-mm) staples are used for the vessels, and the green staples (48-mm cartridge) are used on the fissure and the bronchus. Elevating the vessel with a tie aids placement of the stapler. Articulation of the staplers is unnecessary if the correct angle for the

Table 2. INCISION THROUGH WHICH THE STAPLER USUALLY IS PASSED FOR TRANSECTION OF THE ARTERIES, VEINS, BRONCHI, AND FISSURES

Incision	Tissue to be Stapled
Posterior incision	Superior pulmonary vein
	Anterior trunk of upper lobe artery
	Middle lobe artery and vein
	Left upper lobe bronchus
Utility thoracotomy incision	Minor fissure
	Right upper lobe bronchus
	Inferior pulmonary vein
Midclavicular incision	Inferior pulmonary vein
	Anterior trunk of upper lobe artery
	Major fissure
	Additional left upper lobe arteries
	Lower lobe arteries
	Lower lobe bronchus

stapler is chosen. The incisions that offer the best angle for stapling these structures are shown in Table 2.

Completing the Fissure

The fissure usually is completed after the vessels and bronchus are transected, so completeness of the fissure is not a factor in determining the feasibility of performing a lobectomy by VATS.

Specimen Removal

To minimize the risk for contaminating the incision with the tumor, the lung specimen is placed in a bag for removal through the utility thoracotomy incision. An Endocatch (Ethicon, Cincinnati, OH) is sufficiently large for the middle lobe. Removal of the other lobes or the entire lung requires the LapSac (Cook Urological, Spencer, IN) because it is a larger bag. Some specimens are difficult to remove through the small-utility thoracotomy incision. The lobes usually have a pyramidal shape. Removal of the lobe is easier if the narrow part of the lobe is removed first. Rarely, the ribs may be spread for larger tumors or lobes.

Lymph Node Dissection

Mediastinal node sampling or complete lymph node dissection can be performed by VATS. Paratracheal node dissection is easier if the azygos vein is transected, but that is not required. Posteriorly, a ring forceps lifts the azygos vein for exposure of the tracheobronchial angle node and pretracheal nodes. After the pleura is incised to mobilize the azygos vein, the vein is retracted inferiorly. The posterior ring forceps lifts the pleura and the paratracheal nodes as the surgeon dissects in the planes along the superior vena cava, trachea, and pericardium over the ascending aorta, from the azygos vein to the innominate artery. This exposure is easiest after a right upper lobectomy. After a middle or lower lobectomy, a ring forceps through the midclavicular incision should retract the upper lobe out of the visual field.

Anterior retraction of the lung through the utility thoracotomy incision provides exposure for subcarinal node dissection, which begins at the inferior pulmonary vein and proceeds superiorly. A ring forceps posteriorly lifts the pleura over the nodes so the pleura can be incised, together with the intermediate bronchus. Clips are applied to any tissue that does not easily separate when spreading along the bronchus and pericardium.

Aortic–pulmonary window lymph nodes usually are resected before left upper lobectomy because it makes mobilization of the artery easier. Standard thoracotomy instruments perform this dissection through the utility thoracotomy incision. The pleura is cut parallel to the phrenic nerve and along the superior margin of the superior pulmonary vein from the pericardium and laterally along the apical vein as it crosses the anterior trunk. The nodes and pleura then are lifted to mobilize the tissue from the pulmonary artery. The pleura is incised along the vagus nerve. The recurrent laryngeal nerve is identified and preserved. The lymph node tissue then is dissected off of the aorta.

Simultaneous Stapling Lobectomy

Lewis and Caccavale[12] reported thoracoscopic lobectomy with simultaneous stapling of the vessels and bronchus, rather than individual ligation, as described. This procedure has created considerable controversy when presented at meetings because some surgeons view this as a large wedge resection. With this technique, the lobe is mobilized with partial completion of the fissure. A linear stapler, used for open procedures, is fired across the vessels and bronchus.

RESULTS OF VIDEO-ASSISTED THORACOSCOPIC LOBECTOMY

The results of the larger published series of VATS lobectomy and pneumonectomy (Table 3) compare favorably with the results expected with thoracotomy (Table 4).[7, 8, 12, 18, 20, 21, 23] Seven (0.6%) deaths in 1120 patients were caused by venous mesenteric infarct, myocardial infarction, respiratory failure, or were caused by unknown factors.

Complications occurred in 10.0% to 21.9% of the patients following VATS lobectomy in these series. Complications included prolonged air leak (5–10%),

Table 3. SUMMARY OF MAJOR PULMONARY RESECTIONS

Study	No. Patients	Cancer	Mortality	Length of Stay
Lewis[12]	200	171	0	3.07
Yim[23]	214	168	1 (0.4%)	6.8
Kasada[8]	145	103	1 (0.8%)	NA
Hermansson[7]	30	15	0	4.4
Walker[22]	150	123	3 (2%)	7.2
Roviaro[20]	169	142	1 (0.5%)	NA
McKenna[18]	212	212	1 (0.5%)	4.6
Total	**1120**	**934**	**7 (0.6%)**	**5.28**

Table 4. THE 929 MAJOR PULMONARY RESECTIONS PERFORMED BY VATS IN SIX SERIES

Procedure	No. of Patients
RUL	293
RML	113
RLL	218
BILOB	22
RT PN	6
LUL	234
LLL	277
LT PN	15

RUL = right upper lobectomy; RML = right middle lobectomy; RLL = right lower lobectomy; BILOB = bilobectomy; RT PN = right pneumonectomy; LUL = left upper lobectomy; LLL = left lower lobectomy; LT PN = left pneumonectomy.

arrhythmias, pneumonia, and respiratory failure. Transfusions were necessary in 0% to 3% of patients. Bronchial stump leak requiring surgical repair occurred in four (0.36%) cases.

Conversion to Thoracotomy

Conversion from VATS to open thoracotomy was necessary in 0.0% to 19.5% of the patients in these series. Overall, 119 of 1120 surgeries were converted to open thoracotomy (11.6%). Most commonly, oncologic reasons prompted the conversion, such as centrally located tumors requiring vascular control, a sleeve resection, or unsuspected T3-level tumors (attached to the chest wall, diaphragm, or superior vena cava). Abnormal hilar nodes with granulomatous or metastatic disease adherent to the superior pulmonary vein are evaluated better and more safely resected with thoracotomy. Approximately 30% of the conversions to thoracotomy were for nononcologic reasons, such as pleural symphysis.

Intraoperative Hemorrhage

Bleeding from a pulmonary vessel during VATS can be dangerous because access is limited. Fortunately, this occurs infrequently when experienced surgeons perform the procedure. A sponge stick is always available to immediately apply pressure for controlling hemorrhage if bleeding occurs. With the bleeding controlled, a decision is made as to whether the bleeding can be controlled by VATS or if a thoracotomy is needed.

In these series, bleeding led to the conversion to a thoracotomy in 10 cases (0.9%). No deaths resulted from the bleeding episodes, and not all patients required transfusion. The prevalence and morbidity of this complication, therefore, seem to be small for surgeons experienced with VATS lobectomy. A 1997 survey of VATS lobectomy found only one intraoperative death during 1560 VATS lobectomies, and that death was related to an intraoperative myocardial infarction, not bleeding.[14]

Postoperative Pain

Patients typically seem to have less pain after VATS lobectomy compared with lobectomy by thoracotomy, and some evidence supports this. Walker et al[22] compared the requirement for narcotic pain medicine in 83 VATS resections versus 110 patients who underwent thoracotomy during the same time period. The VATS group averaged less morphine use than did the thoracotomy group (mean, 57 mg versus 83 mg morphine; $P < 0.001$). In a randomized, prospective trial of 70 lobectomies (47 by VATS and 23 by muscle-sparing thoracotomy), postoperative pain was significantly less ($P < 0.02$) after VATS.[5] The prevalence of postthoracotomy pain syndrome after VATS lobectomy (2.2%) was lower than expected after thoracotomy.

Landreneau et al[10] prospectively compared daily narcotic requirements, LOS, and a visual analogue pain scale in 165 patients after muscle-sparing thoracotomy with 178 patients after VATS. The VATS group experienced less pain and greater shoulder strength in the first 6 months postoperatively, although no significant difference was found at 1-year follow-up.

Tumor Seeding of the Incision

Seeding of the VATS incisions occurred in 3 of 934 (0.35%) surgeries performed for cancer, so the risk for tumor recurrence in a VATS incision seems to be low and may be lower with the use of proper bags to protect the incisions for removal of specimens.

Adequacy of Cancer Surgery

A 1997 international survey of 1560 VATS lobectomies by 23 surgeons[14] who had performed at least 20 VATS lobectomies showed that, during these procedures, the biopsy samples were taken from mediastinal nodes with mediastinoscopy alone (22.7%), mediastinoscopy and lymph node sampling (32%), or lymph node dissection (45.5%). Kaseda et al[8] reported that lymph node dissection with VATS lobectomy yielded an average of 23 lymph nodes (range, 10–51 nodes).

Long-term, disease-free survival is the ultimate measure for the adequacy of any cancer surgery. Kaseda et al[8] reported a 94% 4-year survival rate for patients with stage I lung cancer resected with VATS lobectomy. Lewis and Caccavale[12] found 94% 3-year survival for stage I, 57% for stage II, and 25% for stage III cancer. The cure rate for lung cancer does not seem to be compromised when a complete cancer surgery is performed by VATS, so it seems that surgeons can perform that same cancer surgery with VATS or thoracotomy.

SUMMARY

VATS wedge resection and lobectomy can be performed with reasonable morbidity and mortality. A cautious approach is appropriate for VATS lobectomy with proper patient selection, and the completeness of the cancer surgery should not be compromised. Only surgeons with the VATS skills that allow them to perform complex procedures should perform the procedure.

References

1. Bensard DD, McIntyre RC, Waring BJ, et al: Comparison of video thoracoscopic lung biopsy to open lung biopsy in the diagnosis of interstitial lung biopsy. Chest 103:765, 1993
2. Burt ME, Flye WM, Webber BC, et al: Prospective evaluation of aspiration needle, cutting needle, transbronchial and open lung biopsy in patients with pulmonary infiltrates. Ann Thorac Surg 32:146, 1981
3. Downey RJ, McCormack P, LoCicero J, et al: Dissemination of malignant tumors after video-assisted thoracic surgery: A report of twenty-one cases. J Thorac Cardiovasc Surg 111:954, 1996
4. Fry WA, Siddiqui A, Pensler JM, et al: Thoracoscopic implantation of cancer with a fatal outcome. Ann Thorac Surg 59:42–45, 1995
5. Giudicelli R, Thomas P, Lonjon T, et al: Video-assisted minithoracotomy versus muscle-sparing thoracotomy for performing lobectomy. Ann Thorac Surg 58:712–718, 1994
6. Hazelrigg SR, Nunchuck SK, Landreneau RJ, et al: Cost analysis for thoracoscopy: Thoracoscopic wedge resection. Ann Thorac Surg 56:633–635, 1993
7. Hermansson U, Konstantinov IE, Aren C: VATS lobectomy: The initial Swedish experience. Semin Thorac Cardiovasc Surg 10:285, 1998
8. Kaseda S, Aoki T, Hangai N: VATS lobectomy: The Japanese experience. Semin Thorac Cardiovasc Surg 10:300, 1998
9. Kirby TJ, Mack MJ, Landreneau RJ, et al: Lobectomy: Video-assisted surgery versus muscle sparing thoracotomy: A randomized trial. J Thorac Cardiovasc Surg 109:997–1002, 1995
10. Landreneau RJ, Mack M, Hazelrigg SR, et al: Prevalence of chronic pain following pulmonary resection by thoracotomy or video-assisted thoracic surgery. J Thorac Cardiovasc Surg 107:1079–1086, 1994
11. Leaver HA, Craig SR, Yap PL, et al: Phagocyte activation after minimally invasive and conventional pulmonary lobectomy [abstract]. Eur J Clin Invest 26(suppl 1):210, 1996
12. Lewis RJ, Caccavale RJ: VATS lobectomy. Semin Thorac Cardiovasc Surg 10:332, 1998
13. Mack MM: Techniques for the localization of pulmonary nodules for thoracoscopic resection. J Thorac Cardiovasc Surg 106:550, 1993
14. Mackinlay TA: VATS lobectomy: An international survey. Presented at the 4th International Symposium on Thoracoscopy and Video Assisted Thoracic Surgery. Sao Paulo, Brazil, May 1997
15. McKenna RJ Jr: VATS lobectomy with mediastinal lymph node sampling or dissection. Chest Surg Clin North Am 4:223–232, 1995
16. McKenna RJ Jr, Fischel RJ: VATS lobectomy and lymph node dissection or sampling in eighty-year-old patients. Chest 106:1902–1904, 1994
17. McKenna RJ Jr, Fischel RJ, Brenner M, et al: Combined operations for lung cancer and lung volume reduction surgery. Chest 110:885–888, 1996
18. McKenna RJ Jr, Fischel RJ, Wurnig P, et al: VATS lobectomy: The Los Angeles experience. Semin Thorac Cardiovasc Surg 10:321, 1998
19. Roviaro G, Varoli F, Rebuffat C, et al: Videothoracoscopic staging and treatment of lung cancer. Ann Thorac Surg 59:971–974, 1995
20. Roviaro G, Varoli F, Vergani C, et al: VATS major pulmonary resections: The Italian experience. Semin Thorac Cardiovasc Surg 10:313, 1998
21. Walker WS: VATS lobectomy: The Edinburgh experience. Semin Thorac Cardiovasc Surg 10:291, 1998
22. Walker WS, Pugh GC, Craig SR, et al: Continued experience with thoracoscopic major pulmonary resection. Int Surg 81:255–258, 1996
23. Yim APC, Liu H, Izzat MB, et al: Thoracoscopic major lung resections: An Asian perspective. Semin Thorac Cardiovasc Surg 10:326, 1998

Address reprint requests to

Robert J McKenna, Jr, MD
8635 Third, Suite 975W
Los Angeles, CA 90048

SUTURING AND KNOTTING TECHNIQUES FOR THORACOSCOPIC CARDIAC SURGERY

Zoltan Szabo, PhD, G. James Avery II, MD, Andras Sandor, MD,
and Demetrius E. M. Litwin, MD, FRCSC

The range and magnitude of chest disease managed thoracoscopically have widely expanded since videocameras were coupled to endoscopes in the late 1980s.[2, 3] Starting with some simpler procedures relating to the heart and pericardium, investigators have studied the feasibility of performing more complex endoscopic cardiac procedures, including the repair of intracardiac defects, repair or replacement of aortic and mitral valves, surgical correction of atrial arrhythmias, and coronary artery bypass grafting (CABG).

Many aspects of adapting CABG to endoscopy are in the early stages of development. The most surgically challenging aspect of CABG, whether it is performed conventionally, through a minithoracotomy, or totally endoscopically, is the construction of the distal anastomosis. Performing the anastomosis using standard open chest techniques with direct visualization of the surgical site, although challenging, is within the capabilities of skilled surgeons; however, performing this task with totally endoscopic techniques and manually manipulated instruments has challenged even the most skilled surgeons. Numerous anastomotic techniques have been tested for endoscopic application, including tissue glue, vascular staples, laser tissue welding, and endoscopic suturing.[4] Suturing seems to offer the most accurate, expeditious, and reliable technique for an end-to-side anastomosis.

The learning curve is long and steep for endoscopic CABG (E-CABG);

From the Microsurgery and Operative Endoscopy Training Institute, San Francisco (ZS); the Department of Cardiac Surgery, California Pacific Medical Center, San Francisco (GJA), California; the Departments of Surgery (AS), and the Minimally Invasive Surgery Services, and EndoSurgery Center, University of Massachusetts Medical Center (DEML), Worcester, Massachusetts however, cardiac surgeons experienced with the surgical microscope for microvascular anastomosis and endoscopic suturing have already overcome a major hurdle.

APPROACH

Endoscopic Modality

E-CABG is the transfer of conventional open CABG to the endoscopic field. Although similarities exist between the two methodologies, the differences are more striking. Attempting to use standard techniques endoscopically is a daunting task. Cardiac surgeons likely will encounter difficulties in initially adjusting to the endoscopic field. It is one with many restrictions—a visual field bounded by the edge of the endoscope, an image derived from a video system. In addition, access is limited by the location of the instrument ports, and movements are restricted by the narrow space between the heart and the chest wall. Although endoscopic surgery is a form of magnified surgery, it is performed mostly by viewing the image on a television monitor. A cardiac surgeon's experience with surgical loupes, as opposed to an operating microscope, has some, but insignificant, applicability. Movements in the endoscopic field initially are difficult to control, and surgical maneuvers also are difficult to accomplish. Understanding and incorporating a few basic principles governing endoscopic surgery and suturing techniques and applying many of the strategies developed by other surgical subspecialties facilitate cardiac surgeons' development of the skills necessary for successful performance of E-CABG.

From the many endoscopic techniques developed for other surgical specialties, only some elements are applicable for minimal access cardiac surgery. For instance, only intracorporeal knotting should be used because cardiovascular structures are all delicate. Also, some devices, such as circular staplers, although useful (e.g., for the anastomosis in minimally invasive direct coronary artery bypass [MIDCAB], which is accessed through a small thoracotomy) are, however, not yet available for endoscopic application. Even if they eventually become available, a suture or two may be necessary to close the opening through which the stapler is used, and those sutures will probably be made manually. As has been demonstrated in other fields of endoscopic surgery that use staplers and clips, these devices can be challenging to apply correctly, and given that devices fail on occasion, surgeons without manual endoscopic suturing skills might be compelled to convert to open surgery after a considerable amount of time, effort, and material has been expended.

Enabling technologies will be pitched to a specialty new to the endoscopic modality; these include three-dimensional (3-D) video systems and robotic systems. Both are appealing in concept but not a panacea in practice. First, both are in development. Three-dimensional video systems were introduced during the explosive evolution of endoscopic surgery in general surgery to restore the lack of depth perception inherent with current endoscopic video systems. Although the premise was logical, these new systems were found to be suboptimal. Earlier generations of 3-D video systems characteristically had more disadvantages than advantages. With regard to visual clarity and illumination, the 3-D video systems were substantially inferior to the two-dimensional three-chip video systems. General surgeons and gynecologists familiar with this generation of 3-D systems, and even with the newer generation, believed that the addition of depth perception was nonessential compared with the need for high-quality imaging. They had learned sufficient compensatory techniques in circumventing the need for 3-D. Current 3-D systems under development offer greater promise, but their benefit is yet to be proven.

Surgical robotics is an exciting concept. It conjures up visions of machines automatically constructing the anastomosis. Surgical robots are simply a computerized master–slave system, the actions of which are directed entirely by the surgeon.[7] Under ideal circumstances, systems such as these can facilitate and enhance challenging procedures, such as E-CABG, specifically by holding and repositioning the endoscope and by positioning and sustaining the hand instruments as directed by the surgeon. The latter can be helpful because some positions can be awkward for the surgeon to manually sustain and result in significant discomfort and fatigue for the operator. Severe operator fatigue could result in the abandonment of the endoscopic approach to a given procedure; however, the robot is not absolutely essential when a surgeon is particularly skilled. The procedure cannot be accomplished without the surgeon possessing the skills to perform the procedure manually because the surgeon performs the same exact series of coordinated movements with the robot as he or she would perform without it. The robot's role is simply to enhance the surgeon's movements, by filtering out tremor and improving instrument maneuvering. Hence, the following section describes the basic endoscopic surgical and suturing skills needed for the cardiac surgeon to perform E-CABG manually.

ENDOSCOPIC INSTRUMENTATION AND SUTURES

Well-designed endoscopic suturing microinstruments (Karl Storz GmbH, Tuttlingen, Germany), especially those with curved tips, are invaluable in helping to identify the cut edges, position the tissues for entrance and exit bites, and carefully adjust the tension on the suture loops as the approximation progresses.

The suture material that cardiac surgeons typically use is polypropylene, which is dyed dark blue. Although this material has been the suture of choice, nylon might be a better choice in the endoscopic field. Both suture materials are nonabsorbable, but nylon is less brittle and more elastic than is polypropylene, making it stronger and easier to handle. Two new nonabsorbable suture materials have been introduced for cardiac applications: (1) polyhexafluoorpropylene-VDF (Pronova; Ethicon, Somerville, NJ) and (2) polybutester (Vascufil, USS-DG, Norwalk, CT). Both suture materials are also dyed dark blue and are said to offer better handling than polypropylene by virtue of their reduced memory and brittleness and greater elasticity and tensile strength. Another nonabsorbable suture material is polytetrafluoroethylene (Gore-Tex), which has many favorable properties for cardiac surgical application, including great visibility (fluorescent white), manipulability, and tensile strength.

Endoscopic Microvascular Anastomosis

Although vascular surgeons developed vascular anastomoses techniques to a fine art nearly a century ago, such demanding techniques are beyond the reach of the laparoscopic approach. A complete redesign of the anastomosis technique is necessary to maximize efficiency, considering the difficulty of approach.

End-to-end anastomosis is the preferred method of joining equal-caliber and equal-wall-thickness conduits. Depending on function, the number of sutures and the amount of bite are calculated for each situation. It could be fashioned using continuous or interrupted sutures. The interrupted sutures allow for greater precision and control; the continuous technique is more rapid but less forgiving. End-to-side anastomosis permits the union of conduits with disparate lumens and wall thicknesses and is technically easier to accomplish than is an end-to-end anastomosis.

Endoscopic Suturing Techniques

During construction of a suture line, tissue should be mobilized so that the approximation could be accomplished without tension. The length of suture must be calculated and trimmed to the shortest necessary length to avoid tangling in the field. The trocars for the needle driver and assisting grasper should be ideally positioned so that the needle driver is parallel with the suture line; the assisting grasper is offset from the needle driver between 45° and 90°; the trocars are positioned at least 9 cm apart. In the process of preparing the most effective setup, the surgeon should position himself or herself so that the entrance–exit scooping motion follows a 1 o'clock to 7 o'clock direction (if right-handed), relative to the surgeon's frontal plane. Additional details on the angles of setup are described in a subsequent section.

As the suture line is constructed, interrupted sutures may be placed using a suspension slip knot technique[8] to initially approximate tissue that may be under considerable tension, or where visibility is desirable for the placement of subsequent sutures. Sutures should be placed to bring the tissues together evenly, without excessive tension or misalignment of the layers. The number of stitches needed is based on the number needed to complete an adequate suture line or provide adequate tissue edge alignment.

Interrupted Versus Continuous Suturing Technique

In a learning environment, the endoscopic interrupted suturing technique is practiced first to develop the necessary eye–hand coordination, the basic laparoscopic suturing technique, and the proper tissue alignment. The next step is to learn the continuous suturing technique, which is a more rapid but more difficult technique to accomplish than the interrupted suture technique.

During the learning phase, the surgeon should practice suturing on both sides of the suture line, left to right, and right to left, and with both hands, so that ambidextrous skills and increased dexterity are developed.

Interrupted suturing is a more labor-intensive process because knots must be tied and the suture cut after each stitch; however, construction of the anastomosis is more easily controlled because an individual suture can be replaced if an error is detected without adversely affecting the remaining stitches. The tissue edges tend to be more accurately approximated, and this technique lends itself to the solo surgeon.

With continuous suturing, construction of the anastomosis is more rapid, but it is also associated with more technical problems. If the suture breaks during the anastomosis, unraveling of the anastomosis can occur. Also, continuous suturing tends to be less accurate than an interrupted suture line with regard to consistency in the size of each stitch, the spacing between them, the accurate approximation of the tissue edges, and the tension placed on each stitch. Surgeons should avoid placing excessive tension on the suture line because purse-stringing can result and is difficult to detect in the endoscopic environment. The continuous suturing technique is suited to a team approach, with the assistant "following" the surgeon, including maintaining the appropriate tension after each stitch. In this manner, the surgeon is freer to focus primarily on the placement of sutures.

PRINCIPLES

Endoscopic Visual Perception

In open CABG and MIDCAB, direct observation of tissues provides an optimal image and offers an abundance of visual clues. The surgeon is free to shift the focus of his or her attention from one side of the surgical field to the other without hesitation, even when surgical loupes are used. With the endoscope, the visual field is significantly smaller and is limited by the perimeter of the lens of the endoscope. Scanning the surgical field is no longer a simple matter because it requires moving the endoscope around the field slowly and systematically. Also, most endoscopic procedures are performed with a video-camera coupled to the endoscope; as such, the image quality is degraded compared with direct vision of the surgical field or with the surgeon viewing the field directly through the endoscope.

Interestingly, the brain creates an image from the least amount of available visual information. It fills in the gaps from visual memory developed during training. Proper training is important because accumulating a good visual memory, coupled with good reasoning, allows the surgeon to read sketchy visual clues correctly.

Maximizing the image quality is of utmost importance when working with the video visualization derived from the endoscope-and-camera system. After time, sustained concentration on the video monitor can cause eye strain, vibration, and occasional whiteout. Adjusting the sharpness, clarity, brightness, color, and contrast of the image is vital because using a well-tuned, high-quality setup provides the proper video image necessary for endoscopic suturing.

Good visual health, correction to 20/20 vision, and rested eyes are part of the ideal physical and mental conditions necessary to accomplish endoscopic suturing smoothly. Although a surgeon might not always wear corrective lenses for open surgery, especially if the correction is minor, this lack of sharp visual acuity is problematic when looking at the magnified surgical field. A visit to the ophthalmologist is recommended before taking a course or operating endoscopically.

Second to the video monitor, the camera assistant is most instrumental in providing the best visual image. In the surgical team, holding and guiding the camera is one of the most difficult roles. First, the camera assistant must know exactly what the primary surgeon must see, then he or she must provide the view accordingly, making certain that the image is always focused and the objective lens is clean and unfogged. This concentration seems difficult to maintain for more than 0.5 hour, particularly when the procedure is not going smoothly, so it is often helpful for the assisting surgeon, whose role is to retract tissues, and the camera assistant to rotate roles from time to time to facilitate proper concentration.

When performing endoscopic suturing, the need to move the endoscope around the surgical field is reduced because the surgeon typically must have the endoscope zoomed in or out of the suture line area. Therefore, endoscope holders, mechanical or motorized, can be beneficial in holding an image steady and in relieving the strain of an individual sustaining a position over a prolonged time.

Endoscopic Eye–Hand Coordination

Magnification, whether solely optical or coupled with a video system, facilitates a more accurate, precise, and delicate surgical repair. The benefits of the larger image with its greater details are offset by an eye–hand coordination imbalance. Normal movements under magnification appear fast paced and difficult to control.

Re-establishing this balance is accomplished by reducing the speed of one's movements significantly. The surgeon must slow down until proper control is re-established, which is approximately proportional to the magnification factor. The ballistic movements of open surgery are clearly counterproductive.

To place a suture precisely or retrieve a suture tail, the endoscope must be brought in close to the target area; when tying the knot, the endoscope is pulled back to provide the greater field of view needed for knotting and suture handling. When an important decision is required, magnification must be increased and focused on a particular part of the field; the surgeon's movement must slow down further, always proportional to the magnification. By reducing the speed of movement, not only is eye–hand coordination restored but also the brain is given time to compose and formulate the most informative image possible, all of which is needed to proceed correctly. On the other hand, if the surgeon rushes, the quality of the individual sutures and suture line, even if suboptimal, might be accepted for the sake of expediency, which may result in error. This error can be manifested in reduced precision and increased trauma. The wasted time spent making the error, recognizing it subsequently, and then correcting it results in interrupted momentum and less efficiency.

Reduced speed can dramatically lengthen operating time, which of course is counterproductive when considering anesthesia time and operating costs. A means of increasing efficiency can be found in two important principles: (1) the "economy-of-motion" principle and (2) a "choreography of movements." For example, knot-tying movements have been analyzed and choreographed[6] into the least number of necessary movements that flow into one another smoothly. The ultimate goal for the surgeon is to develop a "flawless technique."

In intracorporeal suturing and knot tying, precisely controlled instrument movements are vital. Iatrogenic injury is a constant concern; thus, emphasis on control is imperative. Control can be accomplished through training, supervised practice, and the proper frame of mind. The needle holder and assisting grasper must work together in an orchestrated fashion, like a duet, with each instrument performing its ideal function, taking turns or working simultaneously.

Such choreography is an important technique that should be learned by novices and experienced surgeons, who can appreciate the time-saving and effort-saving features. It is better to carefully grasp an object once than to make several fruitless passes at it.

Besides choreography, another important aspect of endoscopic surgical efficiency is accurate targeting and placement of instruments because sutures, needles, and tissues must be handled repeatedly. Such accuracy is a significant challenge when working in a two-dimensional visual field. Nothing wastes more time and causes more frustration than groping about and missing the intended target. The remedy for the surgeon is to slow his or her movements significantly and narrow his or her focus. He or she should invest the time to touch the

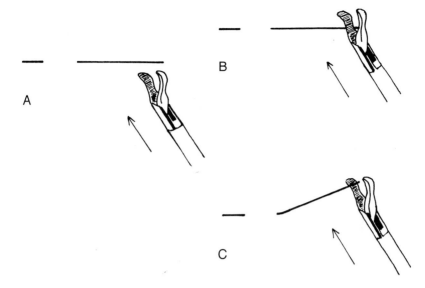

Figure 1. Depth perception can be challenging in laparoscopy. *Touch confirmation* can be applied to save time and effort when grasping a targeted object. *A,* With the instrument jaws open, the surgeon should attempt to touch his target with one of the jaws to confirm that the instrument is in the right plane. *B,* If the target does not move, the instrument is in the wrong plane and should be raised or lowered, and the target sought for again. *C,* If the target moves, the surgeon can complete the maneuver (e.g., grasp the thread).

intended target to confirm its location before committing to grasping it ("touch confirmation"), thus avoiding "a swing and a miss."

This step can be accomplished by opening the instrument jaws and positioning the lower jaw slowly under the target structure, touching it slightly to cause slight movement (Fig. 1). This step confirms accurate location of the target tissue. Afterward, the jaws can be closed and the structure grasped, proceeding with the next task. If no movement is detected, the instrument is positioned incorrectly. The surgeon's goal should be not to miss his intended target, even once, during the procedure, thus attaining a flawless technique.

This slowed choreography requires considerable patience and energy, so the surgeon should abstain from stimulants, such as caffeine, and be in top physical and mental condition. A surgeon at the beginning of a procedure has a limited amount of energy for precision surgery. This limit can be increased by a sportsmanlike lifestyle, conditioning, and discipline. Avoiding mental and physical distractions in the surgical suite and other factors that dilute concentration are also important.

Endoscopic Tissue Handling

The handling of tissues is a major concern in intracorporeal tissue approximation. Because it involves the use of long leveraged instruments, collateral trauma can occur easily, leading to adhesion formation, increased scarring, and poorer postoperative results overall. One of the main areas is in retraction of tissues. Often performed by less experienced assistants, applying tension to tissues is necessary; however, frequent or inattentive handling easily can result in battered tissues.

Most available instruments have jaws with small footprints, which can exert considerable force to a small area of tissue. Endoscopic instruments with larger jaw surfaces, such as traditional bowel clamps (e.g., the Allis or Babcock), are less traumatic in this regard. They provide a greater grasping surface and reduced leverage, thereby, less pressure per square centimeter. The result is fewer crushing and ripping injuries.

It may seem desirable to have universal endoscopic instruments that could handle tissue, needles, and sutures with equal effectiveness, but the more diverse the functions, the less effective each function is. Retractors perform their intended function best. Although a needle driver could grasp the tissue, it was not intended for that purpose. Its powerful jaws could easily cause damage when the surgeon or assistant loses his or her focus on it. When handling tissue with locking instruments, the activation of the locks and ratchets of the instrument also could be dangerous.

Mental concentration also is important. Under the endoscope, the surgeon focuses his or her attention on a small area of the visual field. Known as *macular vision*, it involves a great deal of concentration. While focusing intently on specific areas of the field or the procedure, the surgeon and his or her assistant must be constantly mindful of the instruments in their hands. What often occurs in the heat of battle is that the surgeon or assistant inadvertently applies pressure to tissues, that is, he or she presses down on surrounding tissue or places excessive force on retracted tissue. This problem easily could result in iatrogenic injury. Thus, instruments must be maintained in the field of view at all times.

Another potentially dangerous technique is holding the needle during knot tying to fold the suture material. Unless the suture is short, waving a needle around could lacerate surrounding tissues inadvertently.

The need for delicate tissue handling cannot be overstressed. Tissues must be handled as gently as possible, especially when positioning them for needle passage. Counterpressure should be provided by the jaws of the assisting grasper immediately adjacent to the point of needle entrance or exit. Minor adjustments and initial testing of tissue could be done with the tip of a needle firmly held in the grip of the needle driver.

A good setup makes surgery easier. If tissues to be approximated are brought within close proximity of one another and positioned well, suturing can be a fairly straightforward process. Another set of "hands" may be needed to create the optimal setup; whether they are in the form of another instrument or device can be determined by the surgeon.

Endoscopic Setup and Angles of Approach

The proper placement of trocars is critical to success. The relationship of the suturing instruments (needle driver and assisting grasper) to the camera position and to the suture line is important, especially when an anastomosis is involved (Fig. 2).

The following position follows the natural position of the surgeon, with the endoscope centered, and the needle driver and assisting grasper on either side of it (coaxial alignment; Fig. 2A). This position is the most natural because it does not require the surgeon to spend time recalculating the differences between his or her normal movements and the altered orientation. Alternatively,

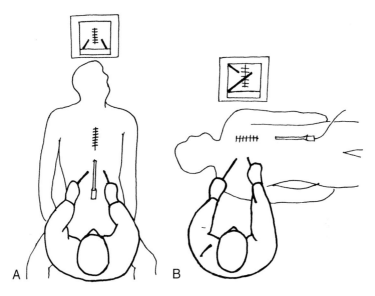

Figure 2. The view, the instrument ports, and the television monitor in relationship to the suture line. *A,* In the coaxial alignment, the surgeon, view port, suture line, and television monitor are all coaxially aligned. This arrangement follows the surgeon's natural position, with the view port in the center, and the two instrument ports on either side of it, 4 to 5 inches behind. These three ports form an equilateral triangle. *B,* The offset (non-coaxial) position involves having the view port placed similarly to the coaxial position, but the two instrument ports, while positioned near each other, are offset (perpendicularly) to the suture line and view port. In this position, the suture line is also perpendicular to the instruments. Note that both instruments approach the suture line from only one side.

the off-set position (Fig. 2*B)* involves both instruments located on one side of the laparoscope or the other. This position is somewhat awkward to use because the suture line is perpendicular to the instruments. In either case, the trocars should be sufficiently far apart, that is, 9 cm, at an angle of separation of 60° to 90°, to avoid a "chopsticks" effect[1] (Fig. 3). After mastering suturing skills, the surgeon will find that either position is feasible, even an upside-down setup with the camera facing the surgeon, although the latter positioning never feels completely natural. A mirror-image setup is the only virtually impossible proposition because the risk for serious error is too great.

Ideally, the needle driver instrument should be lined up parallel with the proposed suture line so that the needle can be held in the instrument jaws in a perpendicular fashion. The needle also must be positioned perpendicular to the suture line. The assisting grasper should be offset at least 60°, set 9 cm or 10 cm apart.

TECHNIQUES

Preparing for Endoscopic Suturing

After the suture is removed from its package, its length is trimmed appropriately. For initial training and practice, that length should be approximately 18

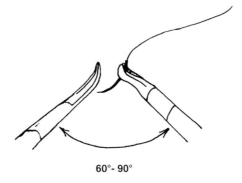

60°- 90°

Figure 3. The ideal angle of separation between the assisting grasper and the needle driver is 60° to 90°.

cm for larger sutures, that is, 2-0 to 5-0. For the E-CABG anastomosis, the length should be 5.5 cm to 7.0 cm. If the curvature of the needle needs altering, such as modifying a half-circle needle to a ⅜-circle curvature, it should be done now by using a standard needle driver or hemostat.

Next, the surgeon suspends the suture by the thread with the fingers of his or her dominant hand; he or she then rotates the thread until the needle faces the direction it is to be driven through the target tissues. With a curved assisting grasper pointing medially (3-o'clock position), the surgeon grasps the suture 2 cm to 3 cm from the end of the needle and prepares it to be introduced through the trocar. Attention is important during the passage of the suture through the trocar because it easily can be "lost" (i.e., the needle pulled off the thread or the suture stuck) in the trocar.

If present, the reducer cap is removed or the valve of the trocar is opened. Then the assisting grasper carefully passes the suture through the trocar, and, under endoscopic visualization, it is brought to the surgical site. The needle driver can then be introduced into the field. While the suture continues to be held by the assisting grasper, the suture is lowered until the bottom of the needle touches the surface of the surrounding tissue to stabilize it (Fig. 4).

If the suture is accidentally released by the assisting grasper, the surgeon should, using the assisting grasper, regrasp the suture 2 cm to 3 cm behind the needle. If the needle is pointing in the wrong direction, the assisting grasper can be rotated around within the surgeon's hand until the needle is properly directed.

The surgeon then approaches the needle with the needle driver, opens its jaws, and grasps the needle at a point approximately two thirds of its length from the tip. Now the needle should be in the correct position, ready for the entrance bite. To confirm this, the needle is brought closer to the camera and the needle driver rotated back and forth (supinated and pronated) to demonstrate and confirm the proper position. If it is correct, the needle can be locked in the needle driver. The correct position is reached when the needle is perpendicular to the needle driver. When the surgeon is well acquainted with the proper basic suturing technique and becomes facile at it, the needle position can be adjusted in a nonperpendicular fashion if needed.

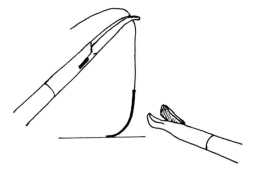

Figure 4. Loading the needle into the needle driver. The assisting grasper holds the suture material approximately 2 to 3 cm from the end of the needle and positions the needle tip on the surface of the surrounding tissue. If the needle is not initially pointing in the correct direction, the assisting grasper can be rotated, pirouetting the needle until it is properly positioned. Afterward the needle driver grasps the needle approximately two thirds of its length from the tip.

Adjusting the Needle and Correcting Deflection

If the needle is positioned incorrectly, that is, pointing in the wrong direction, correcting it can be a fairly straightforward process. The problem usually is the result of the needle swiveling or pivoting out of position within the jaws of the needle driver, especially when the force applied or the needle direction is not perpendicular to the tissue surface. Thus, the solution is to swivel it back into position, which is accomplished by loosening the grip of the needle driver on the needle slightly and then pushing the needle with the assisting grasper (with jaws closed) until it is in the correct position.

Another method is to hook the needle tip into the surrounding tissue, in an avascular area, loosening the grip on the needle without letting it go, then pulling the needle driver away from (or pushing it toward) the tissue surface, and pivoting the needle back into the desired position (Fig. 5). Another method involves slightly loosening the grip on the needle and brushing the back of the needle backward against adjacent tissues. This movement sweeps the point of the needle tip in the opposite direction that it is pushed. When the ideal position has been reached, the grip on the needle is tightened to lock it into this position.

The classically ineffective method of correcting a deflected needle is to hand the needle back and forth between the needle driver and the assisting grasper. Although seemingly logical, no effective change in needle position usually occurs.

Needle Driving

The needle must be held perpendicular to the jaws of the needle driver and it must be passed perpendicularly through the tissue surface. If the needle is directed at the proper angle, the needle passes through the tissue layers with the least amount of resistance, effort, and trauma. In doing so, the needle passes crisply through the tissue and provides the surgeon with some sense of tactile feedback. If the needle is driven at another angle through the tissue, more resistance is encountered, and it is more difficult to distinguish a clean needle

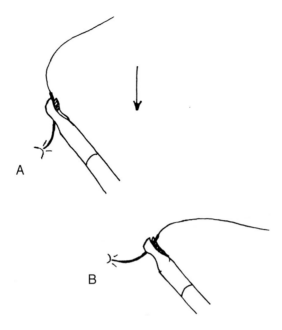

Figure 5. Correcting a deflected needle. While attempting to pass the needle through the tissue, the surgeon may inadvertently push the needle driver down toward the tissue surface, thereby causing the needle to be deflected within its jaws. *A,* To correct this problem, the surgeon should lighten his grip on the needle, and then, with the needle still hooked into the tissue *(B),* the needle driver is pulled slowly away from the tissue surface. In the process, the needle direction is corrected.

passage from one that could be troublesome (e.g., involving inclusion of the posterior wall).

If the needle is pushed in a direction different from which the tip is pointing, needle deflection occurs, with the needle pivoting out of proper position proportional to the difference between the correct and incorrect directions. This occurs most commonly when a novice attempts to place sutures endoscopically in the same manner as he or she does in open surgery. If a strongly grasping needle driver is used, the misdirected force easily could cause inadvertent tissue trauma, such as a laceration, because a rigidly held needle can act like a knife, so the softer grasping technique (or instrument) is recommended, particularly in the early phases of learning endoscopic suturing techniques.

Selecting the Point of Entrance

Properly selecting the first entrance point sets the stage for the remainder of the sutures and should be carefully calculated to create the ideal suture line, taking into consideration critical concerns, such as a hemostatic seal. Mistakes can be made in selecting an entrance bite that is too small or too large, or using a combination of the two, which results in a tortuous suture line and possibly failure of the anastomosis.

Amount of Bite

The size of entrance and exit bites is important because too little may not provide an adequate seal or strength. Then more sutures must be added than would otherwise be necessary, thereby wasting time and potentially inflicting additional trauma. A bite that is too large involves excessive tissue, which results in a bulky suture line, possibly narrowing the lumen of a vessel and possibly resulting in suture necrosis. For the E-CABG anastomosis, the cardiac surgeon essentially can apply the same technique as is used in the conventional approach.

A careful approach is of critical importance during suture placement in the entrance and exit bites, so establishing a proper setup, applying atraumatic technique, including effectively using counterpressure or countertraction when possible, and meticulously checking for errors reduce the risk for including the posterior wall in a stitch and contribute to the overall efficiency of the procedure.

Exit Bite

The exit bite is an easier pass to make than the entrance bite, so double-armed suturing is encouraged where two exit bites could complete the suture. This technique involves cannulation of the lumen with each needle tip individually, and is advantageous when anastomosing blood vessels because it decreases the risk for including the posterior wall in a stitch.

To locate the proper exit point, the needle tip is turned upward (in the external direction), creating an upward tenting of the tissue. If the bite appears too large or small, adjustments can be made. When the correct exit point has been determined, the needle can be pushed forward, exposing the needle tip. The assisting grasper can push the tissue further down against the needle, and then the tip can be grasped with the assisting grasper or needle driver. In either case, the needle is pulled out carefully, applying counterpressure as much as possible to minimize trauma. The suture then is advanced as far as is necessary in preparation for the next suture.

Intracorporeal Knot-Tying Techniques

Intracorporeal knot tying in endoscopic suturing has been considered a formidable challenge, so much so that it has largely taken a back seat to extracorporeal knot tying and the use of substitute devices in other surgical specialties. This has been true especially for surgeons who suture infrequently. The latter approaches are limited in their application, and the need still exists for intracorporeal knot tying; without it, the progress of advanced laparoscopic surgical techniques is hampered.

The ability to competently and confidently tie knots intracorporeally with endoscopic instruments is an essential and fundamental skill because it is based on time-honored, universally adaptable methods that can use readily available materials. Intracorporeal knot tying must be second nature to surgeons. When sophisticated devices fail, or if the surgeon practices in locations where economic conditions deem such devices unfeasible, what remains is the surgeon and his or her skills. Best of all, intracorporeal suturing and intracorporeal knot tying need not be overwhelming challenges because all that is necessary is the proper approach and technique—in particular, the choreographed knotting technique.

First, the ideal knot—one that is simple to tie, hold securely, and adaptable for multipurpose use—must be selected. Such a knot is the traditional square knot (Figs. 6–8) that is familiar to most surgeons, with two added features. The additional benefit of the square knot is that it can be converted into a slip knot that is adjustable and reconvertible into the locking configuration (i.e., square knot) numerous times (Figs. 9 and 10), which permits the use of the slip-knot suspension technique, a practical method for vascular anastomosis. The choreographed sequence that is presented here must be practiced meticulously

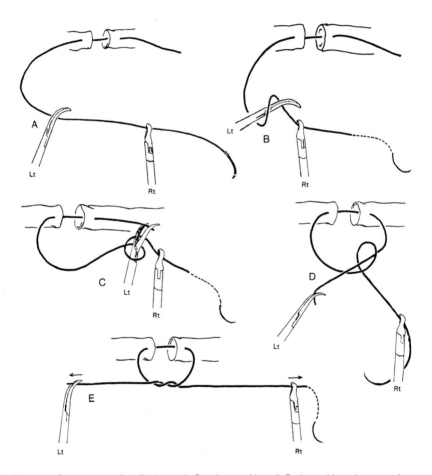

Figure 6. Square knot: first flat knot. *A,* Starting position: A C-shaped loop is created, open to the same side of the field as the short tail. *B,* First wrap: The assisting grasper, with jaws closed, is placed over the loop, and the thread held by the needle driver is wrapped around it once. *C,* Grasping the short tail: Moving together as a unit, the two instruments proceed to the short tail, with the assisting grasper taking hold of the short tail. *D,* Completing the first flat knot: The short tail is pulled through the loop. *E,* Adjusting the knot: The knot can be shifted over, especially if the resulting short tail is rather long. *(From Szabo Z, Berci G: Extra and intracorporeal knotting and suturing technique. Gastrointest Endosc Clin North Am 3:367–379, 1993; with permission.)*

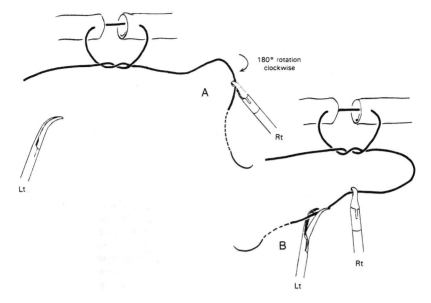

Figure 7. Square knot: preparing for the second flat knot. *A,* The long tail is rotated 180° in a clockwise direction. *B,* it is then passed to the assisting grasper in preparation for tying the second half of the square knot. (*From* Szabo Z, Berci G: Extra and intracorporeal knotting and suturing technique. Gastrointest Endosc Clin North Am 3:367–379, 1993; with permission.)

because the time-saving and effort-saving benefits of this approach are built into its choregraphy.

SURGICAL TECHNIQUE FOR ENDOSCOPIC CORONARY ARTERY BYPASS GRAFTING IN THE BOVINE MODEL

The method described here involves the performance of CABG under total endoscopic visualization with cardiopulmonary bypass (CPB) on a still heart.

Endoscopic Internal Mammary Artery Takedown

Port positions must first be determined for the internal mammary artery (IMA) harvest, then for the anastomosis of the IMA to the left anterior descending (LAD) coronary artery. A 5-mm or 10-mm port is placed for the endoscope in the midaxillary line of the left side of the chest in the third or fourth intercostal space. Two additional 5-mm ports are placed for the hand instruments on either side of the view port, 8 cm to 10 cm apart, creating an equidistant triangular formation. To increase the working space, lower the heart to provide access to the IMA; the mediastinum is bluntly dissected with a 5-mm Babcock and monopolar cautery needle, in a cephalad to caudal direction.

The needed length of the IMA is determined first. The IMA and internal mammary vein are dissected as a pedicle or in a skeletonized fashion, first marking the path of the vessels on the surface of the muscle bed. Intercostal

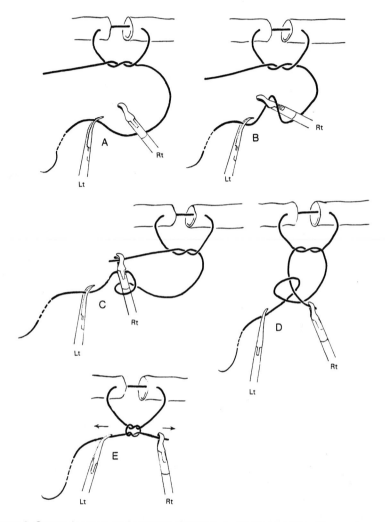

Figure 8. Square knot: second opposing flat knot. *A,* Starting position: The newly created reversed C loop again is open to the side of the field where the short tail is located, with the long tail positioned inferior to it. *B,* Wrapping: The needle driver is then placed over this loop, and the thread is wrapped around it. *C,* Grasping the short tail: Again, both instruments move together as a unit, and the needle driver then grasps the short tail *(D)* and pulls it through the loop *(E)*, and the knot is then tightened. If the knot is snug against the tissue at this point, the knotting process is completed for smaller sutures, such as 6-0 or smaller. For larger sutures, a third throw should be added, accomplished in the same manner as the first flat knot. (*From* Szabo Z, Berci G: Extra and intracorporeal knotting and suturing technique. Gastrointest Endosc Clin North Am 3:367–379, 1993; with permission.)

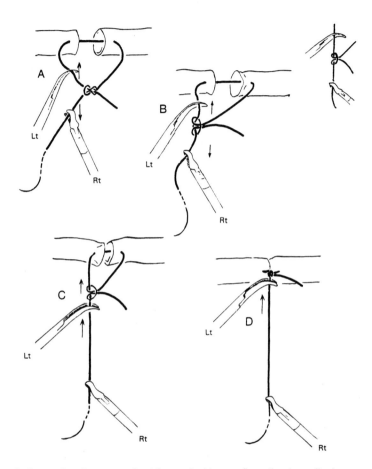

Figure 9. Converting the square knot from a locking configuration to a slipping one. If the resulting knot leaves the tissue edges too loosely approximated, or if the square knot was tied loosely on purpose (such as in a stay suture), the locking square knot can be altered and repositioned appropriately. *A,* Starting position: On the ipsilateral side, the tail and the stitch are pulled in opposite directions, perpendicular to the stitch. *B,* When the knot changes its configuration, a snapping sensation can be felt. *C,* While continuing to put tension on the tail, the other instrument performs the role of a knot pusher and advances the knot toward the tissue *(D),* until the tissue is approximated to the desired tension. (*From* Szabo Z, Berci G: Extra and intracorporeal knotting and suturing technique. Gastrointest Endosc Clin North Am 3:367–379, 1993; with permission.)

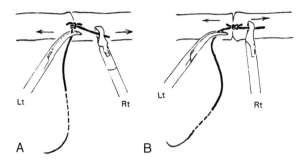

Figure 10. Reconverting the slip knot back to its locking configuration, the square knot. *A,* The tails of the stitch are pulled in opposite directions, parallel with the stitch, in the same manner in which the knot was originally tightened. *B,* The reconversion is complete and the square knot has been recreated. If a third throw is desired, it can now be placed in the same manner as the first flat knot. (*From* Szabo Z, Berci G: Extra and intracorporeal knotting and suturing technique. Gastrointest Endosc Clin North Am 3:367–379, 1993; with permission.)

side branches are coagulated with the monopolar cautery. When the appropriate length of the dissected vessel has been calculated and dissected, the vessel is temporarily occluded at the midportion with a ligature or a clip; it is then cauterized at the distal end.

A pericardiotomy is manually prepared with endoscopic microscissors to determine the location and course of the LAD and to locate the optimal position for the anastomosis to be performed. The IMA then is introduced to the vicinity of the LAD to check for sufficient length. The IMA then is trimmed of excessive tissue around the vessel end and, without twisting, carefully positioned near the anastomotic site. CPB is then prepared in the animal.

Afterward, the view port is relocated to the first, second, or third intercostal space in the most medial position possible. The ideal viewing angle is created so that the LAD can be viewed on the video monitor, running approximately in an 11 o'clock-to-5 o'clock direction. Then the instrument ports are calculated and placed approximately 8 cm to 10 cm apart, recreating an equidistant triangle with the view port.

A temporary ligature is prepared on the LAD just proximal to the anastomotic site in case the anastomotic field is obscured by bleeding. The distal ligature also is prepared but is not tightened until necessary, which follows the creation of the arteriotomy. A ligature is placed around the internal mammary vein, which is still attached in part to the IMA; it is then fastened to pericardium to stabilize IMA in position and in preparation for the anastomosis. A 3-mm to 5-mm arteriotomy is prepared, cutting from proximal to distal directions on the anterior surface of the LAD with microscissors; it is then irrigated. If necessary, the distal ligature is tightened. In the absence of adverse factors, the anastomosis then is begun; however, if adverse factors cannot be eliminated, surgery is halted and considered a CPB failure. Adverse factors include flow or leakage of the cardioplegic solution, movement or filling of the heart, and obstruction of view by the lungs.

Endoscopic Anastomosis of the Internal Mammary Artery to the Left Anterior Descending Artery

A 7-0 or 8-0 polypropylene, polytetrafluoroethylene, or other suture is prepared by cutting it to a length of 5.5 cm to 7.0 cm. This single-armed suture then is introduced to the field. The first suture (Fig. 11) is placed at the heel of the anastomosis (12 o'clock position), first entering from outside of the IMA to inside of the LAD, taking approximately a 1-mm bite on the donor and recipient vessels. The square knot is tied to pull the edges of the donor and recipient vessel together securely.

The right half of the anastomosis (downleg) is completed first, using continuous suturing techniques (entering in the IMA and exiting through the LAD), taking approximately 1-mm bites on either side of the vessel edge, with stitches spaced 0.5 mm apart. When the toe of the anastomosis has been reached (6 o'clock position), the running loops are pulled to the appropriate tension and, if needed, a knot is tied to secure the completed first half.

Without cutting the suture, the anastomosis is continued on the left side (upleg), progressing toward the starting position of the heel stitch (12 o'clock) in a similar fashion as the first half of the procedure, from inside of the IMA to outside of the LAD. Periodically, the suture line is checked for the absence of posterior wall inclusion or stenosis.

When the final stitch is completed and pulled tight and the lumen has been found to be satisfactory, the suture is tied securely to the tail of the toe knot using a square or surgeon's knot. The anastomotic site is then irrigated and checked for irregularity, such as gaps. If needed, additional interrupted sutures are placed to ensure hemostasis. Cardioplegic solution then is allowed to flow to test for hemostasis and to expel air.

If applied, the distal or proximal ligatures of the LAD now are released, retrograde flow is permitted into the anastomotic site, and any air bubbles present are expelled. The IMA occlusion then is released, restoring flow through the anastomosis. Hemostasis is checked again. The anastomotic site then is irrigated. If anastomotic leakage or peripheral hemorrhage is observed during or after CPB discontinuation, additional 7-0 or 8-0 sutures are placed by the thoracoscopic access. After satisfactory inspection, the thoracoscopic instruments are removed. The CPB team takes over to wean the calf from bypass and measure flow in the IMA.

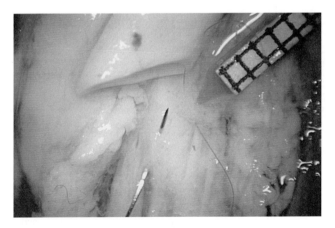

Figure 11. Endoscopic setup of the internal mammary artery-to-left anterior descending artery anastomosis. The anastomosis begins with the heel stitch at the 12-o'clock position and proceeds on the right half of the anastomosis (downleg) to the 6-o'clock position, then continues to the left side (upleg).

SUMMARY

The preceding description of E-CABG may seem excessively detailed, even redundant, for trained cardiac surgeons; however, the authors' extensive experience with training surgeons on endoscopic techniques suggests that, despite a high level of proficiency and dexterity that a surgeon may possess in open surgery, becoming equally proficient and dexterous in the endoscopic environment is not simple. Participating in an in-depth, systematic endoscopic microvascular surgery training program in a laboratory setting is essential before applying the previously described E-CABG techniques in humans.

The E-CABG procedure is one of the most challenging endoscopic techniques. Successful completion of this procedure requires that the surgeon be motivated to succeed and willing to invest the time and effort necessary to develop the new skills. Also critical is the avoidance of the temptation to use devices and systems that promise to obviate the need to bother with learning these difficult endoscopic skills.

Long term results of the minimally invasive approach remain to be defined. However, some early studies of port-access procedures are encouraging.[1] To date, a prospective randomized clinical trial comparing conventional LAD bypass to E-CABG has not been conducted. Although most investigators believe that long term patency of the IMA to the LAD using either technique should be the same, this is as yet unproven. Nonetheless, the adaption of endoscopic skills by the cardiac surgeon will further advance the evolution of this specialty.

References

1. Galloway AC, Shemin RJ, Glower DD, et al: First report of the port access international registry. Ann Thorac Surg 67:51–56, 1999
2. Liu HP, Change CH, Lin PH, et al: Thoracoscopic management of effusive pericardial disease: Indications and technique [abstract]. Ann Thorac Surg 48:1695–1697, 1994
3. Mack JM, Landreneau RJ, Hazelrigg SR, et al: Video thoracoscopic management of benign and malignant pericardial effusions. Ann Thorac Surg 103(suppl 4):390–393, 1993
4. Mack MJ, Landreneau, Yong P, et al: Cardiac applications of video assisted thoracic surgery. Int Surg 82:217–222, 1997
5. Szabo Z: Laparoscopic suturing and tissue approximation. *In* Hunter JG, Sackier JM (eds): Minimally Invasive Surgery. New York, McGraw-Hill, 1993, pp 141–155
6. Szabo Z, Berci G: Extra and intracorporeal knotting and suturing technique. Gastrointest Endosc Clin North Am 3:367–369, 1993
7. Szabo Z, Sackier JM: Laparoscopic fixation and guiding devices. *In* Szabo Z, Kerstein MD, Lewis JE (eds): Surgical Technology International, ed 3. San Francisco, Universal Medical Press, 1994, pp 245–252
8. Szabo Z, Stellini L, Ellis MS, et al: Slip-knot suspension technique: A fail-safe anastomosis technique for small caliber microanastomosis. Microsurgery 13:100–102, 1992

Address reprint requests to
Zoltan Szabo, PhD
MOET Institute
153 States Street
San Francisco, CA 94114

e-mail: MOETinst@aol.com

CORONARY SURGERY
Off-Pump and Port Access

Michael J. Mack, MD

Following in the footsteps of minimally invasive initiatives in other surgical subspecialties, including general surgery and thoracic surgery, late 1995 saw the introduction of minimally invasive cardiac surgery. Two divergent methods to reduce the "invasiveness" of cardiac surgery were introduced virtually simultaneously: (1) Port-access (Heartport, Redwood City, CA) surgery and (2) beating-heart surgery.[22, 23] Port-access coronary artery bypass (CAB) sought to replicate laparoscopic techniques in cardiac surgery by defining a "ports-only" approach to cardiac surgery. Initial attempts were unsuccessful because of several limiting factors, including space inside of the chest, technology, instrumentation, and procedural complexity, and it rapidly evolved to an open procedure, albeit through a limited-access approach.

The same limited-access approach was used for the initial minimally invasive beating-heart procedures. Although beating-heart surgery had been performed selectively during the 1980s,[3, 5, 17] the introduction of stabilizers and limited access redefined beating-heart surgery. The advocates of minimally invasive direct CAB (MIDCAB) believed that cardiopulmonary bypass was the most invasive component of conventional cardiac surgery and that its elimination would do more than just limit access to decrease invasiveness.

At the turn of this century, both procedures have been relegated to a relatively limited "niche" status; however, the events promulgated by these two procedures that were set in motion promise to profoundly change the face of cardiac surgery. Off-pump CAB (OPCAB) now comprises more than 15% of all CAB surgery. Robotics has been introduced to clinical cardiac surgery, and a plethora of enabling techniques is in the "pipeline" with the intent to make totally endoscopic CAB (TECAB) as routine as the laparoscopic cholecystectomy.

This article summarizes each facet of minimally invasive CAB, MIDCAB, port-access CAB, and OPCAB and attempts to put into perspective the relative

From the Cardiopulmonary Research Science Technology Institute, Dallas, Texas

SURGICAL CLINICS OF NORTH AMERICA

roles of each in coronary revascularization and to make some assessment regarding future developments.

MINIMALLY INVASIVE CORONARY ARTERY BYPASS SURGERY

Evolution

The initial clinical experience with MIDCAB was reported by Subramanian et al[23] in 1995. The procedure as initially described was performed through a limited left anterior thoracotomy incision. The left internal mammary artery (IMA) was harvested under direct vision, and an anastomosis was performed to the left anterior descending (LAD) coronary artery on a beating heart. Early procedures were hampered by lack of appropriate instrumentation and the exacting requirement of performing a precise vascular anastomosis without a motionless surgical field. Performance of the procedure was dramatically simplified and results were significantly improved with the introduction of mechanical stabilization. Stabilizers are mechanical feet placed adjacent to the target vessel that accomplish local immobilization while global cardiac function remains relatively unimpaired. The initial device was a nonsuction foot introduced by Cardiothoracic Systems (Cupertino, CA; Fig. 1) and was rapidly followed by a suction stabilizer, the Octopus (Medtronic, Inc., Minneapolis, MN; Fig. 2). User friendliness and results improved dramatically, leading reporting of results to be segregated to the prestabilization and poststabilization eras. Both stabilizers have undergone second-generation and third-generation changes, and numerous disposable and reusable alternatives have been introduced (Figs. 3 and 4).

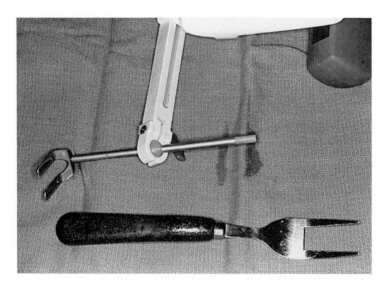

Figure 1. First clinical stabilizer (fork) with first commercially introduced stabilizer.

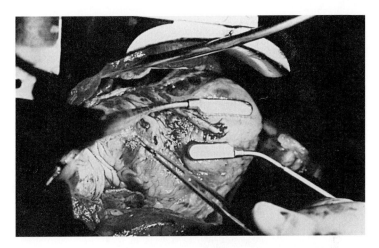

Figure 2. First suction stabilizer with arms attached to table made it difficult to use.

Technique

Most commonly, the procedure is performed through a 6-cm to 7-cm left anterior thoracotomy incision in the fourth intercostal space. Using various available chest wall retractors to elevate the chest wall superior to the incision, the IMA is harvested under direct vision. Thoracoscopic IMA harvest has been described by Nataf et al[16] and seems to cause less chest wall trauma and therefore less pain but has proved to be problematic for cardiac surgeons who have limited endoscopic experience. The use of robotic assistance for IMA harvest also has been described.[14, 19] Although IMA harvest has proved to be a

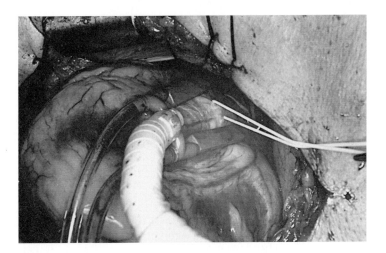

Figure 3. Newest generation Octopus stabilizer (Medtronic, Minneapolis, MN).

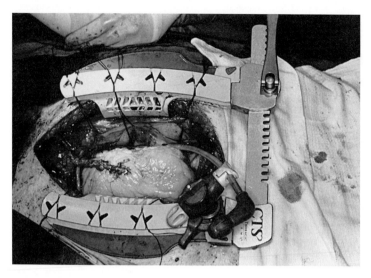

Figure 4. Newest generation Ultima nonsuction stabilizer (Guidant, Menlo Park, CA).

good training and proving ground for the introduction of robotics into cardiac surgery, it has not yet succeeded in significantly facilitating the procedure.

When IMA harvest has been completed, a later-generation stabilization device is placed around the LAD. The author places a snare proximally around only the LAD to occlude blood flow, obviating any concern regarding distal coronary artery injury from snaring. Although intracoronary shunts can be placed to maintain a bloodless field, the author uses a blower of carbon dioxide during the anastomosis and reserves intracoronary shunts for large, dominant, non–totally occluded right coronary arteries during OPCAB surgery.

On completion of the anastomosis, a small drainage tube is placed in the left pleural cavity. A regional intercostal block is given, and the patient is extubated in the surgical suite. Discharge is usually on postoperative day 2 or 3.

Indications

MIDCAB is almost totally limited to revascularization of a single vessel, the LAD. Although multivessel CAB has been performed and the right coronary artery revascularized by a right thoracotomy approach, these procedures are more effectively performed by a sternotomy approach. The most common indications for MIDCAB include restenosis after catheter-based therapy or lesions at high risk for recurrence after catheter-based therapy. Those LAD lesions include complex type C lesions of the proximal LAD, especially those involving the origin or a bifurcation. High restenosis rates after percutaneous transluminal coronary angioplasty (PTCA) or stent therapy in diabetic patients with LAD disease clearly have been demonstrated (BARI trial),[1] so MIDCAB should be considered in these patients, especially if significant local institutional experience with MIDCAB exists. Other low success or high recurrence rate situations for PTCA or stent therapy include chronic total occlusions, saphenous vein graft disease, and small target vessels (< 2 mL),[7] so these patients should be considered for MIDCAB.

Hybrid Procedures

MIDCAB, left IMA to LAD, occasionally has been used as part of a "composite" procedure with catheter-based therapy for multivessel disease. Candidates for this hybrid approach include high-risk patients for multivessel surgery grafting with LAD disease not amenable to PTCA or stent therapy and who have non–LAD disease approachable by catheter-based therapy. Although experience is limited (largest series, <50 patients)[6] this option should be kept in reserve in the revascularization armamentarium for select difficult patients.

Contraindications

Contraindications are relative and depend to some degree on surgeon experience. Smaller target vessels with significant calcification or an intramyocardial location pose greater technical challenges and should be avoided unless the surgeon has significant MIDCAB experience.

Current Results

Many successful series of MIDCAB results have been published with generally good outcomes. Concerns regarding the issue of graft patency have been addressed in multiple series, demonstrating by early angiography with graft patency rates equivalent to those of conventional CAB (Table 1). Direct comparison of left IMA–to–LAD graft patency rates with conventional CAB has been presented in the Patency Outcomes Economics MIDCAB (POEM) study.[13] The primary endpoint of the POEM study was angiographic patency of left IMA conventional CAB compared with MIDCAB at 6-month follow-up. A total of 311 patients were registered (151 in the conventional CAB group and 160 in the MIDCAB group). The mortality and complication rates are presented in Table 2. No statistically significant difference was found between the two groups. Graft patency was 98.6% in the MIDCAB group versus 95% in the conventional CAB group in the first 88 patients analyzed at 6-month follow-up. These results

Table 1. GRAFT PATENCY BY ANGIOGRAPHY OF PUBLISHED SERIES OF MIDCAB PROCEDURES

Author	Year	Studied/ Occupied	Percent Studied (%)	Interval	Graft Patency (%)	Exclusions/Notes
Schaff	1996	15/16	94	Intraoperative	100	3 revised
Calafiore	1998	271/434	62	≤1 y	93.7	4.8% grade B
Subramanian	1997	169/189	89	24–36 h	92	Stenosis = occlusion
					97.5	Additional 19%
Gill	1997	29/29	100	4–6 h		stenosis > 50%
Mack	1998	100/103	97	38, intraoperative	99	Additional 8%
				62 at 48–96 h		stenosis > 50%

From Mack MI: Graft patency in coronary artery bypass grafting: What do we really know? Ann Thorac Surg 66:1055–1059, 1998; with permission.

Table 2. RESULTS OF THE POEM COMPARISON STUDY OF LEFT INTERNAL
MAMMARY ARTERY GRAFT PATENCY

	Conventional CAB	MIDCAB
Immediate		
No. of patients	130	152
Mortality	0.8%	0
Myocardial infarction	0.8%	0
Neurological deficit	4.6%	1.3%
Atrial fibrillation	23.7%	15.1%
Length of stay (d)	8.3	4.5
6 months		
Mortality	1.5%	2.6%
Myocardial infarction	0	0.6%
Target vessel revascularization	0	2.6%
Stroke	0	1.3%
Patency	98.3%	97.4%
	(n = 32)	(n = 88)

confirm demonstration of equivalent patency of MIDCAB with conventional
arrested-heart CAB.

Whether these results translate to longer-term outcomes is being studied.
The author has performed intermediate-term follow-up study on all MIDCAB
procedures performed at his institution. These patients were followed up for
survival and major adverse cardiac events (death, myocardial infarction, need
for target vessel revascularization) at 1 and 3 years after surgery. Follow-up is
98.6% complete (214/217 patients). Survival and cardiac event–free survival
rates are presented in Table 3. Additional analysis of these results demonstrates
that survival is significantly decreased in patients 80 years old or older compared
with the younger cohort but that half of the mortality in this elderly group was
noncardiac in origin.

LATERAL THORACOTOMY CAB

An interesting variation of MIDCAB is performance of a single bypass using
a saphenous vein graft or radial artery placed from the descending aorta to a
branch of the circumflex coronary system.[2] The typical indication is in a patient
who has had previous CAB and has a patent left IMA to the LAD. The circumflex
disease is such that it is not amenable to catheter-based approach or has recurred
despite a previous PTCA. Commonly, the circumflex system is totally occluded
and a wire cannot be passed.

Table 3. INTERMEDIATE TERM FOLLOW-UP OF MIDCAB PROCEDURES

Outcomes	One Year (%)	Three Years (%)
Survival*	91.1	89.7
Freedom from MACCE	94.4	92.5
Freedom from TVR	97.4	96.4

*N = 214/217 (98.6%)
MACCE = major adverse cardiovascular and cerebral events; TVR = target vessel revascularization.

The procedure is performed through a limited thoracotomy with or without video assistance. The lateral and posterior cardiac surfaces usually are remarkably free of adhesions, and commonly, a previously performed saphenous vein graft serves as a marker for the target vessels. A stabilizer is placed, and the distal anastomosis is performed first, followed by the proximal anastomosis to the descending aorta just above the diaphragm. Occasionally, diffuse disease in the descending aorta presents technical challenges to this anastomosis.

The author has experience in 35 cases of this procedure with no surgical mortality. This procedure should be considered when culprit circumflex disease exists but is not amenable to catheter-based therapy.

FURTHER CONSIDERATIONS

Despite considerable success with MIDCAB outcomes, LATCAB remains a "niche" procedure, comprising less than 2% of all CAB grafting. The reasons for this limited application are multiple, including surgical technical difficulty. It is still a relatively challenging technical procedure, so it is not widely available. As more surgeons become conversant with beating-heart techniques with OPCAB surgery, and as MIDCAB improvements are made (video-assisted IMA harvest?), the procedure may become more widely applied. Procedural success rates are high with catheter-based therapy to the LAD, but despite greater use of stents, 6-month restenosis rates remain 25% to 30%. One would anticipate broader application as a complementary revascularization technique to PTCA in single-vessel disease that reoccurs in a stent or de novo disease in patients at high risk for recurrence with stent therapy.

PORT-ACCESS CORONARY ARTERY BYPASS

The original operative "platform" of the port-access approach to CAB was peripheral cannulation of the femoral artery and vein for institution of cardiopulmonary bypass, a catheter-based balloon delivery system for aortic occlusion (cross-clamping) in cardioplegic delivery, and endoscopic IMA harvest and coronary anastomosis. In the early stages of development, this leap from completely open to totally endoscopic CAB proved to be too large to make at once, and instead, appropriate incremental steps were substituted. Following the initial experience at Stanford, several major institutions, including New York University,[9] Munich,[20] and Durham,[25] gained significant experience with single and multivessel port-access CAB and mitral valve surgery.[8]

Evolution

The procedure has been significantly simplified from the original platform, serving to expedite the performance of surgery and decreasing surgical complications. Early results were plagued by complications of the aortic dissection, but this issue has been obviated largely by the definition of proper patient selection, surgical technique, and technical improvements. Intraoperative fluoroscopy has been replaced by transesophageal echocardiography (TEE), significantly simplifying line and cannula placement. The aortic balloon configuration has been changed to more reliable occlusion and less dislodging.

Despite these platform and technique improvements, however, many centers with significant early experience have abandoned the procedure because of early complications, operative length, lack of perceived benefit, and the concomitant increase of beating-heart surgery. Although many centers perform port-access mitral valve surgery or some limited access variation (e.g., the Chitwood micro-mitral procedure), port-access CAB is limited to a few centers (e.g., New York University, Asheville).

Technique

The surgical technique is simplified significantly from the original iteration. Placement of a percutaneous coronary sinus catheter and pulmonary artery vent is performed by the anesthesiologist through the internal jugular vein. Proper placement is ascertained by TEE. The arterial return cannula is placed through the femoral artery (usually the right) or directly into the ascending aorta (Fig. 5). Proper placement of the balloon occluder in the ascending aorta is ascertained by TEE. Venous access is by way of a femoral venous cannula, which can be placed percutaneously. Access for revasularization is through a limited 6-cm to 7-cm left anterior thoracotomy through the third or fourth intercostal space. In the arrested, decompressed heart, all surfaces can be approached for revascularization by this route. Proximal grafts can be placed on the underside of the aortic arch, usually before cardiac arrest.

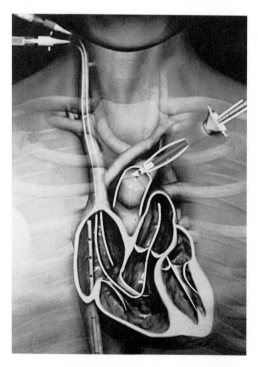

Figure 5. EndoDirect (Heartport, Redwood City, CA) cannulation system.

Extubation can be in the surgical suite or in the first few hours postoperatively, and discharge is usually on postoperative day 4 or 5.

Results

The advantage of port-access CAB is that the optimal surgical setting for performance of a precise anastomosis is recreated from conventional CAB. The motionless, bloodless field, albeit by a limited-access approach, obviates some of the difficulties of the beating-heart approaches. The disadvantages, however, include the use of CPB, which is believed by most cardiac surgeons to be the most invasive component of conventional CAB compared with the median sternotomy incision. Technical challenges and additional expense also have limited the use of this technique. A few large series exist from selected centers (Table 4).[9] Although the results of all of these series are relatively good, they are unhelpful in determining any value added to this approach. All series include selected patients with no risk stratification performed, so no risk-adjusted mortality is discernible. Also, reporting to the registry is voluntary, and it is unaudited so that no firm conclusions can be made regarding these outcomes.

Future Applications

For the near future, port-access techniques seem mostly confined to mitral valve procedures. The breakup of the original platform package (surgeons are able to purchase components separately) and continuing evolution of component parts may simplify the procedure. Alternative systems for peripheral cannulation that deliver arterial return flow centrally and variations of balloon occluders should continue to incrementally improve the technique (Fig. 6).

The road to a totally endoscopic CAB (TECAB), catalyzed by the introduction of robotic systems into cardiac surgery, will continue to use the port-access platform while the technique evolves.

OFF-PUMP CORONARY ARTERY BYPASS SURGERY

CAB was initially performed on a beating heart in the 1960s[12]; however, the introduction of CPB largely made attempts at developing and expanding beating-heart techniques moot. Despite the routine use of CPB in most centers worldwide for CAB, a few investigators, notably Benetti et al[3] in Argentina and

Table 4. RESULTS OF PORT-ACCESS CAB*

Years 1996–1998	Observed (%)	Predicted (%)
Mortality (hospital, 30 d)	0.99	1.2
Reoperate/bleeding	3.3	1.9
Ventilator > 24 h	1.7	3.8
Stroke	1.7	1.2
Myocardial infarction	0	1.3

*n = 302

Data from Grossi EA, Groh MA, Lefrak EA, et al: Results of a prospective multicenter study on port-access coronary bypass grafting. Ann Thoracic Surg 68:1475–1477, 1999.

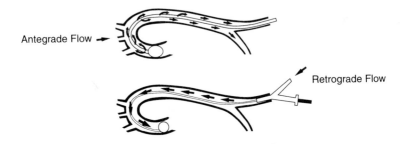

Figure 6. Alternative peripheral cannulation system with central blood return.

Buffolo et al[5] in Brazil, persisted with multivessel, sternotomy OPCAB mainly for economic reasons. Their results and those of Pfister et al[117] in the United States demonstrated that, in selected patients, CAB without CPB could be performed with the results approaching those of on-pump CAB. Numerous other series have been reported, with the results dating back more than 10 years with acceptable outcomes.

With the introduction of MIDCAB in the mid-1990s with the accompanying technology (stabilizers), interest in beating-heart surgery has been renewed. Over the past 4 years, the rate of CAB performed without CPB has doubled. Second-generation and third-generation stabilizers improved techniques to access the posterior circulation (left IMA sutures) and demonstrated equivalency of graft patency, and early results pointing to improved outcomes all have contributed to the intense interest in this aspect of minimally invasive cardiac surgery. If the studies now in progress demonstrate decreased mortality and improved neurocognitive outcomes compared with conventional techniques, one can expect a further expansion of CAB performed with off-pump techniques.[15]

Technique

Although many variations in the standard median sternotomy incision to access the heart for multivessel OPCAB have been described, including partial sternotomies and subxiphoid and intercostal approaches, the full sternotomy incision remains the standard approach for OPCAB. When the sternum has been divided, surgical exposure through the pericardium is the same, with the exception that pericardial stay sutures that can be adjusted to retract or slacken during surgery are placed. During cardiac manipulation, especially to access the posterior circulation, distraction or compression of the right ventricle can occur. Relaxation of the right-sided pericardial sutures and even opening the right pleural space can help to restore right ventricular geometry and hemodynamic stability.

The standard approach is commenced with a full median sternotomy, although the skin incision does not need to extend cephalad as much as previously. The pericardium is opened widely, and the aforementioned pericardial stay sutures are placed. The author usually places three sutures on each side of the pericardial edge. The left side of the pericardium is extended, and the inferior portion of the left pericardium is opened further than usual to allow the apex of the heart to be averted from the pericardial cavity. An additional suture is placed in the posterior pericardium halfway between the apex of the pericar-

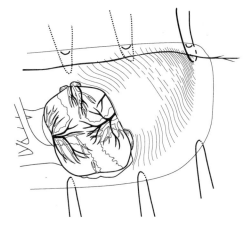

Figure 7. Placement of pericardial traction (Lima) sutures.

dium and the inferior pulmonary vein (Fig. 7). This variation of the left IMA suture is all that the author has found necessary to allow for distraction of the apex of the heart out of the chest cavity to access the posterior circulation (Figs. 8 and 9). Many variations of this technique exist, including the left IMAs, Lima's original description of two more pericardial sutures placed cephalad from the first suture placed. Other variations include placement of a retracting sponge through the suture to allow for rotation of the heart for better exposure.

Harvest and positioning of all conduits are completed before the heart is distracted from the chest cavity. Careful attention to having all grafts ready to be anastomosed minimizes the time that the heart is in a hemodynamically compromised position. The author performs bypass of the LAD first, which usually is performed with the left IMA. The logic behind this choice is that the

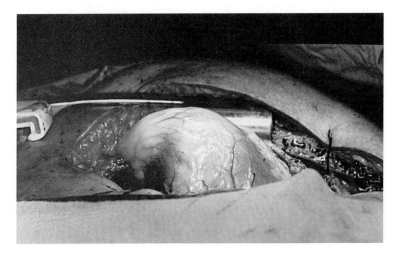

Figure 8. Distraction of heart apex out of chest to access posterior circulation.

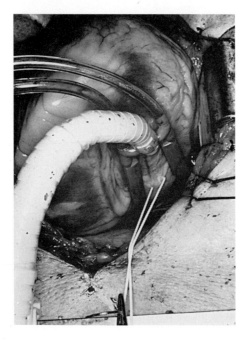

Figure 9. Stabilizer placed to access posterior circulation.

anterior wall and the septum are revascularized with the least amount of distraction possible, and, with this initial revascularization, the heart is able to tolerate more hemodynamically significant maneuvers. The only exception to this is a large, totally occluded right coronary artery filled by collaterals from the LAD. Because the myocardial distribution of two major vessels then is dependent solely on the LAD supply, the author revascularizes the right coronary artery first, followed by the LAD.

To bypass the LAD first, traction is placed on the posterior left IMA sutures, and a stabilizer is placed around the LAD. A Silastic snare on a blunt needle is placed proximally around the LAD and occluded when the vessel is opened. Dissection of the vessel and arteriotomy is performed only after stabilization has occurred. Although an intramyocardial location may make the localization of the LAD somewhat difficult, dissection after the stabilizer has been placed allows an intramyocardial vessel to still be bypassed.

The anastomosis is performed with a single running 7-0 prolene suture, with three sutures placed in the heel of the left IMA and coronary artery and then parachuted down. On completion of this anastomosis, the heart is placed back into the pericardial cavity, and hemodynamic recovery is allowed. The author monitors these patients with a Swan-Ganz catheter and TEE.

Before any more vessels are bypassed, any proximal grafts are placed on the aorta. This is done under partial aortic occlusion, with the systolic blood pressure being maintained at less than 100 mm Hg when the clamp is placed on the ascending aorta. The next easiest vessel to bypass is bypassed next. The logic behind this step is that, at the time that the most difficult vessel bypass is performed, the heart has been revascularized as much as possible. The author's order of sequence of difficulty of vessel anastomosis is listed below, from least to most difficult.

1. Left anterior descending (unless total right coronary artery)
2. Total right coronary artery
3. Diagonal
4. Second obtuse marginal
5. Posterior ventricular branch right coronary artery
6. First obtuse marginal
7. Posterior descending branch right coronary artery
8. Ramus
9. Open dominant right coronary artery

The author usually finds that high obtuse marginal or intermediate branches are the most difficult to bypass because of the compression to the pulmonary artery and right ventricular outflow tract that occurs. Significant hemodynamic consequences can occur when large right coronary arteries that are not totally occluded are bypassed. If the main right coronary artery is bypassed, blood supply to the atrioventricular node is compromised, and a junctional rhythm with distention of the right ventricle can occur. Therefore, if a large, non–totally occluded patent right coronary artery is bypassed, the author places an intracoronary shunt into the vessel after the arteriotomy has been made. The author also places atrial and ventricular pacer wires on the heart before this bypass is performed.

On completion of all anastomoses, heparinization is reversed with protamine and a drainage tube placed. The author does not routinely place pacemaker wires unless they have been placed intraoperatively for the right coronary artery bypass. The author routinely extubates patients in the surgical suite, and discharge is usually on postoperative day 4 or 5, approximately 1 day less than with conventional CAB.

Results

A total of 34 articles have been published that contain data regarding outcomes of OPCAB. Articles by Benetti et al,[3] Buffolo et al,[5] and Pfister et al[17] report their results from the prestabilization era of more than 2000 patients. The mortality rate among these selected patients was less than 2%, and all investigators concluded that OPCAB is safe and effective in selected patients with lower transfusion rates compared with on-pump surgery.

A total of 31 reports of results of OPCAB in the era since stabilization has been introduced have been published. In the largest series, by Tasdemir et al,[24] in Turkey, 2052 cases are reported, with a 1.9% mortality rate. They concluded that OPCAB was safe and effective in selected patients but that incomplete revascularization of the circumflex system resulted in increased mortality in those patients. Numerous other series variously show less blood loss, less need for transfusion, and less inotrope use in OPCAB compared with on-pump surgery; there also is less inflammatory cytokines, specifically tumor necrosis factor-α, interleukin-2, and interleukin-6 levels have been reported.[4, 11] Other reports show a lower risk for myocardial infarction and renal insufficiency and less cognitive dysfunction.

An article by Hart et al[10] reported on a review of 1582 consecutive cases of OPCAB performed with the Octopus stabilization (Medtronics, Minneapolis,

MN) device.[10] The rate of conversion to CPB was 2.6%, the surgical mortality rate was 1%, the permanent stroke rate was 0.6%, and the perioperative myocardial infarction rate was 1.2%. Stanbridge and Hadjinikolaou[21] reported a meta-analysis of 3060 cases of OPCAB performed at 21 centers. The early mortality rate was 2.2% (62/2819). No late mortality occurred, and the perioperative myocardial infarction rate was 1.5%. Some anastomotic problems were evident by postoperative angiography in 5.4% of patients. Their conclusion based on this meta-analysis was that OPCABs are better than early reported results with MIDCAB, and they encouraged further use.

The author's results of CABG in 1999 included 125 consecutive cases performed without CPB. No conversion to CPB was necessary, and no patients were excluded. The surgical mortality was 2.4% (three patients). Death was caused by postoperative graft occlusion (one patient), stroke secondary to atrial fibrillation on postoperative day 2 (one patient), and renal insufficiency (one patient).

Puskas et al[18] reported their results in 200 patients undergoing OPCAB. Eighty-three percent of patients underwent postoperative angiography, with a graft patency rate of 98%. All left IMA–to–LAD grafts were patent. Also, these investigators demonstrated decreased cost, length of stay, and need for transfusion in this series.

Future of Off-Pump Coronary Artery Bypass Surgery

The benefit of OPCAB is the elimination of CPB and left-sided cannulation, shorter operating time, and no hemodilution. Also, global ischemia is eliminated, and instead only regional ischemia is induced during surgery. Less transfusion, less cost, and easier learning curve seem to be involved than with MIDCAB. Also, although still not proven, the neurocognitive outcomes probably are improved by OPCAB. If definitive studies show improved neurocognitive outcomes, and the author believes they will, a stronger push toward OPCAB will be made.

OPCAB still requires a median sternotomy, however, so it is not a limited access procedure. Also, decrease in end-organ perfusion may be associated with OPCAB. Also, some degree of postoperative hypercoagulability seems to lead to complications of graft occlusion, deep vein thrombosis, and embolic cerebral vascular accidents. Objective benefit has not yet been defined clearly, nor has equivalent graft patency.

Several of these concerns, including proper postoperative anticoagulation and fine-tuning of techniques to allow for routine access to the posterior circulations, for most surgeons will become more widespread, and the expansion of OPCAB will continue.

FUTURE OF MINIMALLY INVASIVE CARDIAC SURGERY

In the author's opinion, the most important advances in the immediate future include an increase in procedures performed by a beating-heart approach (i.e., OPCAB) to 25% to 30% of all CAB in the year 2000. Many significant studies will be published demonstrating value added to OPCAB, primarily in neurocognitive outcomes. If these studies indicate a benefit, a further catalyzation of the use of beating-heart surgery will occur. The role of robotics will continue to be defined at many centers in Europe and the United States. As the road to TECAB evolves, numerous anastomotic alternatives to conventional suturing will be the focus of intense investigation, and the interest in the use of right heart assistance with micropumps to facilitate beating-heart surgery will be intense (Fig. 10).

Already established terminology in minimally invasive cardiac surgery includes MIDCAB, OPCAB, and port-access surgery. New terms being described include lateral thoracotomy CAB (LATCAB), transabdominal coronary surgery, TECAB, ventricle to CAB (VCAB), and quick CAB (QCAB). During this march to TECAB, the gold standard has changed. Although the original goal was TECAB on an arrested heart, the success of beating-heart surgery has now mandated that if a limited access procedure is to be successful, it needs to be performed on a beating heart.

A limiting factor of OPCAB is hemodynamic compromise that occurs when accessing vessels on the posterior surface of the heart. The introduction of right ventricular assistance to augment the flow to the right side of heart during these maneuvers may catalyze the transition of more surgeons to beating-heart approaches.

Robotics is an anastomotic facilitator for CAB. The most difficult aspect of TECAB is the suturing of an anastomosis. The precision enhancement of robotics, or computer assistance, is an attempt to facilitate the execution of an endoscopic anastomosis (Fig. 11). Numerous alternatives to conventional suturing and anastomosis are being introduced in additional attempts to facilitate TECAB surgery. The most intriguing of these alternatives includes nitinol sutures that obviate knot tying, chemical bonding with biologic glues, external coupling devices, and internal anastomosic couplers (i.e., covered stents). Also, numerous alternative concepts to conventional coronary artery anastomosis include left ventricle–to–coronary artery shunts, coronary vein–to–coronary artery anastomoses, and percutaneous catheter-based CAB.

The author thinks that minimally invasive cardiac surgery is a breakthrough in coronary revascularization; however, the value of a breakthrough is determined by the refinements and enhancements that occur after the breakthrough.

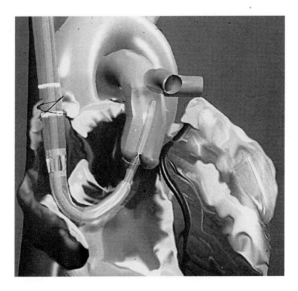

Figure 10. Concept of right heart assistance for beating-heart surgery.

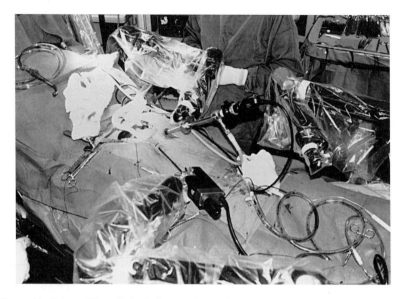

Figure 11. Setup of Zeus Robotic System for endoscopic coronary artery bypass grafting.

One only has to look at the field of portable communications and cellular technology to realize that the universal usage of portable communications required 50 years of enhancements after the introduction to reach the widespread applicability and value of today. Similarly, the success of catheter-based therapy required 20 years of refinements after the original breakthrough. Only 3 years have passed since the introduction of minimally invasive concepts into cardiac surgery, and only the refinements that will occur over the next 5 to 10 years will truly determine the value of minimally invasive concepts.

Pandora's box is open, and there is no going back. Minimally invasive cardiac surgery is a "discontinuous innovation," and incremental improvements will continue to define and enhance value. These technological enhancements and improved surgical techniques will improve user friendliness and applicability. The original goal of TECAB is still a long way off, and the ultimate role of robotics remains unclear. Clear today is that robotics 10 years from now will have little resemblance to current technology.

Minimally invasive cardiac surgery is successfully increasing the value of CAB, and although the continued role will be long-term, the goal is achievable. As W. Edwards Deming said, "It is not necessary to change . . . survival is not mandatory."

References

1. BARI Investigators: Comparison of coronary bypass surgery with angioplasty in patients with multi-vessel disease. The bypass angioplasty reintervention investigation (BARI). N Engl J Med 335:217–225, 1996
2. Baumgartner FJ, Gheissari A, Panagiotides GP, et al: Off-pump obtuse marginal grafting with local stabilization: Thoracotomy approach in reoperations. Ann Thorac Surg 68:946–948, 1999

3. Benetti FJ, Naselli G, Wood M, et al: Direct myocardial revascularization without extracorporeal circulation: Experience in 700 patients. Chest 100:312–316, 1991
4. Boyd WD, Desai ND, Del Rizzo DF, et al: Off-pump surgery decreases postoperative complications and resource utilization in the elderly. Ann Thorac Surg 68:1490–1493, 1999
5. Buffolo E, de Andrade CS, Branco JN, et al: Coronary artery bypass grafting without cardiopulmonary bypass. Ann Thorac Surg 61:63–66, 1996
6. Cohen HA, Zenati M, Contrad Smith AJ, et al: Feasibility of combined percutaneous transluminal angioplasty and minimally invasive direct coronary artery bypass in patients with multivessel coronary artery disease. Circulation 98:1048–1050, 1998
7. Elezi S, Kastrati A, Pache J, et al: Diabetes mellitus and the clinical angiographic outcome after coronary stent replacement. J Am Coll Cardiol 32:1866–1873, 1998
8. Galloway AC, Shemin R, Glower D, et al: First report of the port-access international registry. Ann Thorac Surg 67:51–58, 1993
9. Grossi EA, Groh MA, Lefrak EA, et al: Results of a prospective multicenter study on port-access coronary bypass grafting. Ann Thorac Surg 68:1475–1477, 1999
10. Hart JC, Spooner TH, Pym J, et al: A review of 1582 consecutive Octopus off pump coronary bypass patients. Ann Thorac Surg (in press)
11. Jansen EWL, Borst C, Lahpor JR, et al: Coronary bypass grafting without cardiopulmonary bypass using the Octopus method: Results in the first one hundred patients. J Thorac Cardiovasc Surg 116:60–67, 1998
12. Kolesov VI: Mammary artery-coronary artery anastomosis as method of treatment for angina pectoris. J Thorac Cardiovasc Surg 54:535–544, 1967
13. Mehran R: Results of the POEM Study. Presented at the 11th Annual Meeting of the TCT. Washington, DC; September 28, 1999
14. Mohr FW, Falk V, Diegeler A, et al: Computer enhanced coronary artery bypass surgery. J Thorac Cardiovasc Surg 117:1212–1215, 1999
15. Murkin JM, Boyd WD, Ganapathy S, et al: Beating heart surgery: Why expect less central nervous system morbidity? Ann Thorac Surg 68:1498–1501, 1999
16. Nataf P, Lima L, Regan M, et al: Minimally invasive coronary surgery with thoracoscopic internal mammary dissection: Surgical technique. J Cardiol Surg 11:288–297, 1995
17. Pfister AJ, Zaki S, Garcia JM, et al: Coronary artery bypass without cardiopulmonary bypass. Ann Thorac Surg 54:1085–1092, 1992
18. Puskas JD, Wright CE, Ronson RS, et al: Clinical outcomes and angiographic patency in 165 consecutive off-pump coronary bypass patients. Ann Thorac Surg (in press)
19. Reichenspurner H, Damiano RJ, Mack M, et al: Experimental and first clinical use of the voice-controlled and computer-assisted surgical system Zeus for endoscopic coronary artery bypass grafting. J Thorac Cardiovasc Surg (in press)
20. Reichenspurner H, Gulielmos V, Wunderlich J, et al: Port access coronary artery surgery with the use of cardiopulmonary bypass and cardioplegic arrest: clinical experience with 42 cases. Ann Thorac Surg 65:413–419, 1997
21. Stanbridge R, Hadjinikolaou LK: Technical adjuncts in beating heart surgery comparison of MIDCAB to off-pump sternotomy: A meta-analysis. Eur J Cardiothorac Surg 16(suppl 2):24–33, 1999
22. Stevens JH, Burdon TA, Peters WS, et al: Port-access coronary artery bypass grafting: A proposed surgical method. J Thorac Cardiovasc Surg 111:567–573, 1996
23. Subramanian VA, Sani G, Benetti FJ, et al: Minimally invasive coronary bypass surgery: A multicenter report of preliminary clinical experience [abstract]. Circulation 92(suppl 1):645, 1995
24. Tasdemir O, Vural KM, Karagoz H, et al: Coronary artery bypass grafting on the beating heart without the use of extracorporeal circulation: Review of 2052 cases. J Thorac Cardiovasc Surg 116:68–73, 1998
25. Waston DR, Duff SB: The clinical and financial impact of port-access coronary revascularization. Eur J Cardiothorac Surg 16(suppl 1):103–106, 1999

Address reprint request to
Michael J. Mack, MD
Cardiopulmonary Research Science Technology Institute
8440 Walnut Hill Lane, Suite 705
Dallas, TX 75231

MINIMAL ACCESS SURGERY, PART II   0039–6109/00 $15.00 + .00

REDUCING THE TRAUMA OF CONGENITAL HEART SURGERY

Redmond P. Burke, MD, and Robert L. Hannan, MD

In 1901, Osler[54] wrote, "The most distinguishing feature of the scientific medicine of the century has been the phenomenal results which have followed *experimental investigations.*" Were he able to comment today, Osler might note the equally phenomenal results that have followed *technological applications* at the turn of this century. Endotracheal ventilation and cardiopulmonary bypass (CPB) opened the field of thoracic and cardiac surgery and formed the foundation for a new array of technologies aimed at reducing the physiological and cosmetic impact of thoracic surgical therapy.

Procedures designed specifically to reduce trauma in surgery for congenital heart disease (CHD) have evolved over the past 7 years, beginning with the first report by Laborde et al[44] on video-assisted thoracoscopic (VATS) ligation of patent ductus arteriosus (PDA). Building on advances in endoscopic imaging technology, a limited access approach to various congenital heart lesions has evolved. The spatial and time constraints, anatomic complexity, and technical precision of congenital heart lesion repairs place extreme demands on "minimally invasive" instrumentation and techniques and have resulted in an appropriately slow pace of adoption for new approaches. Also, the small "market" that pediatric patients represent has limited capital investment in technology specifically designed for congenital heart defect repair. Despite these limitations, the goal of reducing surgical trauma in children with CHD remains a compelling grail for surgeons at the opening of the twenty-first century.

AVOIDING THORACOTOMY FOR EXTRACARDIAC CONGENITAL LESIONS

Patent Ductus Arteriosus

Myriad therapeutic alternatives are available for the simplest congenital heart lesion. Posterolateral thoracotomy with ligation or division as described

From the Division of Cardiovascular Surgery, Miami Children's Hospital, Miami, Florida by Gross and Hubbard[27] has been challenged by transcatheter closure techniques, various limited thoracotomy incisions,[67] and VATS.

Transcatheter coil occlusion has been well described as an outpatient procedure requiring no incisions, which usually results in complete ductal closure. Residual flow has been reported as a potential limitation requiring repeat procedures.[31] Six-month closure rates for the Rashkind (USCI/BARD, Tewksbury, MA) device have been reported at 77% compared with 90% for Gianturco (Cook, Bloomington, IN) coils.[38] Femoral vessel size constraints limit the applicability of the transcatheter technique in premature newborns, and patients with larger ducts (>4 mm) have a higher risk for residual flow. Device migration,[55] femoral vessel trauma, hemolysis, radiation exposure, aortic obstruction,[21] and the infectious risk for an intravascular foreign body are other potential drawbacks to transcatheter device closure.

VATS evolved in response to the chest wall trauma of thoracotomy.[63, 65, 66] Applications in adult thoracic surgery soon led to the first pediatric applications. Laborde et al[44] first described pediatric cardiac VATS in his clinical report of VATS ligation in 38 patients with PDA. Patients ranged from 1.5 to 90.0 months of age and from 2.4 kg to 25.0 kg. Successful ductal closure was achieved in all patients. Complications included one recurrent nerve injury. No deaths and no uncontrolled hemorrhage occurred.

VATS uses three or four thoracostomy incisions for insertion of an endoscope (the authors use a 4-mm 30° angled endoscope [Smith and Nephew, Dyonics, Inc., Andover, MA]), and a retractor (Pilling-Weck, Fort Washington, PA). The remaining two ports are used for the surgeon's endoscopic grasper and cautery. Operating with both hands, the surgeon is able to precisely dissect the duct (magnification within the surgical field is 4×) and apply vascular clips or intracorporeal ligatures.[4] Using a similar technique, Laborde et al[43] subsequently have reported excellent results in 332 patients from 1991 to 1996, ranging in weight from 1.2 kg to 65.0 kg.[43] Six patients had residual flow after thoracoscopic clip occlusion. Five of these had successful replacement of the clips (three endoscopically, and two by thoracotomy), and one is being followed up medically. Complications included recurrent nerve dysfunction in six patients (1.8%). Five of these nerve injuries were transient, and one is persistent. No mortality occurred. DeCampli[19] described his experience with VATS for patent ductus arteriosus, with no residual flow, recurrent nerve injury, chylothorax, or transfusion in full-term infants and children.

VATS for PDA also has been effectively used in premature newborns.[7] In 34 premature newborns weighing 0.5 kg to 2.5 kg, the median procedure time was 60 minutes. The operative mortality rate was zero, and trace residual Doppler flow occurred in two patients. Four procedures (12%) were converted to thoracotomy to improve exposure. Hines et al[34] described similar results in their group of 21 neonates undergoing VATS PDA interruption.

Until recently, limited experience with adult patients has been reported. Ho et al,[35] from Taiwan, reported successful closure by VATS in 35 adult patients. No residual flow occurred after double ligation in 32 of 35 cases. In the other three patients, intraoperative echocardiography showed persistent flow, which was obliterated by a third ligature.

Compared with transcatheter device occlusion techniques, VATS allows highly effective ductal closure with no restrictions based on patient size, ductal anatomy, or hemodynamic condition. VATS avoids the risks for radiation exposure, device embolization, left pulmonary artery obstruction, aortic obstruction, and the long-term presence of an intravascular foreign body.

The learning curve is steep for surgeons who have not operated endoscopically, suggesting that experience in an animal or simulation laboratory might be beneficial. It is hoped that long-term assessment of the technique will show that VATS reduces the prevalence of scoliosis,[63, 65, 66] post-thoracotomy pain syndromes,[17] and chest wall deformities,[39] described in pediatric patients after posterolateral thoracotomy. Building on the already extensive literature attempting to identify a cost or efficacy basis for transcatheter or surgical closure will be unproductive because no striking differences have been shown.[23–25, 31] The techniques each have strengths and weaknesses, which vary between institutions. At Miami Children's Hospital, the authors compared the results of VATS and coil occlusion in a consecutive series of patients with patent ductus arteriosus in 1997. The results showed no significant clinical differences in the techniques (Table 1). The authors offer families and referring doctors the option of a VATS approach or a transcatheter device and share the belief that full thoracotomy for patent ductus usually can be avoided.

Vascular Ring

VATS was extended to vascular ring division in 1993.[5] Pediatric patients with vascular ring are approached with the same technique and instrumentation used for VATS PDA interruption. Using the left subclavian artery as a landmark, the vascular ring elements are exposed endoscopically. The atretic arch segment (or the ligamentum) is identified, ligated proximally and distally, and divided, as in an open approach. Intraoperative bronchoscopy confirms relief of tracheal compression, and the thoracostomy incisions are closed. In a report comparing VATS vascular ring division to conventional division by thoracotomy,[9] VATS was used in eight pediatric patients ranging in age from 40.0 days to 5.5 years and in weight from 1.8 kg to 17.1 kg. Clinical success was achieved in all but one patient, who required reexploration by thoracotomy to divide a residual obstruction. Complications included transfusion (one patient) and chylothorax (one patient). These patients were compared with a historical control group of patients undergoing vascular ring division by thoracotomy. The two groups did not differ in age, weight, intensive care unit or postoperative hospital stay, duration of intubation, or hospital charges.

To date, the authors have performed VATS vascular ring division in 20 patients, ranging in age from 8.0 days to 5.5 years. In the past year, procedure times have averaged 2 hours, ranging from 1:25 to 2:30. Length of stay has ranged from 1 to 6 days. Conversion to thoracotomy is not considered a compli-

Table 1. INTERRUPTION OF PATENT DUCTUS ARTERIOSUS AT MIAMI CHILDREN'S HOSPITAL USING EITHER COIL OCCLUSION OR VIDEO-ASSISTED THORACOSCOPIC SURGERY

Observation	VATS (n = 39)	Transcatheter (n = 39)
Thoracotomy	0	0
Recurrent nerve injury	0	0
Transfusion	0	0
Residual flow	1	1
Auscultation	0	1
Doppler	1 trace	1
Applicability	1.6–46.6 kg	5–52 kg

VATS = video-assisted thoracoscopic surgery.

cation but rather the exercise of good clinical judgment, particularly when the ring is formed by large patent vessels. Evidence shows that pulmonary function abnormalities persist in patients with vascular rings repaired after the onset of symptoms.[49] The decreased chest wall incisional trauma of the VATS approach may justify earlier intervention in patients with asymptomatic vascular rings.

Other Extracardiac Lesions

VATS techniques have been applied to various other extracardiac congenital lesions, including pericardial window, epicardial pacemaker insertion, treatment of chylothorax, diaphragm plication,[64] interruption of arterial and venous collaterals, and thoracic explorations for esoteric lesions (i.e., absent left pericardium syndrome).[10] VATS for early treatment of pediatric empyema has been described as a method of decreasing the duration of hospital stay (average postoperative stay was 4.9 d, total stay was 7.3 d).[26]

Thoracotomy for shunt palliation can be avoided in all patients by using a median sternotomy approach.[53] Patients with bilateral thoracotomies and median sternotomy clearly have suffered unnecessary chest wall trauma, when their staged management could have been effectively performed through repeated median sternotomy. Other advantages to the median sternotomy approach for shunts include improved patency, decreased phrenic nerve injury, decreased pulmonary artery stenosis, decreased accidental shunts to the pulmonary vein, better access for conversion to bypass, easier access to the shunt site at reoperation, and decreased chest wall collateral formation in cyanotic patients.

Intraoperative Cardioscopy

Routine video-assisted procedures for extracardiac lesions naturally led to video-assisted endoscopic applications during open-heart surgery.[8] The authors define cardioscopy as the use of endoscopic imaging tools during open-heart surgery to facilitate visualization and repair of remote intracardiac structures and to create visual documentation of cardiac lesions before and after repair. This technique allows surgeons to achieve anatomic visualization without resorting to excessive retraction or extended cardiac incisions, which is an advantage when exposure has been limited by operating through small incisions.

At Miami Children's Hospital, this technique has evolved into the routine use of a 4-mm endoscope in the surgical field as a third eye for the surgical team, exposing remote areas within the ventricles, the left and right ventricular outflow tracts, and the subvalvar apparatus. The pleural spaces also can be easily explored by limited sternotomy using the endoscope. Cardioscopy has been used to facilitate the repair of ventricular septal defects, left ventricular outflow tract reconstructions, complex valvuloplasty, manipulation and placement of septal occlusion devices, and left ventricular thrombectomy.[51]

Video-assisted endoscopic imaging technology also allows for the collection and storage of video and still pictures for immediate and future correlation with other imaging modalities (e.g., angiography and echocardiography). The images also can be digitally stored for long-term reference, allowing surgeons to assess the outcomes of various surgical techniques and to prepare for reoperations. At Miami Children's Hospital, the authors have used routine intraoperative cardioscopy for the past 5 years in 1000 open-heart procedures, with no complications related to the endoscopy. Other investigators have described similar experiences with routine intraoperative cardioscopy.[56]

ALTERNATE APPROACHES TO OPEN HEART SURGERY FOR CONGENITAL LESIONS

Alternatives to Median Sternotomy for Septal Defect Repair

Nearly lost at the end of the last century was the median sternotomy incision for simple congenital heart repairs. Publications on alternate incision approaches for atrial and ventricular septal defects swelled the thoracic literature. Symbolic of the new information age, one of the first alternate approaches was reported on the Internet by Levinson.[45] A lower sternotomy and xyphoid resection was combined with femoral cannulation and fibrillatory arrest to close an atrial septal defect in an adult. A Medline (National Library of Medicine) search for atrial septal defect repair in 1999 revealed a dramatic international repudiation of the median sternotomy, as cardiac centers around the world present their technical variations. Ironically, as we were working to eliminate thoracotomy for extracardiac lesions, many of our colleagues have embraced thoracotomy to avoid median sternotomy for intracardiac lesions.

Thoracotomy

In Dresden, Germany, Kappert et al[41] describe a right lateral chest incision and femoral cannulation using the port-access technology (Heartport, Inc., Redwood City, CA). They describe 13 patients from 17 to 61 years repaired through a 4-cm to 8-cm incision in the fourth intercostal space. Bypass is achieved by femoral cannulation. No mortality occurred, and the median hospital stay was 8 days.[41] Adult cannula size limits the port-access technology in the pediatric population. The anterior thoracotomy is also a cosmetic risk in infants because the breast tissue is unpredictable in location and vulnerable to injury and subsequent deformity.

In India, 37 patients, ranging from 18 to 67 years in age, were approached with a 7-cm right anterior thoracotomy and femoral cannulation, with a centrifugal pump to facilitate cardiac drainage. Aortic clamping was achieved with a special clamp placed through a small midclavicular incision. Hospital stay averaged 4.2 days, and no complications or mortality occurred.[48] Surgeons in Singapore describe a similar technique for atrial septal defect repair by a right anterior thoracotomy with femoral cannulation.[62] In Hannover, Germany, three approaches have been compared, including (1) right parasternal incision with central cannulation, (2) anterior submammary mini-incision with femoral arterial and central caval cannulation, and (3) percutaneous cervical cannulation.[16] In 24 patients, this technique was used with no neurologic complications or mortality, and cosmetic acceptance was described as "high." In Japan, parasternal and partial sternotomy approaches have been advocated.[52, 60]

Partial Sternotomy

In Boston, Byrne et al[12] describe the evolution of their nonsternotomy approach. In this series, 59 adult patients underwent repair through a right parasternal, submammary, or upper hemisternotomy incision. No mortality occurred and four major complications were seen. Also in Boston, del Nido et al[20] describe a similar approach to pediatric atrial septal defect repairs. A consecutive series of 91 patients was divided into sternotomy ($n = 52$) and partial lower sternotomy groups ($n = 54$). Within the partial lower sternotomy group, patients were cannulated centrally ($n = 29$) or femorally ($n = 25$). Findings in the "minimal access group" included no conversions to full sternotomy, no difficulties placing femoral or aortic cannulas, no re-explorations for bleeding, and no wound infections requiring surgical drainage. Echocardiographic follow-up on 19 of 54 partial sternotomy patients showed no residual atrial shunts. No differences were found between the partial sternotomy group and the full sternotomy group in bypass duration or cross-clamp time. No remarkable differences were found between the groups in the incidence of postoperative pericardial effusions, or hospital stay, which averaged 3 days after partial sternotomy and 4 days after full sternotomy.

In San Francisco, Khan et al[42] describe a lower sternotomy approach, which spares the manubrium. Conventional aortic and bicaval cannulation is used. The heart is fibrillated during repair. In this series, 115 patients were repaired through a partial sternotomy starting at the nipple level, with no mortality and a median hospital stay of 4 days.

Sharing the general impression that a full median sternotomy is neither aesthetic nor necessary to safely expose the atrial septum, the authors also have adopted a lower partial sternotomy for atrial septal defect repair. The authors' limited incision technique for atrial septal defect repair was designed to preserve standard CPB, myocardial protection, neuroprotection (deairing and superior vena cava [SVC] drainage), and operative precision, and reduce bypass and operative times. The rationale for a midline approach is multifactorial: (1) central cannulation avoids femoral vessel injury (a risk with the port-access technique), (2) midline incision avoids breast injury and denervation[13] and intercostal and phrenic nerve trauma (a risk with lateral thoracotomy),[33] (3) cardioplegic arrest protects the myocardium and minimizes the risk for air embolism (a risk with fibrillation), and (4) conversion to median sternotomy is rapid to deal with unexpected anatomy or pathophysiology (e.g., left SVC and after repair pulmonary hypertension and right ventricular dysfunction).

Modifications of cardiopulmonary bypass have facilitated these alternate approaches to median sternotomy. An assisted venous drainage circuit using a constrained vortex cone (Biocone, Medtronics, Minneapolis, MN) allows smaller cannulas to be placed centrally or peripherally without compromising bypass flows. The infusion of carbon dioxide into the operative field to displace air may decrease the risk for air embolism and now is used routinely for the authors' open heart repairs. During longer procedures, sweep flows are increased to avoid increases in circulating carbon dioxide. Enabling technology, consisting of operative endoscopes and endoscopic instruments, is used to improve visualization of remote structures through limited incisions.

Cautious observers have rightfully described the many limitations of these variations from established technique for atrial septal defect repair and aver that the only real advantage to the "minimally invasive" approaches is cosmetic.[50]

Alternatives to Median Sternotomy for Other Congenital Lesions

The merits of a limited access incision in most complex congenital repairs, in which surgeons strive to minimize bypass times and maximize dexterity, are difficult to imagine, and these patients are probably best served by a standard median sternotomy; however, several congenital heart lesions can be approached from partial sternotomy incisions. Gundry et al[29] described partial upper and lower sternotomy in a series of 57 pediatric patients, including neonates, for procedures including arterial switch, tetralogy of Fallot repair, atrial and ventricular septal defect repair, aortic and mitral valve replacement, and complex arch reconstruction. Using a T incision in the upper or lower sternum, with aortic and atrial cannulation and conventional bypass and myocardial preservation, direct visualization of the heart is achieved, and repairs are performed using conventional instrumentation. Potential weaknesses of this approach include the lack of effective chest tube drainage of the mediastinum, prolonged bypass times, the possibility of sternal instability from a T incision, and loss of myocardial protection from rewarming by the chest wall.

At Miami Children's Hospital, the authors have used an upper sternotomy routed into the right third interspace for simple aortic lesions, such as subaortic membrane resection. This approach allows for central aortic and venous cannulation and effective deairing. Video-assisted endoscopy improves visualization of the left ventricular outflow tract. To summarize the results of these partial sternotomy approaches, Table 2 compares patients undergoing atrial septal defect repair and subaortic membrane resection at Miami Children's Hospital in 1998 and 1999 using partial or complete sternotomy. The only notable difference between the groups is that the partial sternotomy patients tend to have a shorter hospital stay to complement their shorter incisions.

Alternate incisions for repair of ventricular septal defect have been described, including lower sternotomy and left anterolateral thoracotomy.[15, 46] This approach has not been widely accepted. The disadvantages of these reported techniques for ventricular septal defect repair include: potentially traumatic femoral cannulation, fibrillatory arrest without cardioplegic myocardial protection, loss of precision, highly visible anterior thoracotomy incisions, ventricular incisions to improve exposure, and prolonged operating and bypass times. Although these approaches are technically possible, no data are presented to suggest that they are in any way "minimally invasive" or superior to conventional surgical techniques.

A recent report describes a "minimally invasive" approach to right ventricular outflow tract reconstruction.[36] The investigators effectively used a "left anterior small thoracotomy," with femoral cannulation for bypass, to replace conduits in four adolescent patients. No data are presented to support the assertion that the technique is less traumatic than a repeat median sternotomy. Given the tendency for right ventricular to pulmonary artery conduits to adhere to the left anterior chest wall, the authors are concerned that this approach might increase the risk for conduit entry on opening the chest.

Table 2. COMPARISON OF FULL AND PARTIAL STERNOTOMY FOR SUBAORTIC MEMBRANE RESECTION AND ATRIAL SEPTAL DEFECT REPAIR

Procedure	Weight (kg)	Time (h)	LOS (d)	No. of Patients
SMR (full sternotomy)	24.9	3:16	3.9	11
SMR (upper sternotomy)	25.4	2:34	2.9	31
ASDR (full sternotomy)	20.9	4:10	5.6	181
ASDR (lower sternotomy)	33.6	4:15	3.0	33

LOS = length of stay; SMR = subaortic membrane resection; ASDR = atrial septal defect repair.

Approaches to Minimize Cardiopulmonary Bypass Trauma

Research in CPB technology, blood conservation, neuroprotection, myocardial protection, inflammation, hypothermia, and acid–base management strategy has constituted the basis for reducing the trauma of surgery for CHD. Further modification or ultimately elimination of CPB is an ongoing strategy to further this goal. Whereas in coronary artery surgery, stabilization instrumentation allows surgeons to control and operate on the beating heart, congenital heart lesions present fewer opportunities for repair while avoiding CPB.

Single ventricle palliation for selected patients can be achieved without CPB. Bidirectional cavopulmonary anastomosis can be performed without bypass,[37] although the authors strongly believe that maintaining cerebral perfusion by effective SVC drainage is critical. Extracardiac Fontan surgery also can be performed without the use of CPB[6] by shunting from the inferior vena cava to the common atrium as the extracardiac anastomoses are completed. Patients with more than one source of pulmonary blood flow may be the safest candidates for the off-bypass Fontan procedure. These include patients with bilateral SVC or with native pulmonary artery flow in addition to their bidirectional cavopulmonary anastomosis. Understanding that obstructed caval blood flow could compromise CNS perfusion, the authors have used these approaches sparingly and agree with others[40] that careful neurologic outcome measurements should form the basis for wider application.

Ventricular septal defect repair without CPB has been described, although the limitations in precision are cause for concern. Recent studies suggest that some muscular ventricular septal defects might be closed using a device inserted through the right atrium without the need for CPB. This technique would allow for the use of larger septal occlusion devices, without the risk for vascular trauma from peripheral access, and eliminate the need for CPB.[2]

ROBOTICS

Robotics in cardiac surgery evolved from efforts to create remote-controlled battlefield surgical units. Building on this military application, systems are in development for robotic cardiac surgery. Voice-activated and computer-assisted systems have been used to facilitate endoscopic coronary artery bypass grafting (CABG). One system uses a voice-controlled robotic arm (Aesop, Computer Motion, Inc., Goleta, CA) to control a three-dimensional camera system (Vista System, Vista, Inc., Westborough, MA), and a telemanipulator system (Zeus, Computer Motion, Goleta, CA) for endoscopic suturing.[58]

A truly remote, computer-controlled, robotic surgery system (DaVinci System, Intuitive Surgical, Inc., Mountain View, CA) has been used to perform CABG in humans.[47] With this system, the robotic arms control the surgical instrumentation and the camera. The surgeon manipulates the instruments through a remote virtual manipulator. These techniques have relied on peripheral access bypass systems (Heartport System, Heartport, Inc., Redwood City, CA), which are too large for infant femoral vessels. Adult atrial septal defect repair and mitral valvuloplasty also have been performed with varying degrees of robotic assistance.[14, 22, 57]

Potential advantages of these systems include scaling of the surgeon's hand movements to increase precision and filtering to minimize tremor. By mounting endoscopic instruments on universal joints that can be advanced through small trocars into the thorax, rotational freedom at the tip of the instruments is maximized and may exceed the capabilities of the human wrist, which enhances surgical precision for dissection and suturing, even in confined spaces. The sacrifices include loss of true three-dimensional visualization and the loss of feeling at the fingertips.

Pediatric applications for CHD await resolution of several other limitations in the technology and technique. Current three-dimensional imaging endoscopes (10 mm) are too large to pass through the infant intercostal space without trauma. Available robotic systems require relatively large (7 mm) ports for instrument insertion. Four such incisions would be as large as a standard median sternotomy in infants, negating most cosmetic benefit. The pediatric thorax is also too small for adequate separation of the robotic arms controlling the individual instruments.

Also, a significant difference exists between the nature of most acquired heart operations and most congenital heart defect repairs. To date, robotic systems have been designed for simple anastomotic suture lines, as required for CABG and valve replacement or repair.[57–59, 61] In training simulators, these anastomoses may require 30 minutes to complete 10 suture throws.[28] A typical congenital repair for tetralogy of Fallot requires approximately 100 suture throws, giving surgeons a projected robotic suture time of 300 minutes, which results in a prohibitively long myocardial ischemic time. It is anticipated that, as the instruments are refined and downsized, pediatric applications will be enabled, particularly for simple septal defects. The ultimate downsizing of instrumentation would be the application of nanotechnology and microassemblers to CHD, building molecular level instrumentation for intracardiac repair.

HYBRID PROCEDURES SYNTHESIZING INTERVENTIONAL CARDIOLOGY AND CARDIAC SURGERY

A competitive atmosphere between interventional cardiologists and surgeons treating CHD may impede the development of less traumatic therapy for CHD. A unified field approach, emphasizing the technologic capabilities of both disciplines, might accelerate innovation. To achieve this, the authors envision a multidisciplinary intervention–surgery–diagnostic suite incorporating all existing therapeutic technology into a single procedural suite.

Hybrid Closure of Septal Defects

Transcatheter device occlusion for septal defects is evolving at a feverish pace, limited in the United States only by the constraints of the US Food and Drug Administration regulations on new medical devices. Devices and techniques are available for device closure of atrial[30] and ventricular septal defects. Problems with these devices include intravascular foreign body, residual flow,[1, 18, 32] and vascular trauma. To minimize the risk of these techniques in the authors' center, surgical backup is provided so that patients found in the laboratory to be unsuitable for device closure can be immediately converted to a surgical approach, sparing the child a second anesthetic and saving the family the stress of a failed intervention.

Hybrid procedures are evolving. Building on early cooperative ventures between interventional cardiology and surgery for the management of complex muscular ventricular septal defects,[3] various combined procedures have evolved. Video-assisted cardioscopy has been used to guide the placement of transcatheter septal occlusion devices.[11] Other hybrid procedures include transcatheter closure of extracardiac Fontan fenestrations[69] and emergent placements of transcatheter stents for occluded shunts[68] in which patients have been stabilized with cardiopulmonary support in the catheterization laboratory.

Pulmonary artery stenosis can be managed with hybrid techniques in which surgical cardiac exposure is used to facilitate transcatheter stent placement. The authors have developed several variations of this technique at Miami Children's Hospital in the past 2 years. Most commonly, transcatheter stents have been positioned intraoperatively, on bypass, with video-assisted endoscopic guidance (Fig. 1). Angiographically guided stent placement has been achieved in the catheterization laboratory through sheaths placed directly in the right ventricular outflow tract by the surgical team, with and without CPB. Several advantages exist to these hybrid approaches to pulmonary artery angioplasty. Bypass support minimizes hemodynamic instability, central vascular access minimizes peripheral vascular trauma, large stents can be placed in small patients, stents can be removed and repositioned easily and rapidly, and extensive surgical dissection in the hilum can be avoided.

SUMMARY

While describing the circulatory system in *De Moto Cordis,* in 1628, William Harvey developed precepts for investigation, which could be modified slightly to guide the adoption of new technology and technique in the twenty-first century. Harvey might suggest (1) careful and accurate observation and description of a new technique, (2) a tentative explanation of how the technique

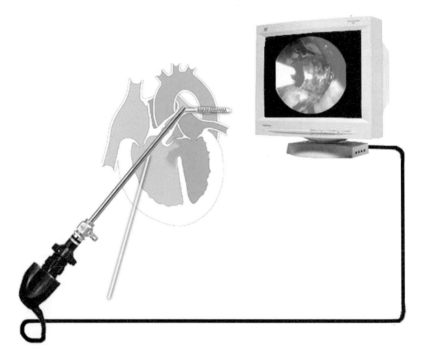

Figure 1. Video-assisted endoscopic stent implantation. A transcatheter stent is positioned in the left pulmonary artery using endoscopic visualization.

improves on existing techniques, (3) a controlled testing of the hypothesis, and (4) conclusions based on the results of the experiments. Also, he might admonish surgery today, with its massively enhanced capabilities for information management, to rigorously test the validity of these conclusions with quantitative reasoning. In the future, precise measurement of the "trauma" of surgery, or even an individual surgeon, may be possible, and the long-term impact of a chest wall incision on a patient's self-esteem may be predictable. Absent such objective measures, justifications for "minimally invasive" deviations from conventional technique in surgery for CHD lack substance. Morbidity, mortality, and physiological endpoints will continue to form the foundation for therapeutic plans; however, the potential for emerging technology to reduce the trauma of these plans remains tantalizing.

References

1. Agarwal SK, Ghosh PK, Mittal PK: Failure of devices used for closure of atrial septal defects: Mechanisms and management [see comments]. J Thorac Cardiovasc Surg 112:21–26, 1996
2. Amin Z, Gu X, Berry JM, et al: Periventricular closure of ventricular septal defects without cardiopulmonary bypass. Ann Thorac Surg 68:149–153, 1999
3. Bridges ND, Perry SB, Keane JF, et al: Preoperative transcatheter closure of congenital muscular ventricular septal defects. N Engl J Med 324:1312–1317, 1991
4. Burke RP: Video-assisted thoracoscopic surgery for patent ductus arteriosus. Pediatrics 93:823–825, 1994
5. Burke RP, Chang AC: Video-assisted thoracoscopic division of a vascular ring in an infant: A new operative technique [see comments]. J Card Surg 8:537–540, 1993
6. Burke RP, Jacobs JP, Ashraf MH, et al: Extracardiac Fontan operation without cardiopulmonary bypass. Ann Thorac Surg 63:1175–1177, 1997
7. Burke RP, Jacobs JP, Cheng W, et al: Video-assisted thoracoscopic surgery for patent ductus arteriosus in low birth weight neonates and infants. Pediatrics 104:227–230, 1999
8. Burke RP, Michielon G, Wernovsky G: Video-assisted cardioscopy in congenital heart operations. Ann Thorac Surg 58:864–868, 1994
9. Burke RP, Rosenfeld HM, Wernovsky G, et al: Video-assisted thoracoscopic vascular ring division in infants and children. J Am Coll Cardiol 25:943–947, 1995
10. Burke RP, Wernovsky G, Van Der Velde M, et al: Video-assisted thoracoscopic surgery for congenital heart disease. J Thorac Cardiovasc Surg 109:499–507, discussion 508, 1995
12. Byrne JG, Adams DH, Mitchell ME, et al: Minimally invasive direct access for repair of atrial septal defect in adults. Am J Cardiol 84:919–922, 1999
13. Cherup LL, Siewers RD, Futrell JW: Breast and pectoral muscle maldevelopment after anterolateral and posterolateral thoracotomies in children. Ann Thorac Surg 41:492–497, 1986
14. Chitwood WR Jr: Video-assisted and robotic mitral valve surgery: Toward an endoscopic surgery. Semin Thorac Cardiovasc Surg 11:194–205, 1999
15. Chu SH, Chou NK, Chou TF, et al: Left anterolateral thoracotomy for simultaneous correction of ventricular septal defect and coarctation of the aorta. Tex Heart Inst J 21:158–160, 1994
16. Cremer JT, Boning A, Anssar MB, et al: Different approaches for minimally invasive closure of atrial septal defects. Ann Thorac Surg 67:1648–1652, 1999
17. Dajczman E, Gordon A, Kreisman H, et al: Long-term postthoracotomy pain [see comments]. Chest 99:270–274, 1991
18. Das GS: Failure of devices used for the closure of atrial septal defects [letter; comment]. J Thorac Cardiovasc Surg 113:426–427, 1997
19. DeCampli WM: Video-assisted thoracic surgical procedures in children. Semin Thorac Cardiovasc Surg 1:61–73, 1998
20. del Nido PJ, Bichell DP: Minimal-access surgery for congenital heart defects. Semin Thorac Cardiovasc Surg 1:75–80, 1998

21. Duke C, Chan KC: Aortic obstruction caused by device occlusion of patent arterial duct. Heart 82:109–111, 1999
22. Falk V, Walther T, Autschbach R, et al: Robot-assisted minimally invasive solo mitral valve operation. J Thorac Cardiovasc Surg 115:470–471, 1998
23. Fedderly RT, Beekman RH III, Mosca RS, et al: Comparison of hospital charges for closure of patent ductus arteriosus by surgery and by transcatheter coil occlusion. Am J Cardiol 77:776–779, 1996
24. Galal O, Nehgme R, al Fadley F, et al: The role of surgical ligation of patent ductus arteriosus in the era of the Rashkind device. Ann Thorac Surg 63:434–437, 1997
25. Gray DT, Fyler DC, Walker AM, et al: Clinical outcomes and costs of transcatheter as compared with surgical closure of patent ductus arteriosus. The Patient Ductus Arteriosus Closure Comparative Study Group [see comments]. N Engl J Med 329:1517–1523, 1993
26. Grewal H, Jackson RJ, Wagner CW, et al: Early video-assisted thoracic surgery in the management of empyema. Pediatrics 103:63, 1999
27. Gross ER, Hubbard JP: Surgical ligation of patent ductus arteriosus. JAMA 112:729, 1939
28. Gulbins H, Boehm D: 3-D vizualisation improves the dryu-lab coronary anastomosis using the Zeus Robotics System. Heart Surgery Forum 4:318–325, 1999
29. Gundry SR, Shattuck OH, Razzouk AJ, et al: Facile minimally invasive cardiac surgery via ministernotomy. Ann Thorac Surg 65:1100–1104, 1998
30. Hausdorf G, Schneider M, Franzbach B, et al: Transcatheter closure of secundum atrial septal defects with the atrial septal defects occlusion system (ASDOS): Initial experience in children. Heart 75:83–88, 1996
31. Hawkins JA, Minich LL, Tani LY, et al: Cost and efficacy of surgical ligation versus transcatheter coil occlusion of patent ductus arteriosus. J Thorac Cardiovasc Surg 112:1634–1638, 1996
32. Hekmat K, Mehlhorn U, Rainer DV: Surgical repair of a large residual atrial septal defect after transcatheter closure. Ann Thorac Surg 63:1456–1458, 1997
33. Helps BA, Ross-Russell RI, Dicks-Mireaux C, et al: Phrenic nerve damage via a right thoracotomy in older children with secundum ASD. Ann Thorac Surg 56:328–330, 1993
34. Hines MH, Bensky AS, Hammon JW Jr, et al: Video-assisted thoracoscopic ligation of patent ductus arteriosus: Safe and outpatient. Ann Thorac Surg 66:853–858, 1998
35. Ho AC, Tan PP, Yang MW, et al: The use of multiplane transesophageal echocardiography to evaluate residual patent ductus arteriosus during video-assisted thoracoscopy in adults. Surg Endosc 13:975–979, 1999
36. Imanaka K, Takamoto S, Murakami A, et al: Minimally invasive extracardiac conduit replacement via a left anterior small thoracotomy. J Thorac Cardiovasc Surg 118:1124–1125, 1999
37. Jahangiri M, Keogh B, Shinebourne EA, et al: Should the bidirectional Glenn procedure be performed through a thoracotomy without cardiopulmonary bypass? J Thorac Cardiovasc Surg 118:367–368, 1999
38. Janorkar S, Goh T, Wilkinson J: Transcatheter closure of ventricular septal defects using the Rashkind device: Initial experience [see comments]. Catheterization and Cardiovascular Interventions 46:43–48, 1999
39. Jaureguizar E, Vazquez J, Murcia J, et al: Morbid musculoskeletal sequelae of thoracotomy for tracheoesophageal fistula. J Pediatr Surg 20:511–514, 1985
40. Jonas RA: Commentary [in process citation]. J Thorac Cardiovasc Surg 118:957, 1999
41. Kappert U, Wagner FM, Gulielmos V, et al: Port access surgery for congenital heart disease. Eur J Cardiothorac Surg 2(suppl 16):86–88, 1999
42. Khan JH, McElhinney DB, Reddy VM, et al: A 5-year experience with surgical repair of atrial septal defect employing limited exposure. Cardiol Young 9:572–576, 1999
43. Laborde F, Folliguet TA, Etienne PY, et al: Video-thoracoscopic surgical interruption of patent ductus arteriosus: Routine experience in 332 pediatric cases. Eur J Cardiothorac Surg 11:1052–1055, 1997
44. Laborde F, Noirhomme P, Karam J, et al: A new video-assisted thoracoscopic surgical technique for interruption of patent ductus arteriosus in infants and children [see comments]. J Thorac Cardiovasc Surg 105:278–280, 1993
45. Levinson M, Fonger J: Minimally invasive atrial septal defect closure using the subxiphoid approach. Heart Surgery Forum 1995, pp 1998–2875
46. Lin PJ, Chang CH, Chu JJ, et al: Minimally invasive cardiac surgical techniques in

the closure of ventricular septal defect: An alternative approach. Ann Thorac Surg 65:165–169, 1998
47. Loulmet D, Carpentier A, d'Attellis N, et al: Endoscopic coronary artery bypass grafting with the aid of robotic assisted instruments [see comments]. J Thorac Cardiovasc Surg 118:4–10, 1999
48. Malhotra R, Mishra Y, Sharma KK, et al: Minimally invasive atrial septal defects repair. Indian Heart J 51:193–197, 1999
49. Marmon LM, Bye MR, Haas JM, et al: Vascular rings and slings: Long-term follow-up of pulmonary function. J Pediatr Surg 19:683–692, 1984
50. Massetti M, Nataf P, Babatasi G, et al: Cosmetic aspects in minimally invasive cardiac surgery. Eur J Cardiothorac Surg 2(suppl 16):73–75, 1999
51. Mazza IL, Jacobs JP, Aldousany A, et al: Video-assisted cardioscopy for left ventricular thrombectomy in a child. Ann Thorac Surg 66:248–250, 1998
52. Murashita T, Hatta E, Miyatake T, et al: Partial median sternotomy as a minimal access for the closure of subarterial ventricular septal defect: Feasibility of transpulmonary approach [in process citation]. Jpn J Thorac Cardiovasc Surg 47:440–444, 1999
53. Odim J, Portzky M, Zurakowski D, et al: Sternotomy approach for the modified Blalock-Taussig shunt. Circulation 92:256–261, 1995
54. Osler W: Medicine in the nineteenth century. New York Sun 1:27, 1901
55. Patel HT, Cao QL, Rhodes J, et al: Long-term outcome of transcatheter coil closure of small to large patent ductus arteriosus. Catheterization and Cardiovascular Interventions 47:457–461, 1999
56. Rao V, Freedom RM, Black MD: Minimally invasive surgery with cardioscopy for congenital heart defects. Ann Thorac Surg 68:1742–1745, 1999
57. Reichenspurner H, Boehm D, Reichart B: Minimally invasive mitral valve surgery using three-dimensional video and robotic assistance. Semin Thorac Cardiovasc Surg 11:235–243, 1999
58. Reichenspurner H, Damiano RJ, Mack M, et al: Use of the voice-controlled and computer-assisted surgical system ZEUS for endoscopic coronary artery bypass grafting [see comments]. J Thorac Cardiovasc Surg 118:11–16, 1999
60. Sawa Y, Matsuda H: [Minimally invasive cardiac surgery: the efficacy of right parasternal approach]. Nippon Geka Gakkai Zasshi 99:825–830, 1998
61. Shennib H, Bastawisy A, McLoughlin J, et al: Robotic computer-assisted telemanipulation enhances coronary artery bypass. J Thorac Cardiovasc Surg 117:310–313, 1999
62. Sim EK, Goh JJ, Grignani RT, et al: Minimally invasive surgical closure of atrial septal defects via a right anterior thoracotomy. Singapore Med J 40:271–272, 1999
63. Van Biezen FC, Bakx PA, De Villeneuve VH, et al: Scoliosis in children after thoracotomy for aortic coarctation. J Bone Joint Surg Am 75:514–518, 1993
64. Van Smith C, Jacobs JP, Burke RP: Minimally invasive diaphragm plication in an infant. Ann Thorac Surg 65:842–844, 1998
65. Westfelt JN, Nordwall A: Thoracotomy and scoliosis. Spine 16:1124–1125, 1991
66. Wong-Chung J, France J, Gillespie R: Scoliosis caused by rib fusion after thoracotomy for esophageal atresia: Report of a case and review of the literature. Spine 17:851–854, 1992
67. Yan D, Xie Q, Zhang Z, et al: Surgical treatment of patent ductus arteriosus (PDA) through mini subaxillary extrapleural approach. Ann Thorac Cardiovasc Surg 5:233–236, 1999
68. Zahn EM, Chang AC, Aldousany A, et al: Emergent stent placement for acute Blalock-Taussig shunt obstruction after stage 1 Norwood surgery [see comments]. Cathet Cardiovasc Diagn 42:191–194, 1997
69. Zahn EM, Chang AC, Burke RP, et al: Transcatheter closure of an extracardiac Fontan fenestration. Ann Thorac Surg 66:260–262, 1998

Address reprint requests to
Redmond P. Burke, MD
Division of Cardiovascular Surgery
Miami Children's Hospital
3200 SW 60 CT, Suite 102
Miami, FL 33155–4069

e-mail: Redmond111@aol.com

0039–6109/00 $15.00 + .00

MINIMALLY INVASIVE SURGICAL TRAINING SOLUTIONS FOR THE TWENTY-FIRST CENTURY

James C. Rosser, Jr, MD, Michinori Murayama, MD, PhD, and Nick H. Gabriel, DO

The issue of surgical training has always been a hotbed of concern and evolution. Over the past 100 years, a concentrated effort to mature, deploy, and standardize training protocols at all levels has occurred.[4] At the medical student level is tangible evidence of effective algorithms. This is not to suggest that shortcomings do not need to be addressed. The need for assistance is more urgent on the resident and postgraduate levels. Placement of a competent strategy for medical students is much easier to accomplish because of the meager goals that must be achieved. Medical students require a knowledge base concerning pathophysiology and diagnosis and a superficial awareness of the proper procedure for a clinical situation. None of this subject matter needs to be taken to any degree of depth. Students at this stage of development need only a foundation that allows them to function competently no matter what discipline they decide to specialize in. The establishment of more sophisticated capabilities is reserved for the postgraduate process.

The challenge associated with resident education is an entirely different adventure because of the limitation of time. Residents have many duties that are related to service and not education. Starting intravenous lines, moving patients to CT scanners, preparing discharge, and planning for patients in long-term care facilities are noneducational tasks that compete for time for structured education. These tasks have been traditionally called *scut* work. This is the dark side of everything that is good about training regimens. Scutage is the source of the term *scut*. In medieval times, the definition referred to a tax levied on a tenant of a knight's estate in place of military service.[14] This time-honored standard of resident education is something that the medical field no longer can afford.

From the Endo-Laparoscopic Center, Department of Surgery, Yale University School of Medicine, New Haven, Connecticut

---

Traditionally, the apprenticeship concept has been the mainstay of educational strategy. As pointed out by Cuschieri[1] and Forde,[2] the apprenticeship system needs revision. The use of Halstedian principles of progressive trainee involvement and responsibility over time has trained tens of thousands of surgeons over the past 100 years. Unfortunately, this educational strategy at times seems to follow the principles of osmosis. A lot is left to happen based on observation and behavior copying. The current system is not ineffective, but because of the numerous burdens now placed on surgical education and health care, modification of the educational strategy is needed. Medical education expenses include not only resident salaries and benefits but also the expense associated with system inefficiencies. For example, surgical suite times are significantly longer than those for community hospitals without training programs, which is a challenge to the future of medical education. In the cost containment and efficiency profiling atmosphere, this fact must be reversed. Structured educational algorithms using objective skill and cognitive development could help to remove the surgical suite from the ranks of being the main surgical maturation conduit. It can be a cost-prohibitive classroom.

Residency training programs suffer from a lack of exposure to cutting-edge, minimally invasive procedures. Nine years after the start of minimally invasive general surgery, opportunities for exposure to advanced procedures vary widely among surgical training programs.[12] This disparity hinders the development of future surgeons. Exposure to advanced procedures must be a high priority of any training program. All attending surgeons do not perform these procedures. Often, at institutions where these procedures are being performed, the volume is insufficient to give ample experience. Also, residents must be ready to participate when the opportunity arises to participate in surgery. Acquisition of two-handed choreography for dissection, nondominant hand dexterity, accurate instrument targeting, and intracorporeal suturing are capabilities that Scott-Conner and Berci[13] have strongly recommended. To reach these goals, residents must work to prepare outside the surgical suite to efficiently and safely participate. The elimination of these challenges can occur only if the acquisition of these skills is firmly entrenched within residency training programs.

After its meteoric entry onto the general surgical scene 9 years ago, minimally invasive surgery stands at a crossroads with regard to the twenty-first century. Many obstacles hamper safe and cost-effective deployment. First, a stabilization and reduction of complication rates associated with laparoscopic cholecystectomy must occur. Common bile duct injuries are twofold to threefold higher for laparoscopic cholecystectomy than for open surgery,[3] which is not a matter for discussion only at local morbidity and mortality conferences or at national meetings: patients are being injured. The surgical community has failed to police itself, and the public knows it. This led in 1992 to New York State health officials setting standards of training and surgeon preparedness for performing laparoscopic cholecystectomy.[9] If surgeons do not handle the problem, the politicians will.

Complications during a laparoscopic cholecystectomy typically are failures of skill or judgment. Video reviews of 10 laparoscopic cholecystectomies from 10 surgeons tell the story. Surgeons are practicing procedural algorithms that fail to protect patients. This is not to say that the only problem is poor technique. When a surgeon struggles with basic tasks, such as two-handed dissection, nondominant hand dexterity, and instrument targeting, inappropriate decisions may be made that ultimately put patients in danger. Skill and judgment deficiencies are intimately intertwined in the cause of common bile duct injury.

Widespread deployment of established advanced minimally invasive procedures by trained surgeons is needed. Advanced laparoscopic procedures have not followed the same rate of adoption as laparoscopic cholecystectomy. For some, this is a source of great elation because they believe that these procedures need more formal and rigid determinations of safety and cost-effectiveness. Others have a sense of urgency that this situation be quickly met with a battle plan that can chaperon these procedures into the surgical mainstream with outcome and patient quality assurance data that will justify their deployment.

Also, a credentialing and continuing education process that is globally deployable, impartial, and accessible to all colleagues is needed to achieve a high level of patient quality assurance associated with these techniques. Historically, the granting of surgical privileges lies solely with individual hospitals. For the process to be maximally effective, a fair and diverse initial evaluation procedure must be used, together with a continuous surveillance program with ongoing educational support. To accomplish this, much effort and many resources must be brought to bear to support an optimal effort, which is a price that many hospitals cannot afford to pay, so wide discrepancies exist in the effectiveness of this process among hospitals. For minimally invasive surgery to advance safely, this shortcoming must be corrected.

The encouragement and requirement of trained surgeons in the United States to pursue continuing education were landmark commitments in the early years of this century. This move was ahead of its time and the rest of the world is just making a similar commitment. Despite the historical commitment to continuing surgical education, posture over the past 50 years has been mainly defensive. The many technique advances have been gradually disseminated, and all have involved the use of basic surgical skills. With the advent of the minimally invasive revolution, surgeons have been faced with the development of new techniques and procedures that require an alien skill set that is difficult to acquire. The unprecedented influence of technology has led to new, swift developments. Also, the increasing involvement of patients in the health care delivery process has cultivated patient demand as a factor that must be addressed. All of these conditions are producing increasing pressure to change the educational strategy from defensive to offensive. To address all of the aforementioned factors, education must harness these new procedures. This task is further complicated by an economic crunch. Managed care has significantly cut reimbursements and decreased productivity time because of bureaucratic algorithms and paperwork. Surgeons do not have the time or money to pursue an aggressive postgraduate education program, so all strategies must be convenient, cost-effective, and continuous. Traditional educational strategies and delivery systems do not address current needs. The medical field must turn to technology to address these issues effectively.

To their credit, the Society of American Gastrointestinal Endoscopic Surgeons (SAGES) and the American College of Surgeons (ACS) have aggressively pursued formulating requirements of all efforts designed to address these challenges. The following sections are summaries of their guidelines.

SAGES REQUIREMENTS

Skills Acquisition for Advanced Laparoscopic Surgery

Examples of skills for laparoscopic surgery include two-handed dissection and intracorporeal and extracorporeal knot tying. Mastery of these skills is encouraged before initiating advanced laparoscopic surgery. Experience in surgery by celiotomy also facilitates mastery of the similar laparoscopic procedure using a minimal access approach.

Until complete integration is possible, SAGES believes that the following measures can help to accomplish the integration of advanced laparoscopic training into general surgery residency: (1) train faculty, (2) train residents, and (3) provide guidelines for postresidency training for prospective faculty.

Basic Laparoscopic Surgery

Most programs provide adequate experience in basic laparoscopic surgery. To ensure ongoing availability of basic training resources, basic laparoscopy courses for residents and faculty are recommended.

Advanced Laparoscopic Surgery

Faculty Training

Courses. Hands-on courses are useful for conveying the techniques of laparoscopic surgery to those who are proficient in the similar open techniques. See subsequent section on resident training courses.

Faculty Mentoring. SAGES believes that faculty who already have acquired the fundamental skills in advanced laparoscopic surgery and who desire to learn a new or modified laparoscopic surgery will benefit from observing and interacting with peers who are skilled and accomplished in that procedure.

Fellowships. With postgraduate training in advanced laparoscopic surgery, faculty or faculty candidates may obtain experience. SAGES believes the main goal of such fellowships should be to train future faculty.

Resident Training

Courses. Appropriate candidates for resident training courses are:

- Residents who plan a career in general surgery
- Residents who already have achieved a mastery of basic laparoscopic surgery
- Residents who are unlikely, based on the practice patterns of their program, to obtain a significant experience in advanced laparoscopic surgical techniques
- Faculty from programs who do not have faculty to teach a procedure

Skills Laboratories. The creation of inanimate and animal training facilities by individual programs is encouraged to provide supplemental teaching of advanced laparoscopic surgical skills.

Needs Assessment. SAGES continues to assess the needs of residency programs in terms of faculty training and overall program needs.

Re-examination of Residency Training. SAGES suggests that the appropriate leadership organizations consider re-examining the flexibility of the general surgery residency training to optimize the availability of such advanced cases for residents planning a career in general surgery.

Educational Resources. SAGEs continues to offer other educational resources, such as postgraduate courses, annual meetings, and an extensive video library.

AMERICAN COLLEGE OF SURGEONS REQUIREMENTS

Guidelines for the evaluation of credentials of individuals for awarding surgical privileges in new technologies include:

- The surgeon must be a member in good standing of the department or service from which privileges are to be recommended.
- A defined educational program in the technology, including didactic and practical elements, must be completed and documented as a postresidency course of instruction or as a component of an approved residency program.
- The surgeon must be qualified, experienced, and knowledgeable in the management of the diseases for which the technology is applied. For example, laparoscopic instrumentation would be applied by surgeons with abdominal or pelvic surgical experience and credentials.
- The qualifications of the surgeon to apply the new technology must be assessed by a surgeon who is qualified and experienced in the technology and should result in a written recommendation to the department or service head. In the case of a resident trained in the technology during residency, recommendation by the program director is acceptable.
- Maintenance of skills should be documented through periodic outcomes assessment and evaluation in association with the regular renewal of surgical privileges.

These suggestions by SAGES and the ACS are excellent starting points. But the difficulty is in working out the details. Formulating mechanisms by which these suggestions can be executed effectively is the dilemma. How can the standards suggested be achieved with similar levels of excellence throughout all the hospitals worldwide? It boils down to a matter of effective deployment of educational content, which can be accomplished only by using technology to achieve these goals that have been set forth by government.

TECHNOLOGIC ADVANCES FOR MEDICAL EDUCATION

A three-point plan for the integration of technology into medical education is suggested. The first component involves the adoption of standardized, objective-based skill development programs that can establish and monitor the progress of skill acquisition (Fig. 1).

Skill-Development Programs

At Yale, such a program has been developed and instituted over the past 8 years (Fig. 2) and involves the development of drills that are correlated with the achievement of a clinically related task—intracorporeal suturing.[6, 7] Three endoscopic tasks were found to correlate with accomplishing intracorporeal suturing, probably the most challenging skill to develop in minimally invasive surgery and a key for advanced laparoscopic surgical procedures and for developing the skills necessary for delicate tissue dissection and manipulation. These drills, together with a detailed suturing algorithm, are taught within a 2-day curriculum that establishes this highly regarded capability in a short time. This program also has a database that allows instructors to rank the participants with more than 4000 surgeons worldwide who have participated in this program. This facet provides an excellent follow-up evaluation tool to give participants an idea of where their abilities stand among those of their peers. This program has proven to be invaluable in achieving basic skill capability simultaneously for trained surgeons and trainees, which is advantageous during this stage of

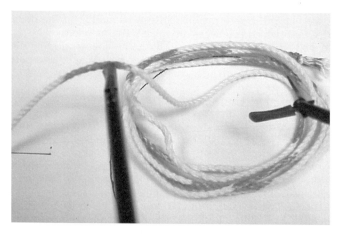

Figure 1. Example of objective-based skill development drill using the Cobra Rope (Yale Endo-Laparoscopic Center, New Haven, CT).

maturation of minimally invasive surgery because trained surgeons and trainees must be up to speed as quickly as possible. Also, this program allows a proctor or mentor to objectively evaluate the capabilities of surgeons in a remote location who must undergo standard and telemedicine enabled proctorships or mentorships, which can help to eliminate the fear of procedural anarchy in this era of telecommunications-assisted surgeon collaboration. Also, this program could be a great advantage in helping to overcoming credentialing and privileges issues.

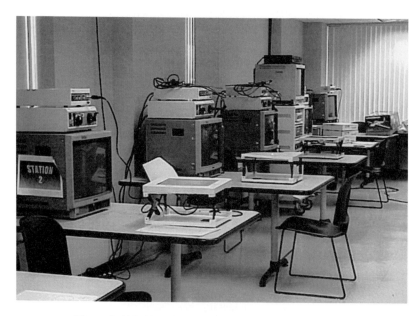

Figure 2. Yale University laparoscopy inanimate laboratory.

To provide a platform to encourage skill development in surgical residency programs, the "Top Gun Laparoscopic Skill Shoot-Out" was started at the 1996 meeting of the ACS in the scientific exhibit section. This event combined fun, excitement, entertainment, competition, perseverance, and sweat (Fig. 3). This concept was designed at Yale University School of Medicine to provide the

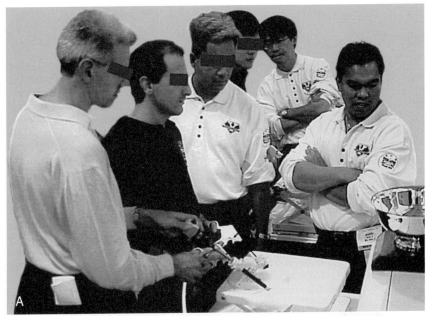

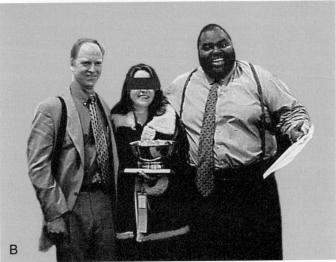

Figure 3. *A*, American College Top Gun participants. *B*, American College of Surgeons Laparoscopic Top Gun Shootout.

ultimate arena for the residents to demonstrate their laparoscopic skill development while promoting friendly competition between academic education centers. The competition uses the previously mentioned tasks and intracorporeal suturing as the challenges that are contested. This event, meant to "give something back" to the residents in an organized and enjoyable format, has been featured for the past 4 years at the ACS, 1996 SAGES meeting, the World Endoscopic Conference, in *Scientific American*, and on the CBS News *Morning Show*.

Internet

Second, the Internet and computer-assisted instruction must play an increasing role in distant education. The Internet offers the convience of content delivery with the click of a mouse. Infectious disease updates, Health Care Financing Administration billing fraud education, and research protocol re-examinations are just a few examples of topics that can be Web based. Regulation review and testing demonstrate how technology and new knowledge-transfer techniques can meet today's stringent patient quality assurance standards. Unfortunately, the level of interactivity that can be delivered over the Internet is limited because of the limit of available bandwidth allotted for the transfer of data. Bandwidth limitations with the current Internet necessitate special countermeasures to deliver robust multimedia content. One such countermeasure is called *video and audio streaming*, which allows multimedia content to be stored and sent over the Internet. Medical educators are challenged to harness the potential of streaming for educational enhancement. Bandwidth represents the ability to transfer bits and bytes from point A to point B in cyberspace. To draw an analogy, if a pipe through which the river of data flows is large, the data flow rapidly, and if the pipe is small, the data flow slowly. The transfer of large multimedia content files through a limited bandwidth conduit was traditionally a slow and painful downloading process. With the introduction of streaming, this hurdle to real-time distribution of multimedia content on demand can be eliminated.

Streaming works by a client-to-server method of communication over the Internet. To understand this concept, one must have a firm grasp of how a local area network (LAN) functions. One of the most common LAN concepts is demonstrated by how numerous computers can be linked to one printer to cost-effectively fulfill the printing needs of an entire office. A LAN physically links several computers to each other and often to a mainframe or minicomputer. This is accomplished with various materials—twisted-wire cables, fiber optics, phone lines, and even infrared light and radio signals.[16] The streaming process is initiated when the computer user's streaming program sends a request for content to a streaming server. After the server receives the request from the client, it starts to send the requested information from the server to the client. As the client begins to receive the content from the server, the client software sends these data to what is known as a *buffer*, which contains the first few seconds of the data stream. Once the client has an adequate amount of media content in the buffer, the software program starts to display the content to the computer user. As the client software continues to play, content is constantly added to the buffer. Thus, if Internet congestion is present during transmission, the buffer allows continuous content display. This process of simultaneous display and reception of media content continues until the media content is finished or terminated by the computer user. If the content is live audio or video, it must be passed through an audio or video capture expansion card, which turns the analog signal into digital information. Fortunately, with the coming of integrated services digital network (ISDN), digital subscriber line (DSL), cable, Internet II, and Internet III, these bandwidth restrictions will be eliminated. Until then, streaming will be the workhorse in delivering multimedia content over the Web.

Broadband connectivity is needed if computer-assisted instruction is to play a powerful role in any education solution package. This instructional platform is not designed to eliminate contact with an instructor; it is designed to assist the educational process and provides mobility to establish a distant learning component to any program. Computer-based instruction, especially in the multimedia mode, offers consistency and increased cognitive knowledge transfer rates.[5] With the multimedia training potential of computer-based instruction, we are now liberated to design programs not only to transfer knowledge but also to help to mature clinical judgment. With CD-ROMs, a student can be placed in a visual environment similar to that in actual cases (Fig. 4). After viewing a video presentation of a clinical situation, the computer challenges the participant to answer questions, such as where to make incisions, what instruments to use, whether or not dissection is indicated, and where to place sutures (Figs. 5 and 6), after which the participant has 15 seconds to answer. The computer instantly gives feedback as to the correctness of a response, and at the end of a challenge, critiques are given for each answer (Fig. 7). This training strategy is called Objective-Based Clinical Competency Evaluation Scenarios and allows clinical judgment to be matured outside of the surgical suite in a more cost-effective environment with greater safety for patients.

The use of CD-ROM computer-based instruction does not end with the surgeons and surgical residents. This type of multimedia instruction will be important in helping to improve obtaining informed consent. With imagery and audio prompting, together with interactive challenges, patients can be instructed on all aspects of their upcoming surgical procedures. The informed-consent

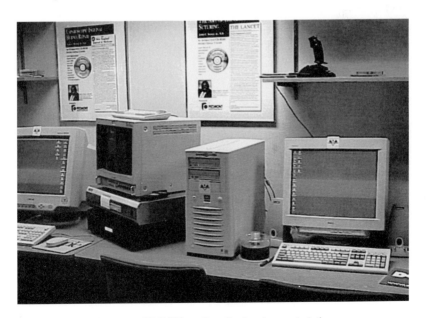

Figure 4. CD-ROM multimedia development station.

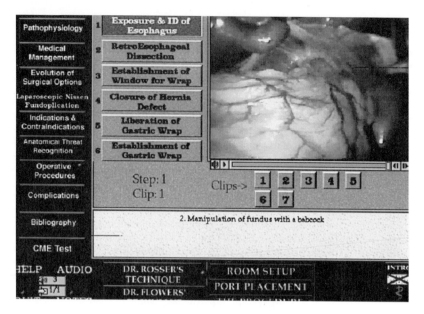

Figure 5. CD-ROM procedure review.

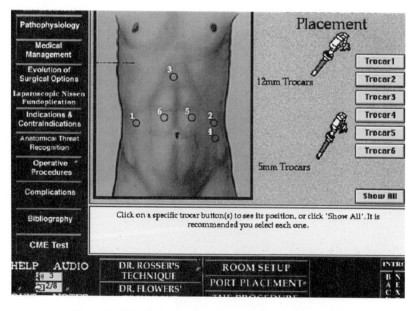

Figure 6. CD-ROM interactive trocar placement simulation.

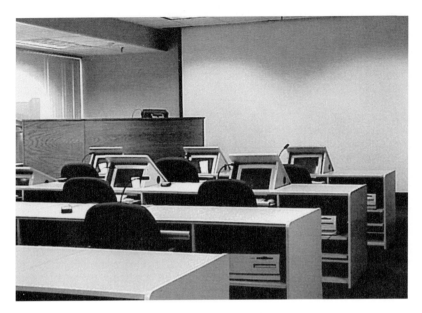

Figure 7. Surgical classroom of tomorrow.

process varies in effectiveness among clinicians. Most patients do not remember what doctors and nurses say during office visits even though appropriate time was taken. Therefore, using technology, we can develop consistency in information transfer with higher retention rates and documentation of a successful effort.

Surgical simulators are another computer-based educational option that will play a major role in the future of surgical education. The use of simulators to speed the transfer of difficult task-performance parameters has been well established in the aerospace industry. In the 1930s, Doolittle, after recognizing the unacceptable accident rate associated with bad weather or night landings, became an advocate of flight simulators. It was amazing how simple recreations of the flight experience could be effective in decreasing accident rates. Surgical simulation had its roots date back to the 1980s, when Delp and Rosen created one of the first virtual reality simulators to teach tendon transplantation procedures for the lower extremity. In 1991, Satava and Lanier created the first abdominal surgery simulator. While impressed by the power of technology, many critics were not impressed by the lack of realism for these early models. But remember the days of early aerospace simulation. The platforms were crude. Often, they were no more than exotic carnival rides. But, despite this, they changed the safety profile of flight. The current generation of simulators still does not have the realism that will eventually come, but they are poised to contribute to the advancement of surgical education. Examples include HT Medical System's (Gaithersburg, MD) central vein catheter placement simulator and the virtual endoscopic simulator. Skill-development simulators, such as the one from Minimally Invasive Surgical Trainer (Virtual Presence Medical, London, UK) have now met cost and ease of use thresholds that will allow them to be deployed in great numbers, which will open the way for traditional studies to validate their effectiveness in assisting the surgical educational process.[10, 11]

Telecommunication

Medical schools must maximize the use of modern telecommunications to share educational content with others in a more timely fashion. Telemedicine is a popular topic because of the prospect of being able to care for individuals who are remote to a caregiver.[15] Most of the accolades associated with telemedicine are based on the provision of clinical services to a distant site. One elementary advantage is the capability of telecommunications to project education. The power of telecommunications must be harnessed to allow health care providers, hospitals, and hospital systems to share in sophisticated continuing medical education programs in cutting-edge arenas, such as minimally invasive surgery. Several projects by the authors have suggested strongly that telecommunications can achieve this goal. Operation Validation was a project that sought to evaluate the effectiveness of deploying the laparoscopic skills and suturing acquisition program to a distant learning mode. A kit that included all of the necessary hardware to perform the exercises, together with the laboratory practical manual, CD-ROM, and laparoscopic trainer, was combined in a package that was sent to several institutions worldwide (Fig. 8). A distant site instructor administered the program. The instructor progressed the CD-ROM for the group using a data projector, administered the precognitive and postcognitive tests, and facilitated the laboratory practical and collected the data. Video telecommunications were

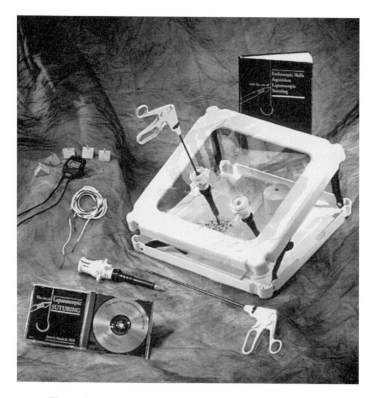

Figure 8. Distant learning laparoscopic skill development kit.

used for the introduction of the goals and objectives of the program and for troubleshooting lectures. Also, video conferencing provided a forum to conduct a final examination by the chief program director at the base site. The purpose of the remote oversight of the final examination was to validate that the data were collected under the same rigid conditions that have been set by the training protocol. The sample data obtained by the program director were compared with the data that were procured by the local instructor. The two data sets were compared, and results showed that the data obtained by the remote instructor and the data obtained by the base instructor had no statistically significant difference. The success of this project demonstrated that a skills-acquisition course could be deployed globally with the same level of effectiveness as if the participants completed this course at Yale University.

All institutions cannot provide the same exposure to advanced minimally invasive cases, so, to equalize experience, a pool of these advanced procedures should be presented to institutions that have a low volume. Video conferencing can allow (1) the sharing of clinical experience from the surgical suite and (2) a lecture series to occur in cyberspace. Surgeons can be guided during their initial procedures with the assistance of telementoring,[8] a technique that involves the remote guidance of a therapy or investigational procedure. Multiple educational and technologic requirements place telementoring in a much more sophisticated and higher-risk category than standard telemedicine applications. These factors dictate that a standard training protocol be formulated, so that quality assurance can be maintained. Operation Outreach was a 3-year program that developed the concept of telementoring. The effectiveness of this technology should not rely solely on electronics; rather, it should be dictated by the human resources commanding it. To apply this technology competently to a clinical situation, educators must proceed within a structured and well-thought strategy with a complete educational agenda that covers four basic aspects:

1. A preprocedural assessment and enhancement of laparoscopic surgical skills to ensure patient safety. A 3-day laparoscopic skills and suturing program should be first conducted for all participating surgeons. The program placed the surgeons through a series of drills and exercises that have a large preexisting database and have been demonstrated to have a high correlation with being able to suture intracorporeally. This provides a yardstick to evaluate each participant's skill capability and generate a checkpoint to document progress. Each participant at the end of the course could competently suture, which greatly increased surgeons' confidence that intraoperative complications could be effectively handled.
2. The establishment of a standardized and tactical approach to the procedure is mandatory to promote a stable and anticipated operative sequence with the mentor and student sharing common ground. This establishes a step-by-step protocol.
3. A telementoring simulation laboratory was developed to introduce participants to the experience of being instructed from a remote site. This laboratory was used during the animate laboratory exercise, in which the students conducted the different procedures on porcine specimens. A telecommunication system similar to the authors' standard setup was used, with the exception of the coder/decoder.
4. To better assist in the guidance of the student surgeon and to establish a standardized, reproducible database for each surgeon who is mentored, the concept of "tactical information deployment" (TID) should be used. This intraoperative support package was made possible by the develop-

ment of procedure-specific CD-ROM multimedia interactive computer programs that can rapidly deploy reference information to the video monitor in the surgical suite. If this preparatory strategy is followed, and the decrease in the cost of hardware and telecommunication utilization prices occurs, telementoring will become a more and more cost-effective option in the future.

Operation Full Court Press, an ambitious distance education project from Yale Laparoscopy, brought all of these aforementioned components together to effectively provide multiple hospitals from Hawaii to Connecticut in multidisciplinary educational content using telemedicine applications. This program provided tele-education programs in orthopedics, gynecology, and primary care and deployed the standardized objective-based skill development courses, CD-ROM and multimedia technology, and patient care clinical content. It demonstrated that technology could enable the existence of a total educational package that could significantly affect challenges in minimally invasive surgery and beyond. All of the technology-empowered strategies previously mentioned allow for the organization of a global credentialing and continuing medical education program in minimally invasive surgery.

"Open architecture" design allows other disciplines to share the same platform. Such a program was realized in the fall of 1998, at Northshore Long Island Jewish University Hospital. A prominent system faced the dilemma of a lack of widespread deployment of advanced laparoscopic surgical procedures in all of their hospitals and quality assurance issues. After assigning these issues a high level of priority, they quickly realized that to generate a complex program to fulfill their needs on their own would be challenging, so they sought a proven program that could be administered and overseen by an academic institution. The highlights of this bold and cutting-edge initiative are as follows:

Goals

The overall goal is to establish a standardized advanced laparoscopic surgery continuing education and support strategy to ensure the penetration of excellence in the minimally invasive surgery arena by all surgeons who are willing to participate in the Minimally Invasive Surgery Tactical Program. This organized, objective-based effort will help to establish superior patient outcomes and quality assurance in an arena that has been plagued with medicolegal controversy and spotty surgeon participation. The deployment of this program will allow surgeons to stay on the cutting edge of the advanced procedural envelope within a resource-sharing educational support system that will be furnished by Yale Laparoscopy.

Laparoscopic Skill Development

A laparoscopic skill curriculum must be established to objectively evaluate the skills of all participating surgeons. This curriculum will allow for (1) a rapid overview of the baseline abilities of the staff and assist in the formulation of a long-range skill development and maintenance strategy and (2) the implementation of the telementoring component of the program. The establishment of intracorporeal suturing capability as a standard will be the first goal for all participating staff. Being able to perform this difficult task will boost morale and establish confidence in the minimally invasive environment similar to the open arena. Attending surgeons will then be capable of participating in the training of the residents in this arena, thus producing a common ground that will nurture team work.

Cognitive Development Program

Skill is important for consistent successful outcomes with minimally invasive procedures, but the key to successful surgery is clinical judgment, which can be accomplished only with a foundation of cognitive knowledge and experience. Therefore, a clinical judgment development program is essential. A yearly schedule of nine tutorials will be given by videoconferencing, including:

1. The Difficult Laparoscopic Cholecystectomy and Avoiding Bile Duct Injuries
2. Difficult Laparoscopic Cholecystectomy Objective-Based Clinical Competency Evaluation Scenario
3. Laparoscopic Common Bile Duct Exploration
4. Laparoscopic Nissen Fundoplication
5. Laparoscopic Nissen Fundoplication Objective-Based Clinical Competency Evaluation Scenario
6. Laparoscopic Hernia Repair
7. Laparoscopic Hernia Repair Objective-Based Clinical Competency Evaluation Scenario
8. Laparoscopic Appendectomy
9. Laparoscopic Appendectomy Objective-Based Clinical Competency Evaluation Scenario

The presentation of these topics will form a core knowledge base that will lead to other topics in the succeeding years that are more advanced or respond to contemporary issues. Also, additional lectures will discuss common issues of other disciplines.

Each hospital should purchase and have available to the surgical staff and residents the Yale Laparoscopy CD-ROM series. The titles include Laparoscopic Cholecystectomy, Laparoscopic Nissen Fundoplication, Laparoscopic Hernia Repair, Laparoscopic Cholecystectomy Pre and Post Operative Tutorials, Laparoscopic Nissen Fundoplication Pre and Post Operative Tutorial, and Laparoscopic Hernia Repair Pre and Post Operative Tutorials. The last three tutorials are also designed for nurses and patients. Four new tutorials will be released each year until all topics are covered, and a yearly almanac in the latest development in minimally invasive surgery will be released each year. Students should be tested on the content of these tutorials, and their grades should be recorded. Also, a set of nursing titles should be available for each hospital for continuing nursing education.

Remedial Education for Quality Assurance

Physicians who have documented quality assurance problems with minimally invasive surgery should not experience disciplinary action without having available a remedial education option. Concerns are primarily related to laparoscopic cholecystectomy and common bile duct injuries, but other emerging procedures, such as the laparoscopic Nissen fundoplication, have quality concerns also. At Yale Laparoscopy, an innovative, objective-based skill and clinical judgment maturation program has been developed to provide a solid foundation to combat the risk for committing injurious complications.

The skill component uses the internationally renowned Top Gun Laparoscopic Skill Boot Camp. Dissection technique challenges are presented, critiqued, and scored. A micellular surgical technique instructional strategy establishes procedural tendencies that avoid trouble. Surgical technique and decision making then are challenged by Objective-Based Clinical Competency Evaluation Scenarios. This modern knowledge-transfer tactic uses digitized video of clinical cases with anatomic, instrument selection, and technical challenges that all must be answered instantly with an interactive keypad system, which places participants in a simulated real-time clinical situation in which they must make a decision rapidly. At the end of the exercise a score is generated that can be used to evaluate current capabilities and follow progress. The course is 5 days long, with a small class size (five-person limit) that ensures a large amount of intimate attention. This unique course offers a twenty-first–century solution to a monumental problem that is continuing to grow.

Tactical Leadership Development

If this program is to work, leaders must be assimilated into this modern knowledge and skill transfer program and become at ease with cutting-edge technology. These leaders will provide support for the surgeons and nurses at the local level to help to ensure the continuity of the Yale Laparoscopy Continuing Education Program in Minimally Invasive Surgery. This will be established by having selected surgeons participate in the Yale Laparoscopy Six Week Advanced Minimally Invasive Surgery and Technology Fellowship. To make it more convenient for the participants and their practices, the program can be divided into 3-week sessions. The cost includes lodging, food, recreation, and educational materials.

Nursing Program

The program must have a nursing education component. Without the parallel maturation of nursing support capabilities, all efforts are doomed to failure. Therefore, the authors strongly suggest that nurses be exposed to the same lecture series as the surgeons. If the surgeon's conference schedule is inconvenient for the nurses, these 1-hour lectures should be given using prerecorded videotapes at an agreed-on time.

A core group of 20 to 40 nurses should attend an 8-hour advanced minimally invasive surgery course. This group should be made up of administrators, circulating nurses, and operative assistants. This course offers a detailed review of all cutting-edge minimally invasive procedures, ergonomic and setup efficiency strategy, and safety tutorials. This group will carry these concepts and capabilities back to their home hospitals.

Telemedicine

One of the most exciting topics on the medical scene is telemedicine, which offers many possibilities to enhance health care delivery. It is subject matter on which administrators and clinicians alike must be up to date. Twenty selected participants representing the total hospital system will attend the Yale Introduction to Telemedicine Program. This 2-day course establishes the technical and application foundation for this new art form. The program includes a day of lectures and a day of hands-on laboratory practicals. This course should provide an excellent foundation to help the health care system to accurately guide its march into the twenty-first century.

SUMMARY

Despite the tremendous impact of laparoscopic cholecystectomy on the practice of surgery over the past 9 years, minimally invasive surgery faces many challenges that must be addressed. SAGES and the American College of Surgeons already have defined guidelines that, if properly implemented, could eliminate most of these challenges. Medical educators must formulate a detailed program as to how these guidelines can be widely deployed with acceptable effectiveness. The current educational philosophies and techniques will not ensure widespread access to a standardized program that would support the achievement of the goals set forth by major surgical governing bodies. Therefore, new educational strategies and techniques that are assisted with the integration of cost-effective technology are needed. Suggested solutions include the deployment of a standardized, objective-based skill-development program that has a large database to evaluate the progress of participants. Next, the Internet, with its ability to transfer content with the click of a mouse, will play an increasing role in distant education. Video and audio streaming techniques will allow the deployment of content previously shackled to a CD-ROM platform. CD-ROM interactive technology also can help in developing clinical judgment with innovative strategies, such as Objective-Based Clinical Competency Evaluation Scenarios. Telecommunications will fuse the components of a coordinated distant learning strategy. Also, telecommunications will allow the availability of new training capabilities in the form of teleproctoring and telementoring to hospitals, no matter what their size or location. All of these components combined enable the realization of a continuing education program in minimally invasive surgery that is readily available to hospitals worldwide. Last, institutions, resident training programs, and individual surgeons must commit the time to partake in these cutting-edge programs for challenges facing us to be completely eliminated. A high priority must be placed on the resolution of these issues.

References

1. Cuschieri A: Shape of things to come: expectations and realism. Surg Endosc 8:83–85, 1994
2. Forde KA: Minimal access surgery: Which path to competence? Surg Endosc 8:1047–1048, 1989
3. Olsen D: Bile duct injuries during laparoscopic cholecystectomy. Surg Endosc 11:133–138, 1997
4. Reznick RK: Surgical education: Teaching and testing technical skills. Am J Surg 165:358–361, 1993
5. Rosser J: CD-ROM multimedia: The step before virtual reality. Surg Endosc 10:1033–1035, 1996
6. Rosser JC, Rosser LE, Savalgi RS: Skill acquisition and assessment for laparoscopic surgery. Arch Surg 132:200–204, 1997
7. Rosser JC Jr, Rosser LE, Savalgi RS: Objective evaluation of a laparoscopic surgical skill program for residents and senior surgeons [see comments]. Arch Surg 133:657–661, 1998
8. Rosser JC, Wood M, Payne JH, et al: Telementoring: A practical option in surgical training. Surg Endosc 11:852–855, 1997

9. Robles AE: Laparoscopy in general surgery: Training, credentialing, and safety. Int Surg 79:266–267, 1994
10. Satava RM: Virtual reality surgical simulator: The first steps. Surg Endosc 7:203–205, 1993
11. Satava RM: Virtual reality. Protocols in General Surgery 1:75–95, 1998
12. Scott-Conner CEH: Integrating advanced laparoscopy into surgical residency training. Surg Endosc 12:374–376, 1998
13. Scott-Conner CEH, Berci G: Unsolved problems in endoscopic surgery. Surg Endosc 7:281–282, 1993
14. Smith CD: Stop considering the unbearable tedium of technology: Resident scut of the 1990s. Int Surg 79:373–375, 1994
15. Swett HA, Holaday L, Leffell D, et al: Telemedicine: Delivering medical expertise across the state and around the world. Connecticut Medicine 59:593–602, 1995
16. White R: How Computers Work, ed 4. Indianapolis, IN, Que, 1998

Address reprint requests to

James C. Rosser Jr, MD
Yale Endo-laparoscopic Center
40 Temple Street, Suite 3A
New Haven, CT 06511

e-mail: james.rosser@yale.edu

INDEX